VASCULAR SURGICAL APPROACHES

Library of Congress Cataloging-in-Publication Data

Voies d'abord des vaisseaux. English
Vascular surgical approaches / edited by Alain Branchereau & Ramon Berguer.
          p.   cm.
     Includes bibliographical references.
     ISBN 0-87993-664-9 (alk. paper)
     1. Blood-vessels--Surgery--Congresses. I. Branchereau Alain, MD. II.Berguer Ramon, MD. III. Title.
     [DNLM: 1. Vascular Surgical Procedures--methods. WG 170 V889s 1998a]
     RD598.5.V6313   1998
     617.4'13059--dc21
          DNLM/DLC
          for Library of Congress   98-43503
                                                                                        CIP

We wish to acknowledge the support of Bard, which has helped to make the English translation of this book possible.

Published by
Futura Publishing Company, Inc.
135 Bedford Road
Armonk, NY 10504-0418

LC #: 98-43503
ISBN #: 0-87993-664-9

Every effort has been made to ensure that the information in this book is as up to date and as accurate as possible at the time of publication. However, due to the constant developments in medicine, neither the author, nor the editor, nor the publisher can accept any legal or any other responsibility for any errors or omissions that may occur.

Printed in the United States of America on acid-free paper.

VASCULAR SURGICAL APPROACHES

Edited by

ALAIN BRANCHEREAU, MD

University Hospital La Timone, Marseille, France

&

RAMON BERGUER, MD, PhD

Wayne State University and Detroit Medical Center,
Detroit, Michigan, USA

Illustrations by JEAN-PIERRE JACOMY

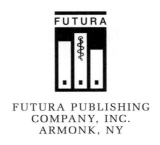

FUTURA PUBLISHING
COMPANY, INC.
ARMONK, NY

CONTRIBUTORS

Bahnini, Amine, MD
Department of Vascular Surgery
Pitié-Salpétrière University Hospital
75651 PARIS
FRANCE

Barral, Xavier, MD
Department of Cardiovascular Surgery
University Hospital (North)
42055 SAINT-ETIENNE Cedex 2
FRANCE

Baudet, Eugène, MD
Department of Cardiovascular
and Pediatric Cardiac Surgery
Bordeaux Heart University Hospital
33604 BORDEAUX-PESSAC
FRANCE

Berguer, Ramon, MD, PhD
Wayne State University Hospital
3990 John R.
DETROIT, MI 48201
USA

Blin, Dominique, MD
Department of Cardiac Surgery
Hôpital Albert Michallon
BP 217
38 043 GRENOBLE Cedex
FRANCE

Brami, Patrick, MD
Department of Vascular Surgery
Pitié-Salpétrière University Hospital
75651 PARIS
FRANCE

Branchereau, Alain, MD
Department of Vascular Surgery
University Hospital La Timone
13385 MARSEILLE Cedex 05
FRANCE

Calligaro, Keith D., MD
Pennsylvania Hospital
700 Spruce St, # 101
PHILADELPHIA, PA 19106
USA

Calvignac, Jean-Louis, MD
Department of Surgery
Hôpital de la Chartreuse
12200 VILLEFRANCHE de ROUERGUE
FRANCE

Chafke, Nabil, MD
Department of Cardiovascular Surgery
University Hospital
BP 426
67091 STRASBOURG Cedex
FRANCE

Chavannon, Olivier, MD
Department of Vascular Surgery
Hôpital Albert Michallon
BP 217
38043 GRENOBLE Cedex
FRANCE

Chevalier, Jean-Michel, MD
Department of Vascular Surgery
Hôpital Edouard Herriot
69437 LYON Cedex 03
FRANCE

Di Mauro, Pascal, MD
Division of Thoracic Surgery
University Hospital.
Hôpital Sainte Marguerite
13009 MARSEILLE
FRANCE

Dougherty, Matthew J., MD
Pennsylvania Hospital
700 Spruce St, # 101
PHILADELPHIA, PA 19106
USA

Dubreuil, Frederic, MD
University Hospital. Hôpital Jean Bernard
86021 POITIERS Cedex
FRANCE

Ede, Bertrand, MD
Department of Vascular Surgery
University Hospital La Timone
13385 MARSEILLE Cedex 05
FRANCE

Enon, Bernard, MD
Department of Vascular
and Thoracic Surgery
University Hospital
49033 ANGERS Cedex 01
FRANCE

Favre, Jean-Pierre, MD
Department of Cardiovascular Surgery
University Hospital (North)
42055 SAINT-ETIENNE Cedex 2
FRANCE

Feugier, Patrick, MD
Department of Vascular Surgery
Hôpital Edouard Herriot
69437 LYON Cedex 03
FRANCE

Fuentes, Pierre, MD
Division of Thoracic Surgery
University Hospital.
Hôpital Sainte Marguerite
13009 MARSEILLE
FRANCE

Gournier, Jean-Paul, MD
Department of Cardiovascular Surgery
University Hospital (North)
42055 SAINT-ETIENNE Cedex 2
FRANCE

Hallett, John W. Jr., MD
Mayo Clinic
200 First St SW
ROCHESTER, MN 55905
USA

Jacobs, Michael, MD
Academic Medical Center
Department of Vascular Surgery
PO Box 22700
1100 AMSTERDAM
The NETHERLANDS

Jausseran, Jean-Michel, MD
Department of Cardiovascular Surgery
Fondation Hôpital Saint-Joseph
13285 MARSEILLE Cedex 8
FRANCE

Kazmers, Andris, MD
Division of Vascular Surgery
Wayne State University
Detroit Medical Center
3990 John R.
DETROIT, MI 48201
USA

Kieffer, Edouard, MD
Department of Vascular Surgery
Pitié-Salpétrière University Hospital
75651 PARIS
FRANCE

Koskas, Fabien, MD
Department of Vascular Surgery
Pitié-Salpétrière University Hospital
75651 PARIS
FRANCE

Kretz, Jean-Georges, MD
Department of Cardiovascular Surgery
University Hospital
BP 426
67091 STRASBOURG Cedex
FRANCE

Laborde, Marie-Nadine, MD
Department of Cardiovascular
and Pediatric Cardiac Surgery
Bordeaux Heart University Hospital
33604 BORDEAUX-PESSAC
FRANCE

Lacombe, Michel, MD
Consultation de Chirurgie
University Hospital. Hôpital Beaujon
92118 CLICHY Cedex
FRANCE

Lucas, Charles E., MD
Department of Surgery
Wayne State University, 6-C UHC
4201 St. Antoine
DETROIT, MI 48201
USA

Magnan, Pierre-Edouard, MD
Department of Vascular Surgery
University Hospital La Timone
13385 MARSEILLE Cedex 05
FRANCE

Mary, Henri, MD
Department of Vascular
and Thoracic Surgery
University Hospital Arnaud de Villeneuve
371, Av. du Doyen G. Giraud
34295 MONTPELLIER Cedex 5
FRANCE

Mathieu, Jean-Pierre, MD
Department of Vascular Surgery
University Hospital.
Hôpital Sainte Marguerite
13009 MARSEILLE
FRANCE

Nicolini, Philippe, MD
Clinique du Grand Large
2, Av. Léon Blum
69150 DECINES CHARPIEU
FRANCE

Perrin, Michel, MD
Clinique du Grand Large
2, Av. Léon Blum
69150 DECINES CHARPIEU
FRANCE

Plissonnier, Didier, MD
Department of Vascular Surgery
University Hospital. Hôpital Charles Nicolle
1, rue de Germont
76000 ROUEN
FRANCE

Ricco, Jean-Baptiste, MD
University Hospital. Hôpital Jean Bernard
86021 POITIERS Cedex
FRANCE

Rosset, Eugenio, MD
Department of Vascular Surgery
University Hospital La Timone
13385 MARSEILLE Cedex 05
FRANCE

Sicard, Gregorio A., MD
Washington University School of Medicine
1 Barnes Hospital P1 5103
ST LOUIS, MO 63118
USA

Soury, Patrick, MD
Department of Vascular Surgery
University Hospital. Hôpital Charles Nicolle
1, rue de Germont
76000 ROUEN
FRANCE

Testart, Jacques, MD
Department of Vascular Surgery
University Hospital. Hôpital Charles Nicolle
1, rue de Germont
76000 ROUEN
FRANCE

Thomas, Pascal, MD
Division of Thoracic Surgery
University Hospital.
Hôpital Sainte Marguerite
13009 MARSEILLE
FRANCE

Thomassin, Jean-Marc, MD
Division of Otorhinolaryngology
University Hospital La Timone
13385 Marseille Cedex 05
FRANCE

Tournigand, Pierre, MD
Department of Vascular Surgery
University Hospital La Timone
13385 MARSEILLE Cedex 05
FRANCE

Toursarkissian, Boulos, MD
Washington University School of Medicine
1 Barnes Hospital P1 5103
ST LOUIS, MO 63118
USA

Veith, Frank J., MD
Montefiore Medical Center
111 East 210th Street
BRONX, NY 10467
USA

Watelet, Jacques, MD
Department of Vascular Surgery
University Hospital. Hôpital Charles Nicolle
1, rue de Germont
76000 ROUEN
FRANCE

FOREWORD

This volume stems from a French book, *Voies d'Abord des Vaisseaux,* published in 1995. It is not a mere translation but rather an extensively reedited version carried out by two friends who share a similar vision of vascular surgery.

Some chapters preserve the same authorship but their translation gave us an opportunity to improve the original version. Other chapters were rewritten by new authors to update information and to balance the European and North American participation. The illustrations were revised by the same artist who did the original work; some were corrected, some added, others omitted. On the whole more than 80 illustrations of this volume are new or modified.

This book is intended as a helpful tool to vascular surgeons in training and in practice. The former will find the elements for basic exposure of vessels that is a first step in surgical training. The latter will profit from the viewpoint of experienced authors on unusual approaches, which may be of great help in special circumstances. It is pertinent to review the extensive array of available vascular surgical appraoches at a time when endovascular techniques are being proposed at most anatomic locations.

The choice of subject headings was dictated by daily practice in vascular surgery. Approaches to arteries such as gluteal or external carotid, usually included in books dealing with vascular exposures, are irrelevant today when balloon occlusion or particle embolization resolve the problems for which these arteries are exposed.

With regard to anatomic nomenclature, we followed the pragmatic rule of common usage. In general, we followed the international notation in the chapters describing limb anatomy, but did not do so in those dealing with the anatomy of the head, neck, and trunk.

The illustrations are the work of medical artist Jean-Pierre Jacomy. To improve this new volume he agreed to extensively revise his original work. We are grateful to Eugenio Rosset, vascular surgeon and anatomist, who helped us with anatomic nomenclature questions. We also thank Futura Publishing Company and its President Jacques Strauss, who encouraged us to do this job to further bridge the practice of vascular surgeons in North America and Europe.

Alain Branchereau
Marseille

Ramon Berguer
Detroit

CONTENTS

1

Carotid Bifurcation

Alain Branchereau, Eugenio Rosset

Description of the Conventional Technique

Patient Position

The patient is placed in supine decubitus with the face turned away from the operative site. The neck should be slightly extended either by inclining the table or placing a medium-size supportive device under the patient's shoulders. The neck should not be overly rotated or extended. Excessive rotation can lead to ischemia by compression of one or both vertebral arteries and/or the contralateral internal carotid artery. To decrease venous pressure in the head, the patient should be placed in a semi-seated position by raising the trunk and lower extremities. The arm on the operated side should be supported by the surgical drape along the trunk. The contralateral arm is placed at a 90 degree angle on an armrest (Fig. 1). The surgeon stands in front of the operative field, the surgical assistant stands beside the surgeon at the head of the table, and the instrument nurse stands on the other side of the surgeon. A surgical drape is placed so that the anesthetist has access to the patient's

face and to the extended arm. In our department we always place the patient in a manner that allows us to harvest the internal saphenous vein from the ipsilateral thigh (Fig. 2) if it becomes necessary.

Skin Incision

A linear skin incision is made obliquely parallel to the anterior edge of the sternocleidomastoid muscle from the end of the mastoid process behind the lobe of the ear to the medial end of the clavicle (Fig. 3). The length of the incision varies from 12 cm to 15 cm. The incision should be centered on the carotid bifurcation defined by the preoperative arteriogram.

Superficial Layer

After dividing the platysma with the electric scalpel, the external jugular vein is divided and ligated. The cervical branches of the superficial cervical plexus are sectioned (this can lead to mild local hypoesthesia). The auricular nerve which generally traverses the upper part of the incision can be dissected and

From Vascular Surgical Approaches, edited by Alain Branchereau and Ramon Berguer. ©1999, Futura Publishing Co., Inc., Armonk, NY.

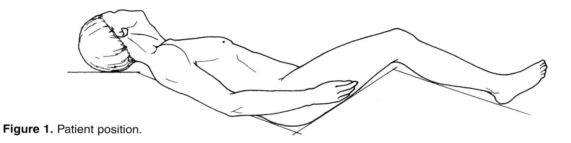

Figure 1. Patient position.

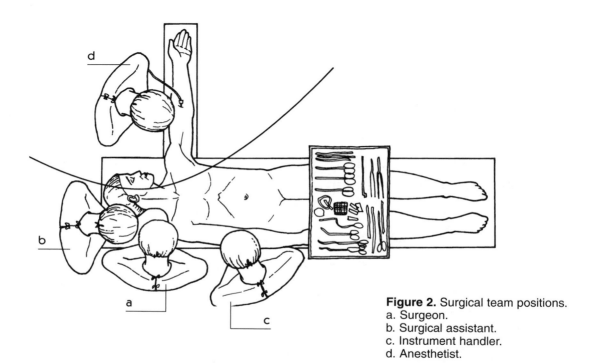

Figure 2. Surgical team positions.
a. Surgeon.
b. Surgical assistant.
c. Instrument handler.
d. Anesthetist.

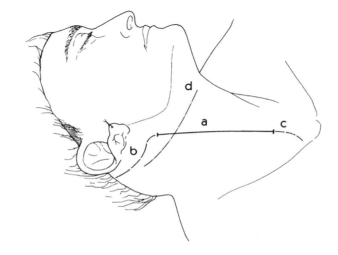

Figure 3. Incisions.
a. Standard incision.
b. Upward extension.
c. Downward extension.
d. Transverse incision.

mobilized but we prefer to cut it; the resulting mild numbness in the ear lobe regresses within a few months. The superficial cervical fascia is incised along the anterior border of the sterno-cleidomastoid muscle and the latter is retracted posteriorly. At the top of this incision, the parotid gland which often overlaps the anterior edge of the sternocleidomastoid muscle is detached from the latter and retracted upward. Injury of the parotid gland can lead to heavy bleeding and hemostasis can be difficult. This mishap is a major cause of local edema and inflammation during the postoperative period. If the incision is carried too far anteriorly at this level, one risks injuring the cervicofacial branch of the facial nerve.

Middle Layer

After the sternocleidomastoid muscle has been retracted posteriorly, a self-retaining retractor is placed between the muscle posteriorly and the superficial cervical aponeurosis anteriorly. The middle cervical aponeurosis should be incised, using Mayo scissors, from the posterior half of the digastric muscle at the top to the tendon of the omohyoid muscle at the bottom. Dissection of the anterior edge of the internal jugular vein allows exposure and ligation of the anterior facial vein (Fig. 4). The anatomy of this venous trunk is highly variable. There can be two or three veins of various sizes entering separately the internal jugular vein in which case each one must be dissected and ligated. It is always necessary to divide all branches along the anterior edge of the internal jugular vein up to the point where the vein crosses the digastric muscle. The loose connective tissue between the facial vein and the digastric muscle is rich in lymph nodes (subdigastric group). This packet of lymph nodes can be divided using the cautery or freed from its anterior adhesions and folded

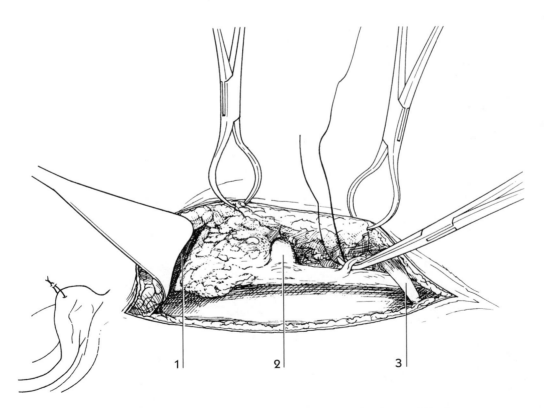

Figure 4. Ligation of a superior thyroid vein after mobilization of the anterior edge of the sternocleidomastoid muscle.
1. Posterior belly of digastric muscle.
2. Thyrolinguofacial vein trunk.
3. Intermediary tendon of the omohyoid muscle.

backward (Fig. 5). During this maneuver to dissect this lymphatic tissue from the vein, it is important to follow the anterior border of the jugular vein in order to avoid injury to nearby nervous structures.

Vascular Layer

Arterial dissection begins in the internal carotid artery distal to the diseased segment. Prior to this the hypoglossal nerve and its descending branch must be identified. In most cases access to the internal carotid artery requires dissection and ligation of the occipital artery or one of its branches, the upper sternocleidomastoid artery, which loops and holds down the XII cranial nerve (Fig. 6). After identifying the vagus nerve in the space between the jugular vein and carotid artery, the descending branch of the ansa of the hypoglossal can be safely divided near its origin. Division at a lower level[1] can result in paralysis of the infrahyoid muscles. The division of the ansa and the upper sternocleidomastoid artery permits mobilization of the hypoglossal nerve upwards and exposure of the internal carotid artery above the plaque where the artery is normal. This can be recognized by its bluish tinge. To avoid vagal reflexes 1-3 ml of Xylocaine® are injected in two spots behind the origin of the internal carotid arteries close to the vagus and between the internal and external carotid arteries. The lower part of the common carotid artery can be easily dissected

after isolating the vagus nerve and the lower portion of the hypoglossal loop. Gentle palpation of the common carotid artery a few centimeters below its bifurcation establishes the level where the arterial wall is normal.

After systemic heparinization, the internal carotid artery is clamped in a normal zone near the level of the XII nerve in order to avoid embolization from the bifurcation plaque (Fig. 7). The posterior aspect of the carotid bifurcation can then be easily and safely dissected. All structures located between the posterior aspect of the carotid bifurcation and the deep cervical fascial layer should be divided using scissors taking care to locate and preserve the superior laryngeal nerve which is visible behind the bifurcation (Fig. 7). The origin of the external carotid artery is dissected as well as the superior thyroid artery. The glomic vessels are located for possible temporary ligation in case they backbleed after the arteriotomy. When the dissection is complete, the external and common carotid arteries can be clamped and the arteriotomy carried out.

Alternative Techniques

Upward Extension

Extension of dissection of the internal carotid artery upwards into the subparotid

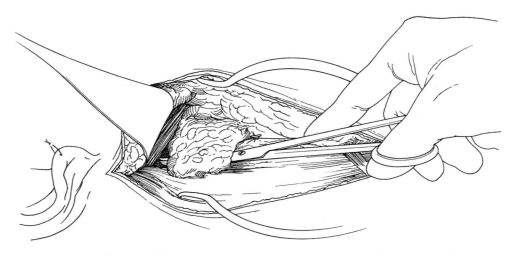

Figure 5. Dissection of the lymph nodes under the digastric muscle.

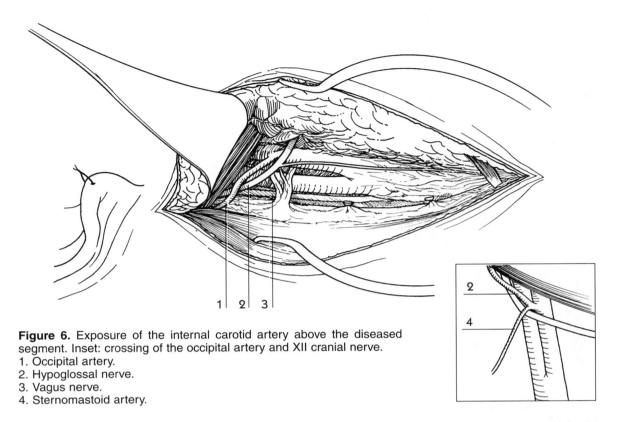

Figure 6. Exposure of the internal carotid artery above the diseased segment. Inset: crossing of the occipital artery and XII cranial nerve.
1. Occipital artery.
2. Hypoglossal nerve.
3. Vagus nerve.
4. Sternomastoid artery.

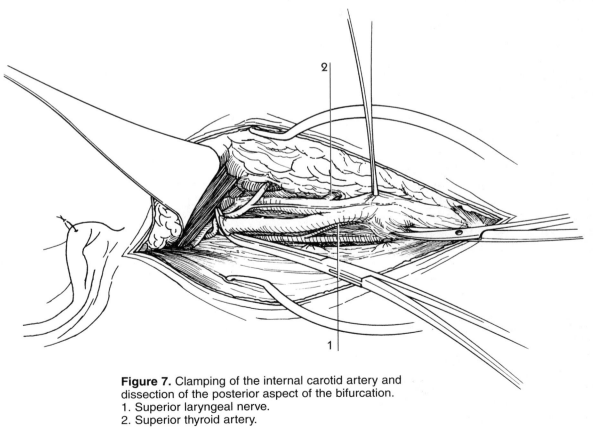

Figure 7. Clamping of the internal carotid artery and dissection of the posterior aspect of the bifurcation.
1. Superior laryngeal nerve.
2. Superior thyroid artery.

space may be necessary to expose an additional 2 or 3 cm of the internal carotid artery or to do the distal anastomosis of a bypass at the level of C1, 3 cm below the base of the skull. If an upward extension is anticipated before the procedure, nasal intubation should be performed and the jaw should be subluxated anteriorly, maintaining the subluxation by a wire between the jaw and the nasal wall.[2] These maneuvers increase the distance between the mastoid apophysis and the ramus of the mandible thus increasing the angle of inferior aperture in which the internal carotid artery is exposed.

For this upward extension, the skin incision must be extended downwards along the posterior edge of the mastoid apophysis (Fig. 3). The intermediate tendon of the digastric muscle is divided and the posterior ventral aspect is released and then folded back and secured using a suture. Careful upward retraction, using a Richardson retractor, shows the styloid muscles. Care must be exercised to avoid injury to the cervicofacial branch of the facial nerve. Using this extended incision, an extra 1 to 2 cm of the artery can be exposed by resecting the tip of the styloid apophysis with a small rongeur and detaching the styloid muscles or, more simply, by fracturing the apophysis with the finger in order to relax the styloid muscles and allow upward and forward retraction using a long thin malleable retractor (Fig. 8, inset). During dissection of the hypoglossal nerve, its adhesions to the plexiform node of the vagus nerve must be divided with care to avoid paralysis of the vocal cords.[3] To avoid injury of the XII cranial nerve itself, the posterior hypoglossal loop (ansa) should be divided 1 cm beyond its origin and its stump is used for traction as the XII nerve is freed. Once the XII nerve is mobilized the internal carotid artery can be exposed. A loop is usually passed around the internal carotid artery to continue the distal dissection of the latter without injuring the arterial wall. Hemostasis should be achieved using thin bipolar coagulation forceps. Further up, the glossopharyngeal nerve can be identified (Fig. 8) as it crosses in front of the internal carotid artery and runs across towards the pharynx. Only under exceptional circumstances can this nerve be divided. Using this extended technique it is possible to expose the internal artery above the IX cranial nerve. When bypass or transposition is to be per-

formed at this level, a useful maneuver may be the division of the internal carotid artery at its origin. In this way the artery can be transposed anterior to the IX and XII nerves and a high anastomosis can be safely made.

Downward Extension

The opening can be extended a few centimeters downward without risk. The major limitations are the clavicle and the top of the sternum. The skin incision is extended a few centimeters (Fig. 3). The platysma can be incised down to its lower attachments and with it the substernal branch of the cervical superficial plexus. During division of the anterior belly or of the intermediary tendon of the omohyoid muscle it is necessary to control the omohyoid vessels and the branches of the superior thyroid artery. ·

Transverse Incision[4]

An oblique transverse incision through a skin fold of the neck is used mainly for cosmetic purposes (Fig. 3) in women and younger patients. Before surgery, arteriography without bone subtraction should be performed to precisely locate the carotid bifurcation and limit the extent of the subcutaneous dissection. For best cosmetic results the neck fold in which the incision is to be made should be chosen and marked before the procedure. The skin and platysma should be incised at the same level in order to obtain a flap with a superomedial concavity. The anterior edge of the sternocleidomastoid muscle is used as a landmark as previously described. The rest of the procedure is the same as in the standard technique except that exposure of the lower part of the common carotid artery is more limited.

Retrojugular Approach[5]

The skin incision for the retrojugular approach is the same as for the standard technique; the sternocleidomastoid muscle is freed up to its mastoid attachment. After locating the spinal accessory nerve, the internal jugular vein is retracted forward. This maneuver

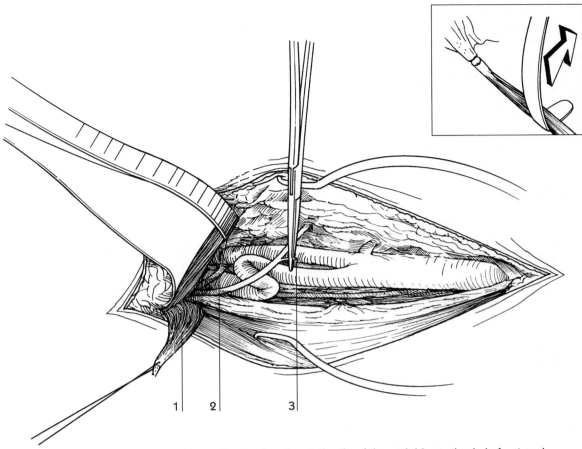

Figure 8. Upward extension. Inset: the tip of the styloid apophysis is fractured and the styloid muscles are retracted using a thin malleable retractor.
1. Posterior belly of the digastric muscle after division of its intermediate tendon.
2. Glossopharyngeal nerve.
3. Divided origin of the posterior ansa of the XII nerve.

requires ligation of some small posterior branches of the internal jugular vein. The vagus and hypoglossal nerves are retracted upward and medially, taking care to identify the superior laryngeal nerve which runs across the back of the internal carotid artery. This technique achieves satisfactory exposure of the carotid bifurcation. Upward extension of the retrojugular approach is also possible by dividing the posterior belly of the digastric muscle near its mastoid attachment. After this maneuver the transverse apophysis of the first cervical vertebra as well as the styloid apophysis can be easily palpated.

Discussion

Patient position is an important factor for the comfort of the surgeon. In this regard several points should be emphasized. The patient's head should be placed at the end of the table with the face turned away from the operative side. This allows the surgeon to remain seated and the surgical assistant to stand over the head of the patient. The neck is always rotated and extended, but neither of these movements should be exaggerated and no restraining device should be used to avoid occlusion of the vertebral artery or of the contralateral internal carotid artery.

The approach that we describe is more time-consuming but achieves wider exposure than the frequently used and more direct alternative consisting of simply directly dissecting the carotid bifurcation. The present technique has two advantages. The first is to reduce the risk of embolization by allowing access and clamping of the internal carotid artery in a nondiseased segment before dissecting the carotid bifurcation. The additional clamp time is, in our opinion, negligible. The second advantage of the present technique is to provide excellent exposure and allow carrying the arteriotomy of the distal internal carotid artery well above the diseased area. Good exposure and proper control are essential for a successful reconstruction. The present approach also facilitates changes in strategy during the procedure if it becomes necessary to enlarge the arteriotomy, place a patch, or perform bypass.

The need for an upward extension may occur intraoperatively, e.g. to do a bypass after an intraoperative angiogram demonstrates a defective endarterectomy, or electively as in the presence of a severely kinked carotid artery. Upward extension as presented in this chapter allows endarterectomy to be performed safely up to the level of the first cervical vertebra. The maneuvers described include resection of the posterior belly of the digastric muscle, resection of the styloid muscle, and subluxation of the mandible. Division or partial resection of the ramus of the lower mandible does not improve upon the described exposure. As stated by Mock, et al this approach leaves an average of 12 mm of the internal carotid artery unexposed between the upper limit of the controllable zone and the point of penetration in the temporal canal.[6] Exposure of the intrapetrosal carotid artery requires mobilization of the facial nerve in association with removal of the central wall of the carotid artery foramen. This type of procedure is performed in collaboration with an ENT surgeon[7] as described in Chapter 3.

In clinical practice the surgeon is seldom confronted with a situation in which he must choose between the standard approach with or without upward or downward extension, and either the horizontal or retrojugular approach. In our experience the horizontal approach has been used for cosmetic purposes in a few cases and in patients who have undergone radiation therapy or laryngectomy. We have used the retrojugular approach for two indications. The first is restenosis of the carotid artery to avoid the risk of injury of the cranial nerves associated with repeated dissection in a fibrotic zone. The second indication for the retrojugular approach in our experience is carotid reconstruction associated with elective distal vertebral bypass. The retrojugular approach provides the best pathway for a distal vertebral bypass, and we prefer to perform the carotid bypass through the same exposure rather than to dissect and mobilize completely the internal jugular vein.

References

1. Sundt TM Jr. Techniques of Carotid Endarterectomy. In: *Occlusive Cerebrovascular Disease: Diagnosis and Surgical Management.* Philadelphia, Saunders, 1987, pp 191-225.
2. Sandmann W, Hennerici M, Aulich A, et al. Progress in carotid artery surgery at the base of the skull. *J Vasc Surg* 1984; 1: 734-743.
3. Pech A, Mercier Cl, Thomassin JM, Piligian F. L'abord chirurgical de la partie haute de la carotide interne cervicale. *Journal Français d'Oto-Laryngologie* 1983; 32: 401-406.
4. Wylie EJ, Stoney RJ, Ehrenfeld WK. Carotid atherosclerosis. In: *Manual of Vascular Surgery. Vol I.* New York, Springer-Verlag, 1980, p 55.
5. Berguer R, Kieffer E. Repair of the internal and external carotid arteries. In: *Surgery of the Arteries to the Head.* New-York, Springer-Verlag, 1992, pp 108-137.
6. Mock CN, Lilly MP, McRae RG, Carney WI Jr. Selection of the approach to the distal internal carotid artery from the second cervical vertebra to the base of the skull. *J Vasc Surg* 1990; 6: 846-853.
7. Magnan PE, Branchereau A, Cannoni M. Traumatic aneurysms of the internal carotid artery at the base of the skull. *J Cardiovasc Surg* 1992; 33: 372-379.

2

High Internal Carotid Exposure

Ramon Berguer

Distal Exposure Between C1 and C2 for Reoperations (Retrojugular Approach)

This approach is used preferentially for carotid operations when the surgeon chooses to avoid the previous operative field and needs to expose the internal carotid artery at a higher level than the one reached in the previous operation.[1] In this situation the reoperation will consist of an exclusion bypass between the common carotid artery (CCA) and the internal carotid artery (ICA). The retrojugular approach described below avoids the dissection and mobilization of the vagus and hypoglossal nerves and allows the surgeon to work in a previously undissected field, reaching the upper cervical ICA at the level of C1.

Following the opening of the scar from the previous operation the dissection is directed between the internal jugular vein (IJV) anteriorly and the sternomastoid muscle posteriorly. The accessory spinal nerve is identified at the point where it penetrates the sternomastoid muscle. The nerve is then slung with a silastic loop and followed distally under the digastric muscle, until the point where it

rests on the IJV as they both lie on the transverse process of C1. The digastric muscle may be retracted or cut. The transverse process of C1, once identified, becomes the upper limit of the distal dissection.

At the lowest level of the operative field the IJV and the vagus nerve are mobilized anterior to and over the common carotid artery, and the latter is exposed and slung. This presents no difficulty since the common carotid artery is usually exposed proximal to the previous dissection. Enough CCA is exposed to carry out an end-to-side anastomosis to a bypass.

Distally, the IJV and vagus nerves are mobilized forward. As the vagus nerve is mobilized anteriorly the hypoglossal nerve is displaced ahead of it. The latter does not block the surgeon's path with this approach and in fact is mostly hidden from view behind the vagus. When dissecting the vagus nerve high in the neck the surgeon identifies the superior laryngeal nerve (Fig. 1). The latter emerges from the vagus and passes beneath the ICA to run deep and medial to the carotid bulb against the larynx. As the IJV and vagus are lifted distally the superior laryngeal nerve is seen hugging the ICA and disappearing below it.

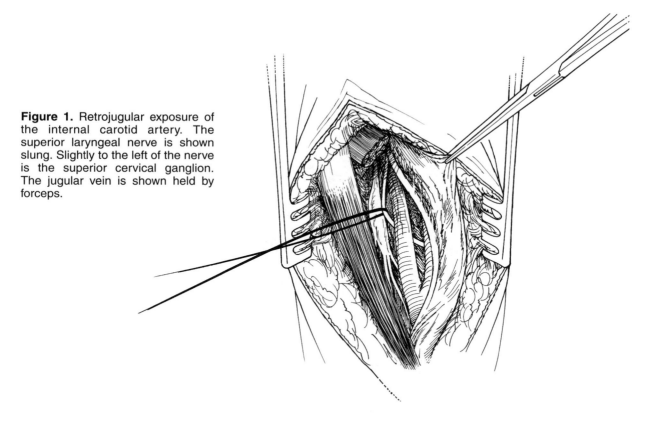

Figure 1. Retrojugular exposure of the internal carotid artery. The superior laryngeal nerve is shown slung. Slightly to the left of the nerve is the superior cervical ganglion. The jugular vein is shown held by forceps.

The superior laryngeal nerve is already under some tension when the vagus is elevated over and in front of the ICA and cannot be mobilized further safely. The ICA is identified and dissected generally below, but sometimes above, the superior laryngeal nerve. At this point the bulging large superior cervical (sympathetic) ganglion is seen subjacent to the ICA. The close anatomic relationship between the distal cervical ICA and the underlying transverse process of C1 is obvious during exposure of the artery at this level.

Distal Exposure Between C1 and the Temporal Canal

The most frequent need for extended exposure arises during a standard carotid endarterectomy when an unsuspected high plaque or a technical problem with the endarterectomy requires a higher exposure. In other instances the need for a high (C1 or above) exposure is anticipated by the arteriographic findings. In the latter case the high exposure will be facilitated by nasotracheal intubation and anterior subluxation of the jaw preoperatively. The subluxated mandible is held in position by a wire around the mandible and through the anterior nasal spine as described by Fischer.[2]

In the course of a carotid operation that needs to be extended cranially, the first obstacle to a higher dissection of the ICA is the hypoglossal nerve. This nerve is tethered posteriorly by the sternomastoid artery and vein, and often by the occipital artery. Division of the sternomastoid vessels allows anterior mobilization of the hypoglossal nerve (Fig. 2). Further anterior mobilization of the hypoglossal nerve is obtained by division of the occipital artery. Dissection can then proceed up to the point where the sheaths of the vagus and hypoglossal nerve come together. At this point the dissection of the ICA is continued above the hypoglossal nerve. The hypoglossal nerve is gently tethered down with a nerve hook, the digastric muscle is retracted or, more commonly, cut and the ICA is isolated and dissected free above the hypoglossal nerve (Fig. 3). If the ICA dissection proceeds distally

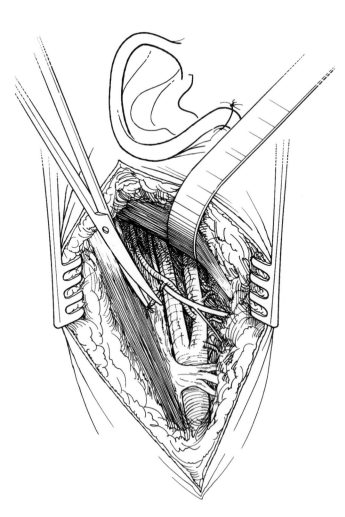

Figure 2. Division of the sternomastoid artery to mobilize the hypoglossal nerve cranially and ventrally.

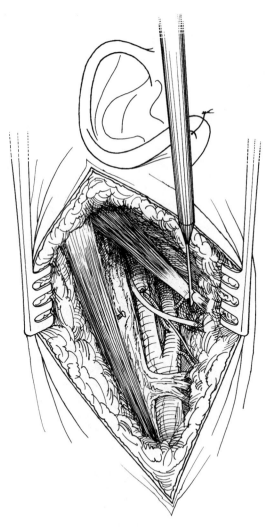

Figure 3. Division of the digastric muscle to increase distal carotid exposure.

enough above the level of the hypoglossus the glossopharyngeal nerve will be encountered as it crosses the ICA (Fig. 4). The glossopharyngeal nerve runs on top of the ICA and below the external carotid artery (ECA). This nerve may be a single or a double trunk. It is dissected,

freed and elevated with a nerve hook to continue the dissection of the ICA. This cranial extension of the dissection of the ICA usually permits mobilizing some length of it into the operative field (Fig.5).

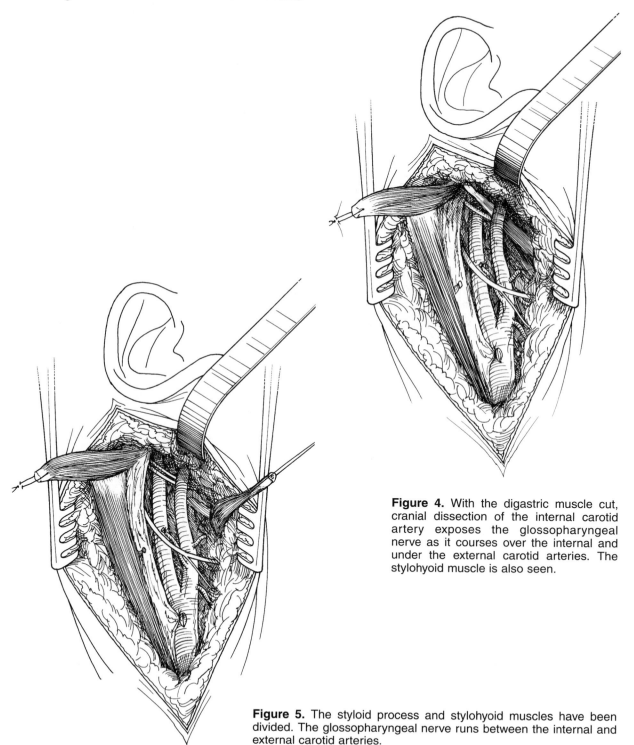

Figure 4. With the digastric muscle cut, cranial dissection of the internal carotid artery exposes the glossopharyngeal nerve as it courses over the internal and under the external carotid arteries. The stylohyoid muscle is also seen.

Figure 5. The styloid process and stylohyoid muscles have been divided. The glossopharyngeal nerve runs between the internal and external carotid arteries.

The next steps depend on the technique chosen for carotid reconstruction. If the surgeon chooses (a) a standard carotid endarterectomy with a longitudinal arteriotomy, he may be able to access the distal ICA by lifting the hypoglossal nerve, or he may have to do the endarterectomy and the closure by working first above and then below the nerve; or, (b) if a carotid bypass has been chosen, the graft is made to lie above the hypoglossal nerve and the distal anastomosis is done as an end-to-side eventually occluding the ICA below the anastomosis to *terminalize* it. Finally, (c) if an eversion endarterectomy has been decided upon, the ICA is amputated at its origin, the ICA is transposed anterior to the hypoglossal nerve, and the eversion endarterectomy performed. The artery is eventually anastomosed to its origin or lower to the CCA, allowing it to lie on top of the hypoglossal nerve.

The maneuver of dividing the origin of the ICA and transposing it anterior to the hypoglossal nerve permits continuation of the dissection on the ICA up to the level of entrance of the temporal canal (Fig. 6). At this point the surgeon needs to do some unroofing to continue the dissection distally. This generally requires the division of the digastric muscle, as indicated above. As the dissection of the ICA proceeds distally the next obstacle is the glossopharyngeal nerve running on top of the ICA and below the ECA.

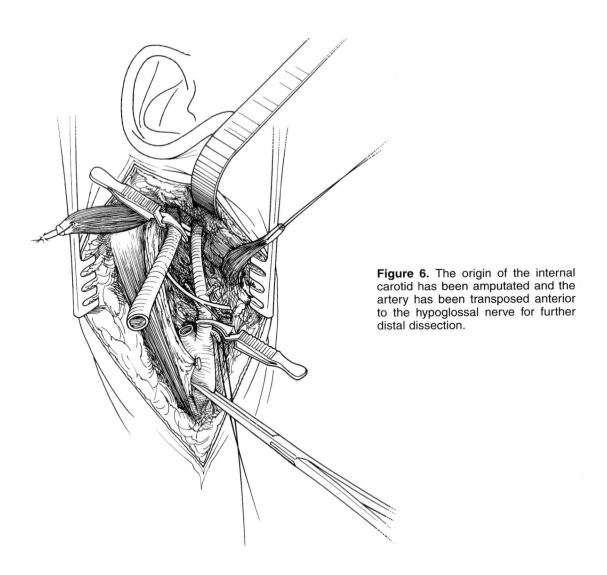

Figure 6. The origin of the internal carotid has been amputated and the artery has been transposed anterior to the hypoglossal nerve for further distal dissection.

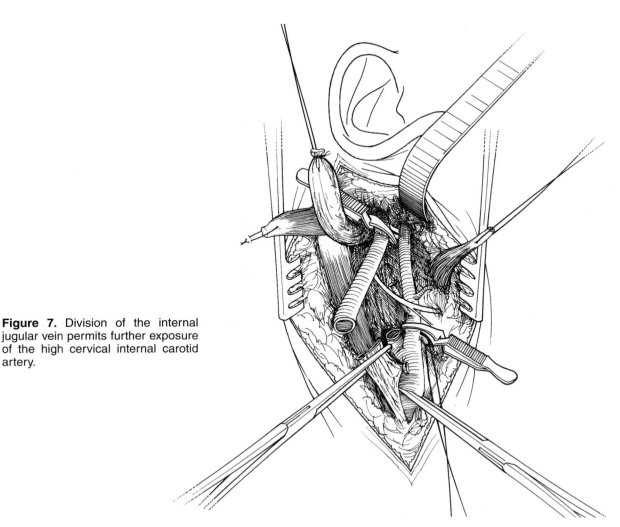

Figure 7. Division of the internal jugular vein permits further exposure of the high cervical internal carotid artery.

The IJV partially overlaps the ICA and obstructs the operative field. If it becomes a problem it can be divided and securely ligated as high as possible to clear the field (Fig. 7). Before this maneuver is done one should make sure that the opposite IJV is patent. This information is usually available in the delayed views of the preoperative angiogram.

Further exposure at this point requires clearing some bone either anteriorly (angle of the mandible) or posteriorly (mastoid). The angle of the mandible can be resected below the entrance point of the inferior alveolar nerve, as shown by Goldsmith.[3] This requires clearing the masseter and pterygoid muscles and the use of a pneumatic saw.

Increasing exposure at the skull base by a partial mastoidectomy is best done by prolonging the incision with an anterior

auricular branch. The facial nerve is dissected and elevated and the mastoid tip is amputated as described by Purdue.[4] The ICA can be dissected free up to its entrance in the carotid canal of the petrous bone.

References

1. Berguer R. Retrojugular approach for exclusion bypass of carotid bifurcation: A useful method for recurrent or high carotid disease. In: Veith F, ed. *Current Critical Problems in Vascular Surgery. Vol 4.* St. Louis, Quality Medical Publishing, 1992, pp 403-406.
2. Fischer DF, Clagett GP, Parker JI, et al. Mandibular subluxation for high carotid exposure. *J Vasc Surg* 1984; 1: 727-733.
3. Goldsmith MM 3d, Postma DS, Jones FD. The surgical exposure of penetrating injuries to the carotid artery at the skull base. Otolaryngol Head Neck Surg 1986; 95: 278-284.
4. Purdue GF, Pellegrini RV, Arena S. Aneurysms of the high internal carotid artery: A new approach. *Surgery* 1981; 89: 268-270.

3

Intrapetrosal Internal Carotid Artery

Jean-Marc Thomassin, Alain Branchereau

Repair of dysplastic, aneurysmal, or traumatic lesions of the internal carotid artery at the base of the skull requires exposure of the vertical portion of the intrapetrosal segment of this artery. In our opinion the anterior infratemporal approach without displacement of the facial nerve is the most suitable route. The procedure is carried out jointly by otolaryngologists and vascular surgeons.

Anatomic Review

The aperture of the carotid canal is located on the inferior surface of the temporal bone. The canal can be divided into three parts: a short, vertically ascending segment no more than 5 mm in height, a 90 degree elbow in contact with the anterior wall of the tympanic cavity, and a long horizontal segment whose medial aspect runs closely parallel to the auditory canal. The auditory canal must be sacrificed to expose the vessel. The exit of the canal, called the foramen lacerum, is located in the skull near the apex of the temporal bone.

Relations of the Carotid Canal in the Infratemporal Fossa (Figs. 1 and 2)

The aperture of the carotid canal is located 10 mm medial to the styloid process in contact with the internal jugular vein in the back. The narrow portion of the jugular canal (jugular foramen) and the exit of the cranial nerves are medial and deep.

The vertical portion of the canal is separated from the tympanic cavity by the tympanic plate. The posterolateral wall of the vertical segment of the carotid canal can be opened by drilling the vagina of the styloid process. The lateral wall of the horizontal segment of the carotid canal is in direct relation with the glasserian or petrotympanic fissure and therefore with the auditory canal (eustachian tube). The pterygoid plate is located immediately in front of the vagina of the styloid process and constitutes a reinforcement on the lateral side of the middle meningeal artery as it enters the small round hole. The vagina of the styloid process must be resected with care towards the front and the middle

From Vascular Surgical Approaches, edited by Alain Branchereau and Ramon Berguer. ©1999, Futura Publishing Co., Inc., Armonk, NY.

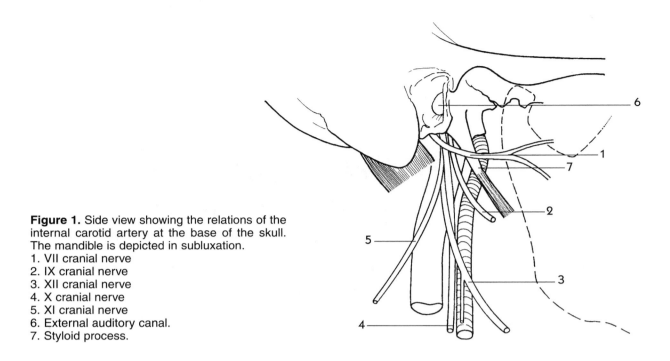

Figure 1. Side view showing the relations of the internal carotid artery at the base of the skull. The mandible is depicted in subluxation.
1. VII cranial nerve
2. IX cranial nerve
3. XII cranial nerve
4. X cranial nerve
5. XI cranial nerve
6. External auditory canal.
7. Styloid process.

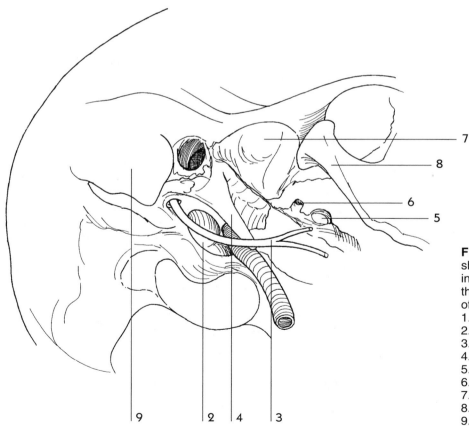

Figure 2. Bottom view showing relations of the internal carotid artery and the facial nerve at the base of the skull.
1. External auditory canal.
2. Jugular foramen.
3. Facial nerve.
4. Styloid process.
5. Foramen rotundum.
6. Small round hole.
7. Glenoid cavity.
8. Mandible.
9. Mastoid process.

meningeal artery must be identified before its entry into the bone canal. The foramen ovalis which contains the inferior maxillary nerve is located more anteriorly.

Exposure of the Vertical Intrapetrosal Segment

Position of the Patient

The scalp should be thoroughly washed using betadine and then a band about 4 cm wide, should be shaved over and behind the ear. In the operating room the scalp should be washed again using betadine. The patient's hair should be combed up and waxed to keep it in place. The patient is placed supine with the head on a headrest or directly on the surface of the operating table. Because the procedure is long, it is important to protect all pressure points using water or silicone gel bags. A heating pad may also be useful. The patient's face should be turned away from the operated side. The surgeon sits on the operated side directly over the mastoid region. The operative field involves the temporal and upper cervical regions (Fig. 3).

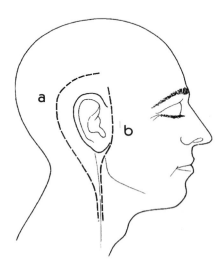

Figure 3. Skin incisions.
a. S-shaped cervicomastoid incision.
b. Vertical preauricular incision.

Skin Incision[1]

An S-shaped skin incision is made starting in the temporal region down to the neck (Fig. 3A). Most of the incision is above and behind the ear. On the neck the incision stops at the anterior border of the sternocleido-mastoid (SCM) muscle at the level of the hyoid. At the top it runs 3 cm above and behind the retroauricular groove. At the temporal level the incision is down to the bone and the soft tissue flap is folded back in the direction of the external auditory canal (EAC). After dividing the EAC the dissection continues to the level of the mandibular condyle. The tissue flap is secured in place using sutures and is covered with a moist lap.

A variation of this approach uses a preauricular skin incision down to the anterior border of the SCM muscle (Fig. 3B).[2]

Vascular Exposure

The dissection anterior to the SCM muscle opens the carotid sheath. The SCM muscle is detached from muscle the end of the mastoid with a musculoperiosteal flap to allow its reattachment at the end of the procedure. The internal carotid and jugular veins are identified as well as the X, XI, and XII cranial nerves.

The retroparotid trunk of the facial nerve, which is located in the angle formed by the anterior wall of the mastoid and the inferior wall of the EAC, is dissected up to its bifurcation in the parotid gland and into its cervicofacial branch. The intraparotid vein is divided and the deep parotid space is entered. The digastric muscle is detached from its insertion and pushed forward. The deep lobe of the parotid gland is released taking care to preserve the mandibular branch of the facial nerve which is freed upwards. The external carotid artery can be preserved or divided; the latter option has the advantage of allowing greater mobilization of the parotid gland forward. The styloid process is divided after several bites with a rongeur. The styloid muscles are retracted taking care not to damage the glossopharyngeal nerve.

The next step is the luxation of the temporomandibular joint (TMJ). This maneuver begins by dissecting the anterior wall of the EAC and the zygomatic arch. The subperiosteal dissection of the glenoid cavity is performed using a rasp above and behind the meniscus of the TMJ. Although bleeding can be substantial, the subperiosteal dissection is essential to obtain the maximal luxation to gain access to the interjugulocarotidian space. A ratchet-type retractor can be used to maintain the field open. During this part of the procedure care must be taken to avoid traction on the facial nerve.

The next step is the exposure of the infratemporal fossa. The tip of the mastoid process is drilled using the microscope (Fig. 4). Drilling stops at the digastric ridge which marks the level of the third portion of the facial nerve. The vagina of the styloid process can now be removed from the tympanic plate. The trunk of the facial nerve is freed up to its exit from the stylomastoid foramen. The deep lobe of the parotid gland is resected. The dissection exposes the inferior wall of the EAC and continues forward to expose the vagina of the styloid process up to the pterygoid plate of the sphenoid. The middle meningeal artery is identified at the point where it penetrates the skull through the round hole (Fig. 5).

The upper part of the internal carotid artery is located above and in front of the glossopharyngeal nerve. At this level the dissection is often hindered by the aneurysmal changes that may exist in the carotid artery. The canal should be used as a landmark to achieve dissection of the vertical segment of the intrapetrous internal carotid artery up to its elbow (Fig. 6). After stripping the anterior, inferior, and posterior aspects of the EAC, petrosectomy of the vagina of the styloid process is resected from the tympanic plate bone resection passing above the facial nerve which crosses the field. The petrosectomy is performed under the microscope using a cutting and a diamond drill to open the lateral wall of the vertical segment of the carotid canal up to the opening of the eustachian tube. Drilling continues forward to the sphenoid wing to expose the internal carotid artery on the anterior wall. The small round hole which contains the middle meningeal artery is spared.

While drilling, the surgeon must take care not to injure the trunk of the facial nerve. Some groups use a long sheathed burr.[3] Another possibility is the use of a small malleable blade to protect the nerve. Drilling of the anterior wall of the tympanic plate must preserve the tympanic cavity but be sufficient to allow mobilization of the intrapetrosal carotid artery.

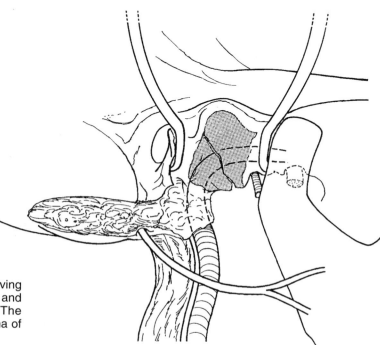

Figure 4. Partial petrosectomy removing the tip of the mastoid (operative view) and the root of the styloid process. The shaded area corresponds to the vagina of the styloid process.

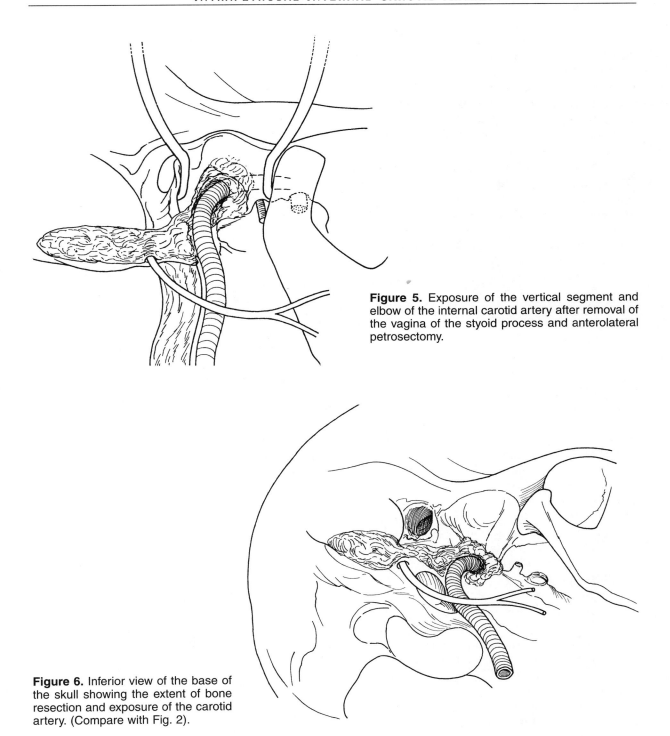

Figure 5. Exposure of the vertical segment and elbow of the internal carotid artery after removal of the vagina of the styoid process and anterolateral petrosectomy.

Figure 6. Inferior view of the base of the skull showing the extent of bone resection and exposure of the carotid artery. (Compare with Fig. 2).

Technical Variations

Exposure of the intrapetrosal internal carotid artery can be achieved by other techniques.

Two alternatives are available to approach the infratemporal fossa described by Fisch.[1] The type A approach allows exposure of the vertical segment and the elbow of the intrapetrosal internal carotid artery. It requires transposition of the second and third portion of the facial nerve and sacrifice of the middle ear. The type B approach allows exposure of the horizontal portion of the intrapetrosal internal carotid artery. It requires lowering of the mandibular condyle after detachment of the temporal muscle, drilling of the middle ear, and transposition of the facial nerve. In this technique, drilling is carried on the glenoid fossa and the major wing of the sphenoid. Division of the middle meningeal artery and of the mandibular nerve allows further lowering of the condyle using a retractor to increase exposure. Care must be taken not to overstretch the retroparotid trunk of the facial nerve. When drilling is completed the horizontal portion of the internal carotid artery at the level of the foramen lacerum is exposed.

Discussion

The high cervical internal carotid artery penetrates deep inside the skull, and its exposure is difficult. Unlike other techniques,[1,2] the procedure described here allows exposure of the vertical portion and the elbow of the carotid canal without sacrificing the middle ear which results in conduction deafness, and without displacement of the second and third portions of the facial nerve and the neural deficits that follow. Quality of exposure depends on two essential factors. The first is luxation of the TMJ to obtain direct access to the interjugulocarotid space and the vagina of the styloid process of the tympanic plate. At the end of the procedure the subperiosteal dissection of the glenoid cavity permits the restoration of the joint. In contrast with techniques that require resection of the mandibular condyle this method does not impair mastication. The second essential point for exposure is the drilling and exposure of the upper and intracranial portions of the internal carotid artery on both sides of the retroparotid trunk of the facial nerve.[3] All parotid gland tissue must be removed from the nerve in order to avoid any risk of stretching the latter with the retractor.

Exposure of the internal carotid artery in the intrapetrosal canal allows access to and surgical management of lesions considered inoperable until recently. Using this approach it is possible to treat traumatic lesions and aneurysms located at the base of the skull and even in the proximal vertical segment of the carotid canal.

It has been clearly established that reconstruction is preferable to carotid ligation for these indications.[4,5] Proximally, the internal carotid artery can be approached either in the subparotid space or at its origin. The second solution is preferable whenever possible since it limits dissection of the cranial nerves (IX, X, XII). We have observed that the dissection of these nerves, even if the trunks remain intact, often leads to impairment of laryngeal mobility and paresis of the IX cranial nerve that may not regress completely.

These procedures must be carried out in collaboration with an experienced otolaryngology team. They extend the indications for reconstruction of the internal carotid artery.

References

1. Fisch U. Infratemporal fossa approach to tumours of the temporal bone and base of the skull. *J Laryngol Otol* 1978; 92: 949-967.
2. Magnan PE, Branchereau A, Cannoni M. Traumatic aneurysms of the internal carotid artery at the base of the skull. *J Cardiovasc Surg* 1992; 33: 372-379.
3. Zanaret M, Giovanni A, Cannoni M, et al. Approche chirurgicale du segment vertical pétreux et cervical haut de la carotide interne. *Ann Oto Laryngol* 1994 ; 111: 211-216.
4. Rosset E, Roche PH, Magnan PE, Branchereau A. Surgical management of intracranial internal carotid artery aneurysms. *Cardiovasc Surg* 1994; 2: 567-572.
5. Moreau P, Albat B, Thevenet A. Traitement des anévrysmes de l'artère carotide interne extra-crânienne. *Ann Chir Vasc* 1994; 8: 409-416.

4

Proximal Vertebral Artery

Ramon Berguer

The first inch of the vertebral artery (VA) is the most frequent site for atherosclerotic disease of this vessel. The plaque that involves the origin of the VA is often contiguous with a subclavian plaque. The approach to revascularize the artery of this segment is straightforward, although it varies depending on the type of procedure that has been chosen. The most common approach is the interjugulocarotid approach which is used for transpositions of the VA to the carotid artery. Reconstructions of the VA based on the subclavian artery require exposure of the retroscalene portion of the subclavian and are also discussed below.

Anatomic Review

The proximal segment of the VA (segment V1) is that segment of the VA extending from its origin in the subclavian to the point where it penetrates the foramen transversarium of the sixth cervical vertebra. In 4% of cases the entry occurs sooner in the transverse process of C7, in 7% of cases the entry is higher at the level of C4-C5.[1] In the latter case as the artery ascends into the neck mostly parallel to the vertebral bodies, it must turn in a sharper manner to enter the transverse process of C4-C5. This acute angulation under the tendinous fibers of the longus colli may result in a point of compression or kinking. In 7% of the patients, the left VA arises independently from the aortic arch.

There are variations in size and dominance. The left VA tends to be larger than the right in 63% of cases. In 5% of cases one VA joins the basilar while the other is hypoplastic and terminates in the posterior inferior cerebellar artery. In the neck viewed frontally, the VA lies behind and deeper than the common carotid artery (Fig. 1). In front of the VA lie the sympathetic chain, the vertebral vein, the carotid artery, and the sternocleidomastoid muscle. The vertebral vein runs in front of the artery and is an important anatomic point of reference.[2] The VA is generally encircled by a sympathetic loop through which the artery runs. The components of the loop exit from the intermediate ganglion above and join the stellate ganglion below. On the left side the thoracic duct crosses in front of the artery as it

From Vascular Surgical Approaches, edited by Alain Branchereau and Ramon Berguer. ©1999, Futura Publishing Co., Inc., Armonk, NY.

emerges from behind the common carotid artery to join the jugulo-subclavian venous confluent. On the right side the recurrent nerve loops the subclavian inferiorly and proximal to the origin of the VA but not far from it. The origin of the VA in the subclavian wall is posterolateral. Lateral to it is the origin of the thyrocervical trunk. The inferior thyroid artery, the more medial branch of the thyroid cervical trunk, crosses in front of the VA to reach the inferior border of the thyroid. As it crosses the VA the inferior thyroid artery often goes through a small loop of the sympathetic chain. The internal mammary artery arises from the opposite subclavian wall slightly lateral to the VA. The VA runs in the deep space of the neck and after being crossed by the superior thyroid artery it deepens under the musculotendinous fibers of the longus colli, which covers its last millimeters like a small lid, to enter the transverse process of C6.

Patient Position

The patient is supine with a roll under the shoulders and the neck slightly extended. The head is rotated away from the operator and the shoulder is held down by a sheet around the arm and tucked under the patient. The position is similar to the one used for carotid endarterectomy.

Anterior or Interjugulocarotid Approach

The incision is oblique, almost transverse, extending from the prominence of the head of the clavicle outwards for about 6 cm (Fig. 2a). After dividing the platysma the two heads of the sternomastoid are exposed. It is advan-

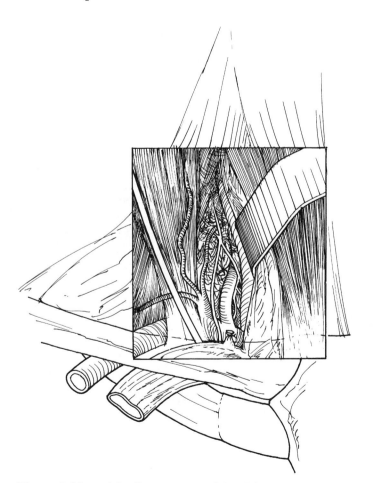

Figure 1. View of the first segment of the right vertebral artery and its anatomic relationships.

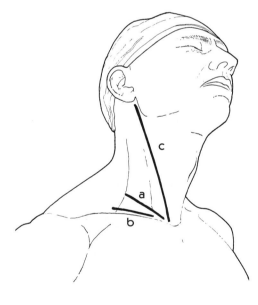

Figure 2. Skin incisions.
a. Oblique incision for anterior (interjugulocarotid) approach to the vertebral artery.
b. Supraclavicular incision for subclavian-vertebral bypass.
c. External carotid incision for simultaneous carotid bifurcation endarterectomy and proximal vertebral transposition to the common carotid artery.

tageous to lift a flap above the sternomastoid muscle of about 2 cm around the entire incision to facilitate mobilization and exposure of the latter muscle. The two sternomastoid heads are separated through their anatomic plane. Some small vessels run between them and are cauterized. The separation between the two heads is completed downwards towards the clavicle and upwards to the limit of the incision. The internal jugular vein is identified and its medial edge dissected. The vein is retracted laterally with the vagus nerve and the common carotid artery is identified medially. The dissection proceeds between the common carotid medially and the internal jugular and vagus laterally, upwards as far as the incision permits, and downwards into the mediastinum. For this the surgeon switches positions temporarily in order to mobilize the common carotid into the mediastinum as far down as possible. As this mobilization proceeds on the left side the fatty bulge caused by the thoracic duct is identified exiting behind the common carotid artery and running laterally and a bit anterior towards the jugulo-subclavian confluent. It is a large structure, generally a single channel between 4-6 mm in diameter with a faint greenish hue. Occasionally two or three individual ducts may be found.

Once the thoracic duct is identified, it is ligated proximally and distally. After division, its proximal end will retract and distend visibly. The separation of the space between the vagus and jugular vein laterally and the common carotid artery medially is completed for identification of the VA.

On the right side, the approach to the deep plane where the VA is located may be crossed by one or two accessory lymph channels which are dealt with in the same manner as described for the main thoracic duct on the left. The presence of lymph channels of substantial size in the right side is frequent.

At this point the inferior thyroid artery which runs transversely in the neck is identified. It is dissected approximately 1 cm and then divided between ligatures. The sympathetic chain is usually medial to the point of division of the inferior thyroid artery. The next step is the identification of the vertebral vein which is slightly larger in size than its accompanying artery and, with few exceptions, lies on top of the VA and therefore permits identification of the latter.

The vertebral vein, unlike the accompanying artery, has some branches that have to be dealt with. Normally the vein is ligated low in the segment that has no branches as it crosses over the origin of the VA. Occasionally the artery is covered at this point by part of, or the entire intermediate sympathetic ganglion, and it is best to isolate the artery above or below this structure which must be protected during dissection to avoid a Horner's syndrome.

As soon as the VA is identified, it is dissected free of surrounding structures, usually sympathetic fibers, and encircled with a vessel loop. The dissection then proceeds both proximally and distally identifying the sympathetic trunks usually above the point of isolation. When this is done we prefer to isolate the artery again above the sympathetic trunks and loop it there as well. The artery is then dissected towards its origin from the subclavian artery and the take-off of the VA from the subclavian artery is exposed. In those cases where the artery arises from the arch, the former is dissected proximally enough to provide a good length for transposition. Distally it may be that the artery appears to have an inappropriate length as it disappears under the longus colli. If this is so, the overlying longus colli is lifted with a right angle clamp and divided with cautery. There is a branch of the vertebral vein running along the lower edge of the fibers of the longus colli that is best individually ligated before cutting the muscle fibers. Once the overlying longus colli is divided, the artery can be pursued until it disappears under the transverse process of C6 (Fig. 3).

After systemic heparinization, the VA is prepared for its transposition to the common carotid artery. The VA is clamped at the level of the longus colli. A transfixion ligature is used to occlude the VA proximally. This ligature generally involves part of the adventitia of the subclavian artery around the origin of the VA. With its proximal end ligated and a microclamp placed below the longus colli, the VA is

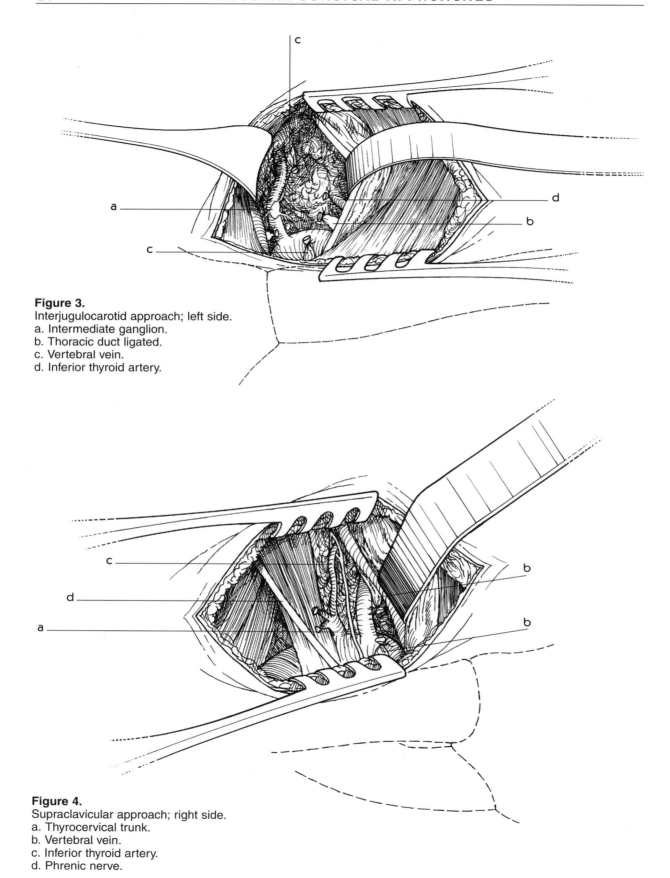

Figure 3.
Interjugulocarotid approach; left side.
a. Intermediate ganglion.
b. Thoracic duct ligated.
c. Vertebral vein.
d. Inferior thyroid artery.

Figure 4.
Supraclavicular approach; right side.
a. Thyrocervical trunk.
b. Vertebral vein.
c. Inferior thyroid artery.
d. Phrenic nerve.

divided above its origin and pulled through the sympathetic ring until it is completely free. The sympathetics then remain posterior and the artery is brought into continuity with the posterior lateral wall of the common carotid artery for its transposition to it.

Technical Variations

If the VA enters the transverse foramen at the level of C7, the extraforamenal segment of the artery is generally too short to do a transposition to the common carotid artery. In this case one may opt to increase the available length by dividing the tendon of the longus colli as it overrides the VA, dividing the venous collateral that contributes at this level to the vertebral vein and, using a fine rounger, unroofing the anterior lip of the transverse process of C7 to expose further length of the VA. The surrounding vertebral vein plexus may result in substantial bleeding. Elevation of the head of the patient to decrease venous pressure, compression, and electrocoagulation with bipolar cautery are the elements for control of perivertebral venous bleeding.

Supraclavicular Approach

The supraclavicular approach to the VA[3] requires exposure of the first segment of the VA and of the retroscalene segment of the subclavian artery. Generally this is an approach used to do a bypass from the subclavian to the VA with the bypass taking origin in the superior wall of the subclavian, lateral to the origin of the vertebral, and the distal anastomosis constructed on the VA where the latter disappears under the longus colli. This technique is used in no more than 5% of all proximal vertebral reconstructions. It is the best alternative when a direct transposition to the carotid artery is not feasible because of inadequate length of VA (such as when the artery enters the foramen transversarium of C7), or in those cases where it is not desirable to clamp the carotid and VA on the same side in order to do a transposition, i.e. in cases with contralateral internal carotid occlusion.

Technique

The position is the same as the one described for the interjugulocarotid approach. The incision is a bit more lateral and runs parallel to the upper border of the clavicle, approximately 1 1/2 cm above it (Fig. 2b). The incision runs laterally up to the level of the external jugular vein. The platysma is divided with cautery. The clavicular head of the sternomastoid is identified and divided with cautery. The superficial part of the prescalene fat pad comes into view. The fat pad is dissected around its periphery leaving a hinge of undissected attachments laterally so that the pad can be replaced in situ later to cover the operative site during closure. As the prescalene fat pad is dissected, the transverse scapular artery and vein are identified in the lower third of the field and divided between ligatures. The anterior scalene muscle is identified by palpation. The dissection of the prescalene pad starts medially and as the pad is lifted off the scalene muscle the phrenic nerve is identified running from lateral to medial and covered by thin fascia. Once the liberation of the superior, inferior, and medial portions of the scalene pad is completed, it is flipped over the hinge left on the lateral edge of field and pushed away with a self-retaining retractor. Medially, the lateral edge of the jugular vein is dissected and retracted using a self-retaining retractor. The phrenic nerve is freed from the thin cellular tissue that binds it to the scalenus anticus muscle and is encircled with a silastic loop to permit its mobilization (Fig. 4).

For this part of the dissection it is generally not necessary to expose and divide the thoracic duct. The scalenus anticus is surrounded with a right angle clamp while maintaining the phrenic nerve separated by a soft, malleable brain retractor. The scalenus anticus is divided with cautery between the blades of the right angle clamp and the subclavian artery is identified below it. The subclavian artery is dissected around its circumference. This may require division of some small posterior or inferior branches. For these small branches of the subclavian artery we prefer a suture ligature with 6-0 polypropylene affixed to the adventitia of the subclavian. The thyrocervical trunk is then identified. Its inferior thyroid branch can be seen running transversely and will eventually cross the VA more medially. Dissection continues medially over the subclavian artery until the vertebral vein is identified as it crosses over the artery to empty into the subclavian vein. Below the vein the VA is identified. The latter is often covered by part of the intermediate cervical ganglion. The inferior thyroid artery is divided in its horizontal portion to dissect the vertebral vein. Once the artery is identified, the dissection proceeds distally towards the lower border of the longus colli. It is not necessary to dissect the artery back to its origin to do a subclavian-vertebral bypass since the distal anastomosis will be done to the most distal portion of the exposed VA. Sometimes it is difficult to find the VA in the deeper plane in which it lies; one may need to follow the superior or superomedial edge of the subclavian artery to identify the origin of the VA as it comes off the former. In order to do that it is generally necessary to divide the thoracic duct on the left side. The carotid artery, jugular vein, and vagus nerve are all retracted medially. Using the same precautions described above to protect the sympathetics, a suitable length of 2 cm of VA is obtained. The VA is looped and freed of adventitia to prepare the site of the distal anastomosis of the bypass.

Proximally, attention turns to the subclavian artery to identify a spot for the proximal anastomosis of the bypass which will be in the superior wall of the artery and generally lateral to the origin of the thyroid cervical trunk. If the artery is calcified or grossly atheromatous except for the origin of the thyroid cervical trunk, the latter can be amputated and its ostium used for the proximal anastomosis of the bypass.

Combined Carotid Endarterectomy and Vertebral Reconstruction

In some patients it is advisable to reconstruct simultaneously the VA and the carotid bifurcation on the same side. This can be done in the same operation using a single incision. The incision is then anterior to the sterno-

mastoid, as is normally used for a carotid endarterectomy, except that it is prolonged inferiorly following the edge of the sternal head of the sternomastoid muscle (Fig. 2c). The anterior edge of the sternomastoid is dissected in its entirety down to the inferior limit of the incision. The first part of the operation is the standard exposure for carotid endarterectomy, retracting the sternomastoid posteriorly and freeing the anterior edge of the jugular vein before retracting it laterally. Once the exposure for the carotid endarterectomy is completed (see Chapter 1) attention is turned to the lower part of the incision. The omohyoid muscle is divided. Occasionally the upper portion of the sternohyoid muscle needs to be divided too. The jugular vein continues to be retracted laterally with the vagus attached to it. The common carotid artery is dissected into the mediastinum encircled with a silastic loop and retracted medially. Using the same approach as was described for transposition the interjugulocarotid space is entered and the VA is isolated. Normally the VA transposition is done first and the carotid endarterectomy follows. In patients who have a contralateral carotid occlusion, the arteriotomy for the carotid endarterectomy is done first, a shunt is inserted low into the common carotid artery proximally and into the internal carotid artery distally. Flow is reestablished through the shunt into the internal carotid artery. At that point the VA is clamped, divided, and transposed to the lowest portion of the common carotid artery which is already bypassed by the shunt. Once the transposition of the VA is completed the shunt is moved distal to the site of transposition and inflow is reestablished into the transposed vertebral artery proceeding with the standard endarterectomy distally.

References

1. Kline R, Berguer R. Vertebral artery reconstruction. *Ann Vasc Surg* 1993; 7: 497-501.
2. Berguer R, Kieffer E. *Surgery of the Arteries to the Head.* New York, Springer-Verlag, 1992.
3. Berguer R, Bauer RB. Vertebral artery reconstruction: A successful technique in selected patients. *Ann Surg* 1981; 4: 441-447.

5

Distal Vertebral Artery (C2-C1): Anatomic Features and Surgical Approach

Eugenio Rosset, Alain Branchereau

Vertebral artery (VA) surgery did not evolve as rapidly as carotid artery surgery. The diagnosis and surgical treatment of vertebral artery disease is hindered by the difficulty of diagnosing vertebrobasilar ischemia and the small size and complex course of the vertebral arteries.

Following the leadership of Thevenet[1] most vertebral surgery performed in France has involved the proximal segment which is both the most accessible and the most common site of atherosclerotic involvement. A few reports describing the approach to the second segment have been published by orthopedic surgeons and neurosurgeons primarily interested in treating osteophytic vertebral compression.[2,3] More recently, several groups[4-6] have emphasized the value of reconstruction of the third segment of the vertebral artery and advised against reconstruction of the VA in its second segment (C6-C2).

Anatomic Review

The course of the VA can be divided into four segments: V1 to V4. The V1 segment extends from the subclavian artery to the foramen of the transverse process of the sixth cervical vertebra. The V2 segment runs from the foramen of the transverse process of the sixth cervical vertebra to that of the second cervical vertebra.[7] Segment V3 extends from the upper limit of the V2 segment to the point where the artery penetrates the dura mater, at which level the V4 begins (Fig. 1). The distal ends of both VA unite to form the basilar artery. Exposure of segment V1 is described in Chapter 4; exposure

From Vascular Surgical Approaches, edited by Alain Branchereau and Ramon Berguer. ©1999, Futura Publishing Co., Inc., Armonk, NY.

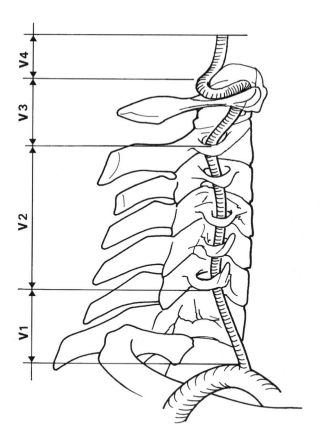

Figure 1. The four segments of the vertebral artery.

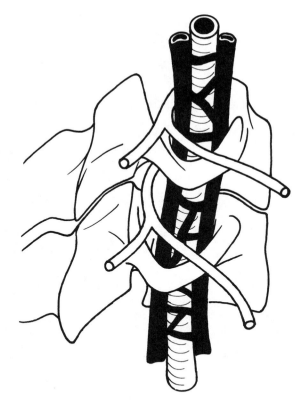

Figure 2. Relations between the vertebral artery, the periarterial venous plexus and the cervical nerve roots, between C3-C6.

of V4 was not included in this chapter because the indications for surgical treatment at this level are exceedingly uncommon and not in the realm of our experience.

Intertransverse Segment of the Vertebral Artery (V2)

The VA is the main element running through the foramen transversaria. The diameter of the foramenal canal varies from 5.6 to 7 mm.[7] The artery lies in the anteromedial part of the canal in contact with the anterior tubercle of the transverse process. The course of the VA in this segment is usually straight but some winding can be observed. The artery is surrounded by a network of veins, the main component of which is a venous trunk in the anterolateral part of the canal (Fig. 2). Since the venous system is adherent to the arterial adventitia as well as to the periosteum, surgical

exposure of the artery at this level may lead to substantial blood loss. Due to the richness of collateral veins, this system has been referred to as the vertebrotransverse sinus.[8] During its entire course, the VA is in close relation with the nerve roots arising from the intervertebral foramina located behind the transverse processes. These roots divide into a posterior ramus that innervates the musculocutaneous tissues and an anterior ramus which will form the cervical and brachial plexi. The anterior rami are in close relation to the VA which they cross horizontally first to the outside and then eventually turning anteriorly before uniting to form the cervical plexus (C1-C4 cervical roots) and the brachial plexus (C5-C6 cervical roots) (Fig. 2). The VA passes near the uncovertebral joints which are located inside and behind the transverse canal. Since the distance between the uncus and the artery is only one millimeter, osteophytes associated with osteoarthritis of this joint may cause compression of the VA.

The VA has branches to the surrounding musculoskeletal walls, to the brain, and to the spinal cord. Spinal branches classically have a metameric disposition and accompany each nerve root over the whole length of the cervical spine. They contribute to the spinal cord circulation by supplying the anterior and posterior spinal systems via their anterior and posterior spinal branches.[9] Recent studies[10-12] have shown that only a few spinal arteries arising from the VA contribute to the blood supply of the cervical cord either by their anterior branches (anterior spinomedullary artery) or by their posterior branches (posterior spinomedullary artery). Lazorthes[11] showed that there are three to five anterior spinomedullary arteries at the cervical level that supply the anterior spinal pathway. They are almost always distributed between the fourth and eighth cervical roots and only two originate from the VA. The others arise from branches of the subclavian artery; i.e. cervicointercostal, deep cervical, and ascending cervical arteries. There are also three to five posterior spinomedullary arteries at the cervical level but they are of lesser size and functional importance. They are found preferentially on the lower roots (C4-C5) although there is often a posterior spinomedullary artery at the level of the second cervical vertebrae. The network of anterior and posterior spinomedullary arteries arising from the vertebral artery is connected with branches of the cervicointercostal artery, occipital artery, and ascending and deep cervical arteries which also contribute to the blood supply of the spinal cord (Fig. 3).

The movement of the cervical spine between the second and sixth cervical vertebrae essentially involves flexion and extension (150 degrees). The C5-C6 cervical disk is the most mobile. Lateral movement is more limited (25 degrees to either side).[13]

Alantoaxial Segment (V3)

The V3 segment of the VA has a winding course (Fig. 4). In the intertransverse space between the first and second cervical vertebrae it makes an upward and outward turn in order to join the transverse foramen of the atlas. The extra length of artery necessary for this turn provides a reserve for rotation of the atlanto-

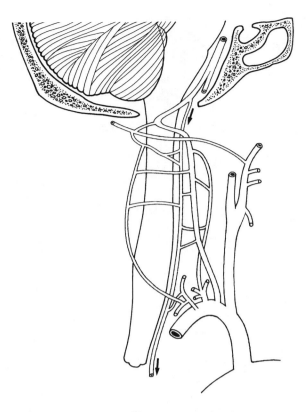

Figure 3. Arterial blood supply of the cervical spine (according to Lazorthes[11]). Note the presence of numerous anastomoses between the vertebral artery, the cervical branches of the subclavian artery, and the occipital artery.

axial joint which can move up to 40 degrees to either side. After passing through the foramen, the artery makes an outward turn that brings it into the vertebral groove of the atlas and then another turn that brings it into the posterior surface of the atlanto-occipital joint until it reaches the atlanto-occipital membrane. At this level the VA is covered by the rectus capitis posterior medially and the obliquus capitis superior laterally. The V3 segment is surrounded by veins and crossed by the occipital nerve. The veins of the base of the skull form the suboccipital plexus which drains mainly into the posterior jugular vein located near the midline.[14] The trunks of origin come from the space between the first and second cervical vertebrae and from the posterior side of the transverse process of C1. Most join to form a posterior vein trunk that hinders the posterior approach to the VA. The greater occipital nerve

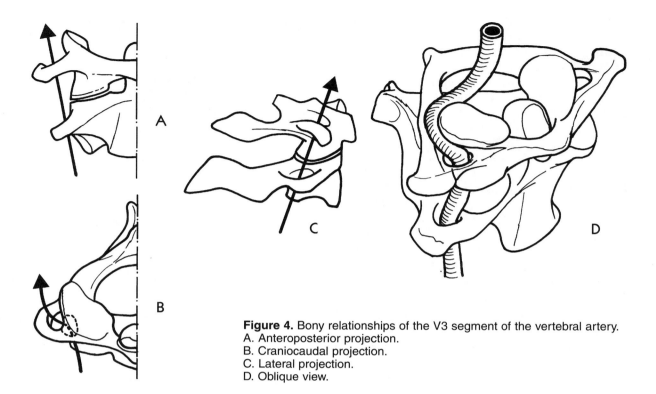

Figure 4. Bony relationships of the V3 segment of the vertebral artery.
A. Anteroposterior projection.
B. Craniocaudal projection.
C. Lateral projection.
D. Oblique view.

is the posterior branch of the second cervical nerve just after the latter crosses the posterior atlantoaxial ligament. The greater occipital nerve gives off motor branches to the nuchal musculature but it is mainly a sensory nerve for the posterior scalp from the base to the top of the skull. Two arterial branches of particular importance at the V3 level are the atlantoaxial branch and the posterior cervical branch which fans out in the area of the Tillaux triangle. These two collaterals connect with the post-vertebral subclavian artery and with the external carotid artery, with the latter via branches of the occipital artery and with the former via the deep cervical artery and the ascending cervical artery. This complex network explains why the V3 segment usually remains patent after proximal occlusion of the VA. As stated above, the presence of a posterior spinomedullary collateral at the level of the second cervical vertebra is common but its functional role seems minimal (see below).

Approach Between First and Second Cervical Vertebrae

The small size of the VA and the narrow operating field warrant the use of magnifying operating loupes, microsurgical instruments (dissecting forceps, scissors) and bipolar electrocoagulation. The patient is placed decubitus, with the neck in extension and rotated slightly to the opposite side avoiding excessive stretching of the sternocleidomastoid (SCM) muscle. A semi-seated position helps to reduce venous pressure in the neck (Fig. 5). The positioning of the patient's arms as well as that of the surgical team is almost the same as for surgery of the carotid artery bifurcation. Access to the saphenous vein in the thigh is provided routinely. The ear lobe is folded up and attached in front of the ear (Fig. 6).

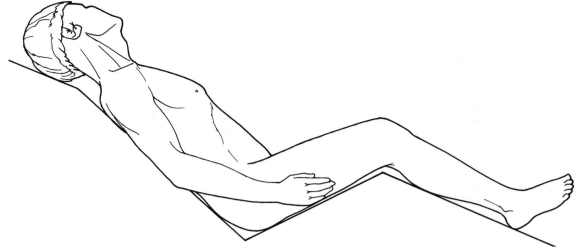

Figure 5. Patient position.

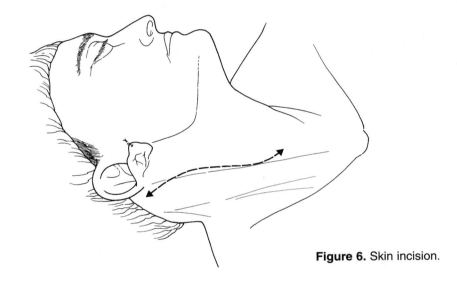

Figure 6. Skin incision.

Skin Incision

An oblique incision, similar to the one used for carotid endarterectomy, is made along the anterior border of the SCM muscle. At the top, the incision is extended up to the tip of the mastoid process. At the bottom, the incision should be made to curve slightly towards the horizontal to avoid unsightly scarring. The common carotid artery should be accessible through the bottom of the incision.

Superficial Layers

The platysma muscle is opened with cautery and the branches of the superficial plexus as well as the external jugular vein are divided. The tip of the parotid gland is separated from the SCM muscle and retracted anteriorly. Complete separation between these two structures is necessary to provide access to the underlying space and to avoid injury of the gland.

Middle Layers

A spreader retractor is placed. The superficial cervical aponeurosis is incised to expose the lower border of the posterior belly of the digastric muscle which is retracted upwards and forward. The wall of the internal jugular vein is dissected free and retracted forwards. The external branch of the accessory spinal nerve is identified between the SCM posteriorly and the internal jugular vein anteriorly. Because of the position of the neck, the nerve is distended and makes a groove on the lateral wall of the internal jugular vein. The nerve can usually be located by palpation but if necessary the SCM muscle can be pulled backward to stretch the nerve so that it appears as a taut string in the operative field. This traction method is particularly useful for the 25% of patients in whom the nerve presents a more internal and posterior interjugulo-carotidian course[15] and is consequently more difficult to locate (Fig. 7). Once identified, the nerve is mobilized as far as possible: proxi-mally up to the point where it disappears under the posterior belly of the digastric muscle and distally to the point at which it enters the SCM muscle (usually 4 cm below the insertion of the muscle on the mastoid process).[16] A silastic tape should be used to manipulate the nerve.

The operator can palpate the transverse process of the first cervical vertebra in the space between the posterior border of the internal jugular vein and the anterior border of the SCM muscle or through the vein itself. This transverse process protrudes below the spinal nerve and serves as the point of attachment for the levator scapula, splenius cervicis, and inferior oblique muscles (Fig. 7). The limit between the prevertebral muscles and the anterior border of the levator scapula muscle can be located by the passage of the anastomotic branch uniting the cervical sympathetic chain and the anterior ramus of the second cervical root.[17] The muscles attached to the transverse process of the first cervical vertebra are divided over a dissector at

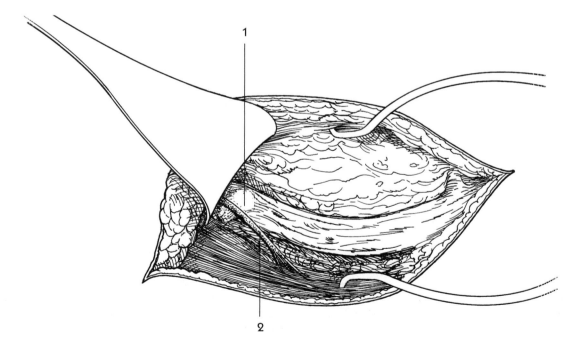

Figure 7. Middle layer. Note the taut spinal nerve between the internal jugular vein and the SCM muscle, as well as the outline of the transverse process of the first cervical vertebra.
1. Transverse process of the first cervical vertebra.
2. Spinal nerve.

their insertion on the transverse process of the first cervical vertebra using cautery. Generally, dividing the fibers of the levator scapula is sufficient (Fig. 8).

Vascular Layer

Microsurgical instruments and magnifying glasses are mandatory at this level. The division of muscle fibers results in exposure of the intertransverse space through which the VA runs roughly in a vertical direction. The upper insertions of the muscle fibers are rongeured and resected in order to enlarge the opening. The lower end of the divided muscle is retracted inferiorly. The anterior ramus of the second cervical nerve crosses the VA to the outside and then in front of this space (Fig. 9). It can be cut to improve exposure without noticeable penalty thanks to the numerous anastomoses between the first three cervical nerves.[17] We attach a thread to both ends of the second cervical nerve after a section in order to open the space containing the artery and facilitate access (Fig. 10). Since the VA is highly susceptible to traumatic injury it is dissected at the subadventitial level taking great care not to grasp it with dissecting forceps. The most frequent problem encountered is bleeding from the periarterial venous plexus. A fine silastic tape is placed carefully around the artery to allow electrocoagulation of the veins at a safe distance from the artery. Should hemorrhage occur before the silastic tape can be placed, the assistant must continually aspirate blood using a fine atraumatic nozzle as the operator continues dissection of the lateral and posterior sides of the VA. As soon as the artery has been sufficiently mobilized, it is encircled with a loop using a small right-angled clamp. The whole length of the artery in the intertransverse space is dissected using the loop for traction. When the dissection is complete, the veins are coagulated at a safe distance from the artery (Fig. 10). Any collateral arteries encountered during dissection are divided and cut between two ligatures of 8-0 monofilament suture.

This method exposes 2 cm of VA, sufficient for clamping and anastomosis.

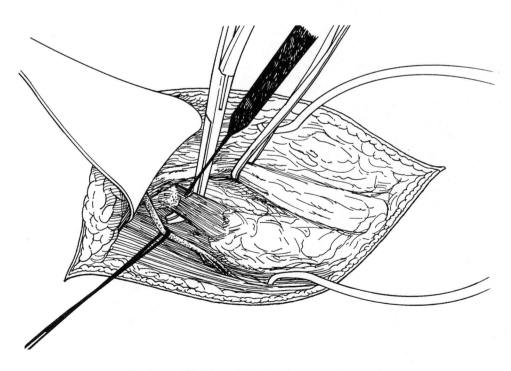

Figure 8. Division of the levator scapula muscle at its point of attachment to the first cervical vertebra.

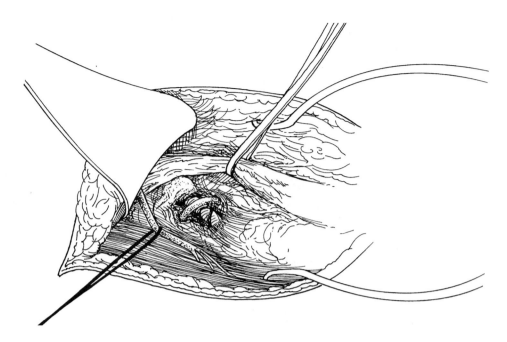

Figure 9. The vertebral artery crossed in front by the anterior ramus of the second cervical nerve is exposed in the space between the first and second cervical vertebrae.

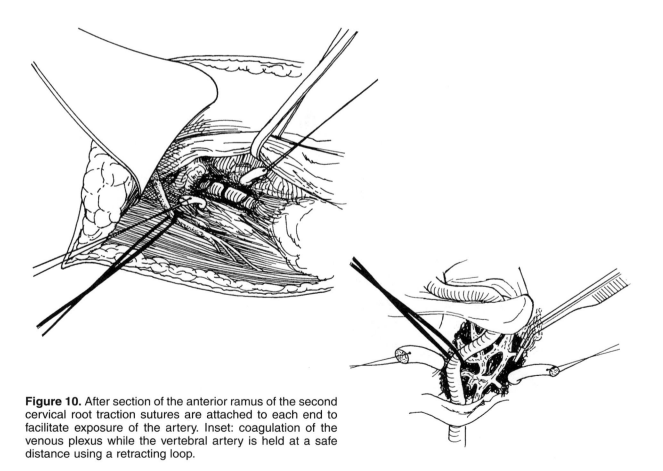

Figure 10. After section of the anterior ramus of the second cervical root traction sutures are attached to each end to facilitate exposure of the artery. Inset: coagulation of the venous plexus while the vertebral artery is held at a safe distance using a retracting loop.

Discussion

The majority of atherosclerotic lesions of the VA involve the V1 segment. However, dysplastic and extrinsic compression lesions of the V2 segment which have been overlooked or left untreated are not uncommon. Exposure of segment V3 offers the possibility of treatment of these lesions because the anatomic accessibility of the V3 segment makes surgical exposure at this level relatively easy. The length of exposed artery obtained between the first and second cervical vertebrae is greater than at other vertebral levels (Fig. 4).[15] Since the vertebral venous plexus is less dense here than at other levels, hemostasis is easier. Although large vertebral arterial branches can be found between the first and second cervical vertebrae, branches supplying the spinal cord are uncommon and involve only the posterior spinal pathway. The blood supply to the cord is abundant at this level and this practically rules out the risk of ischemic cord complications, which we have never observed in our experience and which have not been reported in the literature. We prefer the V3 approach to the V2 approach in which damage of collateral vessels can theoretically lead to spinal ischemia since there are always spinomedullary branches at the latter level.

The most frequently used approach is between the first and second cervical vertebrae. This method allows treatment of dysplastic or compressive lesions generally located between the third and sixth cervical vertebrae.

The V3 approach as described has no major morbidity. A sensory deficit in the region of the auriculotemporal nerve (numbness of the earlobe) is common. Section of the anterior branch of the second cervical root causes no symptoms. The external branch of the spinal nerve is not divided although if it is traumatized it may result in transient paralysis of the trapezius muscle. The presenting signs of this complication are pain in the acromioclavicular joint and slumping of the shoulder. In our experience paralysis of the trapezius muscle resolves in 1 to 3 months with appropriate physical therapy.

The size of the VA is an important factor in determining the success of its surgical reconstruction. A minimum size of 3 mm is needed and this must be ascertained by preoperative angiography. Since the walls of the vertebral artery are among the most fragile that a vascular surgeon has to deal with, microsurgical instrumentation is indispensable to allow safe exposure and handling.

References

1. Labauge R, Thevenet A, Crouzet G, Nivolas M. Insuffisance vertébrobasilaire d'incidence chirurgicale (à propos de 87 malades opérés). *Rev Neurol* 1967; 117: 373-389.
2. Jung A, Kehr P. *Pathologie de l'artère vertébrale et des racines nerveuses dans les arthroses et les traumatismes du rachis cervical.* Paris, Masson, 1972.
3. Huguet JF, Louis R, Nazarian S, Courjaret P. L'artère vertébrale et la chirurgie de la colonne cervicale. A propos de 64 cas opérés de cervicarthrose. *Ann Radiol* 1980; 23: 241-244.
4. Kieffer E, Rancurel G, Richard T. Reconstruction of the distal cervical vertebral artery. In: Berguer R, Bauer B, eds. *Vertebrobasilar Arterial Occlusive Disease: Medical and Surgical Management.* New York, Raven Press, 1984, pp 265-289.
5. Branchereau A, Magnan PE. Results of vertebral artery surgery. *J Cardiovasc Surg* 1990; 31: 320-326.
6. Berguer R. Reconstruction of the distal vertebral artery. In: Berguer R, Caplan LR, eds. *Vertebrobasilar Arterial Disease.* St. Louis, Quality Medical Publishing, 1992, pp 236-247.
7. Argenson C, Francke JP, Sylla S, et al. Les artères vertébrales (segments V1 et V2). *Anatomia clinica* 1979; 2: 29-41.
8. Louis R, Argenson C. Les veines vertébrales. *Travaux Inst Anat Marseille,* 1962; 21: 21-25.
9. Paturet G. *Traité d'Anatomie humaine.* Tome IV. Paris, Masson, 1958, pp 82-87.
10. Lazorthes G, Gouaze A. Les voies anastomotiques de suppléance (ou système de sécurité) de la vascularisation artérielle de l'axe cérébro-médullaire. *Bull Assoc Anat* 1968; 53: 1-230.
11. Lazorthes G, Gouaze A, Djindjian R. *Vascularisation et circulation de la moelle épinière.* Paris, Masson, 1973, pp 41-104.
12. Francke JP, Dimarino V, Pannier M, et al. Les artères vertébrales (arteria vertebralis). Segments atlanto-axoïdien V3 et intra-crânien V4 - Collatérales. *Anatomia clinica* 1980; 2: 229-242.
13. Bouchet A, Cuilleret J. *Anatomie topographique, descriptive et fonctionnelle.* Tome 2. Lyon, Simep, 1983, pp 630-632.
14. Berthelot JL, Andreassian B, Hureau J. Abord chirurgical du troisième segment de l'artère vertébrale par voie postérieure paramédiane. *Press Med* 1983; 12: 1423-1425.
15. Paturet G. *Traité d'Anatomie humaine.* Tome III, fascicule 1. Paris, Masson, 1958, pp 325-343.
16. Rouvière H, Delmas A. *Anatomie humaine.* Paris, Masson 1991. Tome 1, 13ème éd., pp 293-295.
17. Kieffer E. Chirurgie de l'artère vertébrale. Encycl Med Chir, Paris, France. Techniques chirurgicales, *Chirurgie Vasculaire* 43130, 4-9-12, 34 p.

6

Suboccipital Approach to the Vertebral Artery

Ramon Berguer

Most reconstructions of the distal vertebral artery (VA) are done at the C2-C1 level. Occasionally the lesion extends up to the transverse foramen of C1 or beyond it and in order to revascularize the VA the latter has to be accessed above this level. To approach the pars atlantica of the vertebral artery we use the suboccipital approach described below.

Anatomic Review

As the VA emerges from the transverse process of C1 it follows a trajectory which is first posteromedial and then turns anterior to penetrate the dura mater and enter the foramen magnum. The artery exits the transverse process of C1 and as it surrounds the lateral mass of the atlas to turn anterior it overhangs the posterior lamina of the atlas by about 5 mm.[1] It then crosses an oblique groove in the posterior lamina, passes through the atlanto-occipital membrane and penetrates the dura. The VA has radiculomuscular branches that tether the artery to the short posterior nuchal muscles. The ventral ramus of the C1 root is located below the VA and lies between the latter and the posterior arch of the atlas. Throughout its atlantal course the VA is covered by a dense plexus of veins contributed by veins that originated in the jugular foramen, the hypoglossal canal, and the condyloid emissary vein. The plexus of veins surrounding the VA at this level is denser than at any other level throughout its cervical course. The artery is covered first by the short suboccipital muscles that run between the atlas and the occipital. In a more superficial plane the semispinalis capitis and the splenius capitis muscle cover the VA.

Operative Technique

The intubated patient is placed in the *parkbench* position. The temple contralateral to the operative site rests on the forearm. The

From Vascular Surgical Approaches, edited by Alain Branchereau and Ramon Berguer. ©1999, Futura Publishing Co., Inc., Armonk, NY.

surgeon stands on the side of the VA being operated on with the first assistant above him and the second assistant across. The relevant bony reference points are the external occipital protuberance, the tip of the mastoid process and the angle of the jaw. The incision (Fig. 1) is racket-shaped: first horizontal below the occipital protuberance from the midline to the tip of the mastoid where the incision bends to follow the posterior edge of the sternomastoid. The thick subcutaneous tissue is incised. The upper fibers of the trapezius, the stout semispinalis, and the splenius capitis muscles are cut (Fig. 2). Below the splenius the longissimus capitis is also divided. The sternomastoid muscle is disinserted and reflected

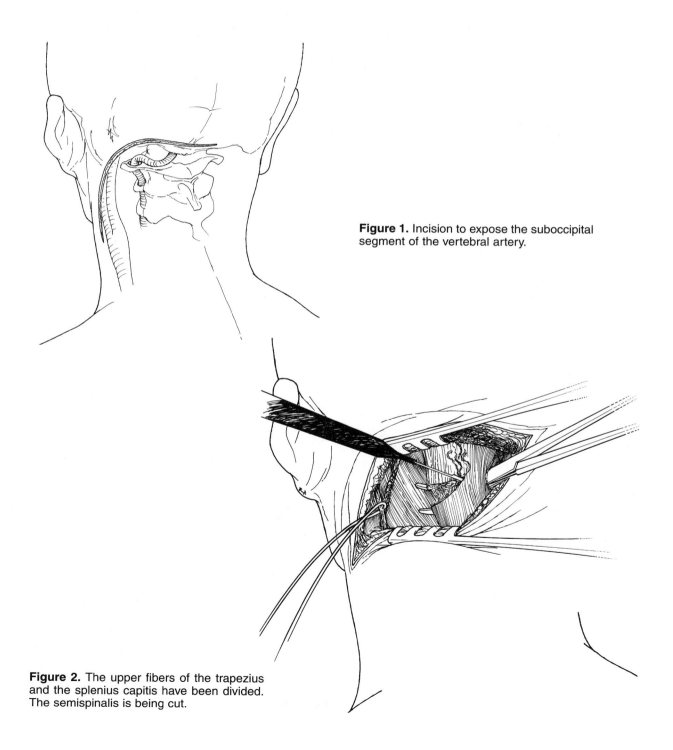

Figure 1. Incision to expose the suboccipital segment of the vertebral artery.

Figure 2. The upper fibers of the trapezius and the splenius capitis have been divided. The semispinalis is being cut.

inferiorly. The jugular vein is visible and the accessory spinal nerve is identified and tagged for safety. The suboccipital muscles are now exposed. The condyloid emissary vein or one of its large contributors inside the medial edge of the obliquus capitis superior is divided between ligatures. The obliquus capitis and rectus capitis posterior major muscles now come into view. The former is divided; usually only the lateral half of the rectus capitis posterior is cut (Fig. 3).

The VA now appears as a blue cylinder because of the dense plexus of veins that covers it at this level (Fig. 4). An anastomotic nerve branch between the suboccipital and the

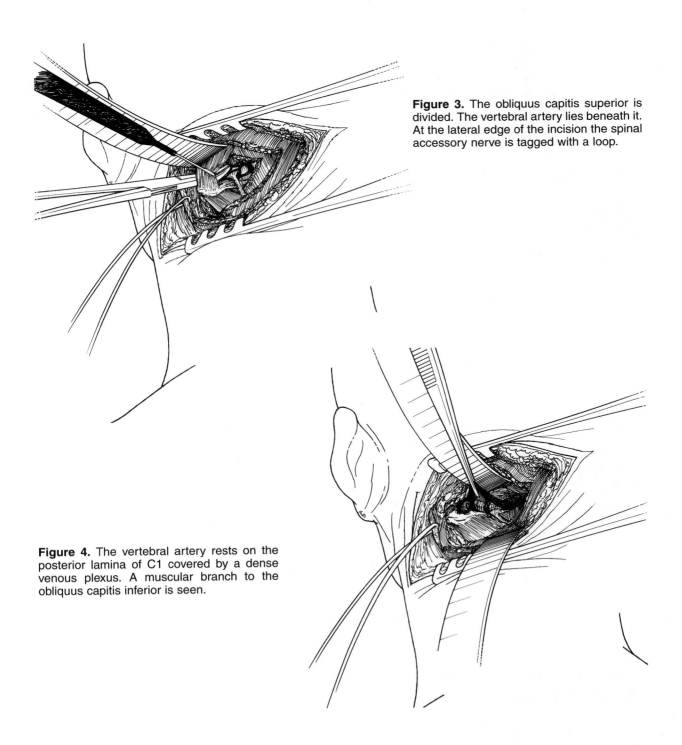

Figure 3. The obliquus capitis superior is divided. The vertebral artery lies beneath it. At the lateral edge of the incision the spinal accessory nerve is tagged with a loop.

Figure 4. The vertebral artery rests on the posterior lamina of C1 covered by a dense venous plexus. A muscular branch to the obliquus capitis inferior is seen.

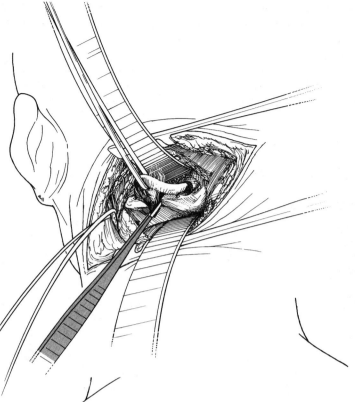

Figure 5. Part of the venous plexus is coagulated with bipolar cautery. The suboccipital vertebral, held by a loop, is dissected up to the atlanto-occipital membrane.

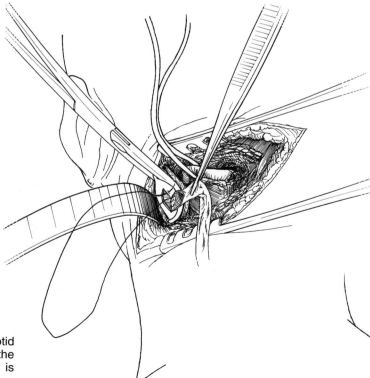

Figure 6. The distal cervical internal carotid has been isolated by retracting medially the vagus and hypoglossal nerves. A vein graft is anastomosed to the internal carotid artery.

greater occipital nerves is divided. One or two of the VA branches supplying the deep nuchal musculature are divided to release the artery from the anchoring affect of these branches. The venous plexus is approached by lifting some obvious vein bridges and dividing them between 8-0 polypropylene sutures passed around the veins using fine needles. Some veins are elevated away from the artery and coagulated with bipolar cautery (Fig. 4). This is a tedious process.

The VA is dissected up to the level of the atlanto-occipital membrane (Fig. 5). At this level the bulging of the dura mater can be seen. The ventral ramus of the C1 root runs below the VA.

Once an appropriate length of VA has been obtained, attention is directed towards the distal cervical internal carotid artery which will be used as inflow. The infratemporal portion of the internal carotid artery is medial to the sternomastoid muscle and is covered posteriorly by the vagus and hypoglossal nerves. These two nerve trunks are carefully isolated and retracted medially. The distal cervical internal carotid artery can be dissected and encircled with a silastic loop. Traction on the loop permits dissection of a segment of 1-1.5 inches in length. The internal carotid artery has no branches at this level and the dissection is reasonably safe. Once an appropriate length is obtained, the bypass can be constructed between the internal carotid (Fig. 6) and the distal vertebral artery passing over the arch of the atlas.

For closure the sternomastoid is reinserted at the mastoid process and the splenius capitis and the semispinalis are approximated.

References

1. Lang J, Kessler B. About the suboccipital part of the vertebral artery and the neighboring bone-joint and nerve relationships. *Skull Base Surg* 1991; 1: 64-72.

7

Surgical Access to the Subclavian and Axillary Arteries

John W. Hallett Jr., Henri Mary

Exposure of surgical lesions of the subclavian or axillary arteries can be problematic. Some of the difficulties arise from surrounding bony structures such as the clavicle and rib cage. In addition, the bulky pectoralis major muscle can limit midaxillary artery exposure. Adjacent nerves must also be avoided (e.g. phrenic, vagus, and cords of the brachial plexus). In the left neck, the thoracic duct may also complicate adequate subclavian artery exposure. Depending on the site of arterial pathology or trauma, a variety of surgical approaches can be used and will be discussed later in this chapter.

The vast majority of subclavian surgical reconstructions are performed for proximal atherosclerotic occlusive disease of the left subclavian artery. Aneurysms related to cervical ribs and thoracic outlet syndrome are another common indication. In busy trauma centers, stab or gunshot wounds require expeditious exposure and control of injured vessels. In contrast, the axillary artery is rarely involved by atherosclerosis. More commonly, it becomes the donor artery for an axillofemoral bypass performed for aortoiliac arterial occlusive disease. Occasionally, an axillary artery aneurysm is still seen and related to chronic crutch use by patients afflicted by polio at an early age. Because trauma may require extensive exposure of both the subclavian and axillary arteries, the exposure of these two vessels will be discussed further in this chapter.

Approach to the Subclavian Artery by a Transverse Cervical Surgical Incision

The patient is placed in supine dorsal decubitus with the head turned 45 degrees toward the contralateral side. A towel roll or small pillow may be placed transversely under the shoulders to permit slight extension of the neck. Caution must be taken so that the neck is not hyperextended with the resulting potential for cervical disk compression. The ipsilateral arm is placed along the side of the body; it can

From Vascular Surgical Approaches, edited by Alain Branchereau and Ramon Berguer. ©1999, Futura Publishing Co., Inc., Armonk, NY.

also be included in the operative field and placed on a table at 90 degrees of abduction. The neck, shoulder, and thorax are prepared. If the surgeon anticipates the need for a vein graft, a groin or thigh site is prepared for harvest.

Superficial Planes

The horizontal supraclavicular incision is made one fingerbreadth above the clavicle. Measuring approximately 6-8 cm in length, it extends from the middle of the clavicle to the internal border of the sternocleidomastoid (SCM) muscle (Fig. 1). The platysma muscle of the neck and the superficial cervical aponeurosis are incised. The external jugular vein can be ligated. The surface of the SCM muscle is exposed, and the sternal and clavicular heads are identified individually. The clavicular head of the SCM muscle is sectioned either partially or completely (Fig. 2). In the lateral or external commissure of the incision, the superficial cervical plexus must be identified and preserved if possible (Fig. 2). Division of the plexus results in a cutaneous prethoracic anesthetic or paresthetic area that can be bothersome to the patient. A Beckman retractor helps to open and hold the exposure. Another retractor can be used to retract the sternal head of the SCM muscle.

Middle Plane

In this layer, one encounters the omohyoid muscle which is sectioned. Medially, the internal jugular vein is identified and mobilized

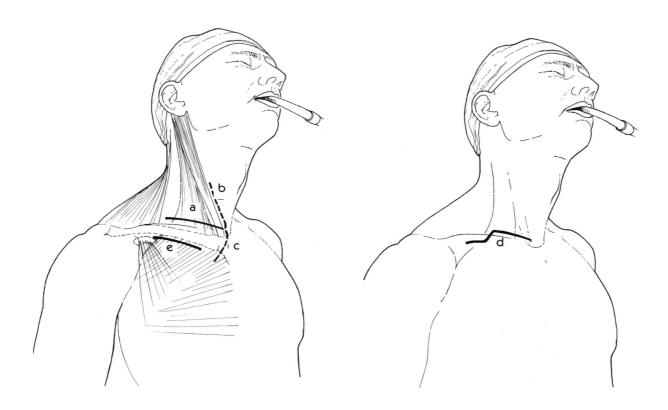

Figure 1. Cervical incisions to expose the subclavian artery.
a. Supraclavicular transverse cervicotomy.
b. Cervical "L" extension from the preceding incision.
c. Medial extension to perform a medial partial claviculectomy.
d. Combined supra- and infraclavicular incision.
e. Horizontal infraclavicular incision.

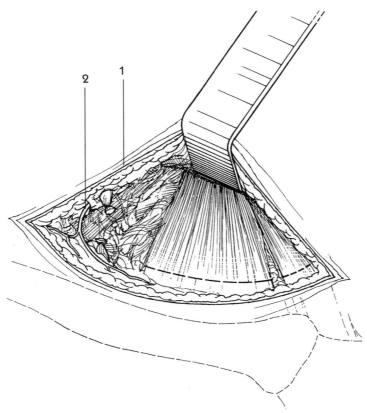

Figure 2. Superficial planes of the supraclavicular incision.
1. External jugular vein.
2. Superficial cervical plexus.

so that it can be retracted in several directions, depending upon the need for more proximal subclavian exposure. Ligation of middle thyroid veins and other local branches may be necessary. Generally, a rubber vascular loop is passed around the jugular vein to assist in its retraction.

Retro- and Postscalene Access

The subclavian artery that lies behind the anterior scalene muscle is approached lateral to the internal jugular vein. The internal jugular vein and adjacent vagus nerve are carefully retracted medially. The scalene fat pad is mobilized superiorly away from the scalene muscle. On the left side, one must be careful not to injure the thoracic duct as it enters the subclavian vein in this area.

The anterior scalene muscle is a fundamental landmark. In front of it, the phrenic nerve courses obliquely from top to bottom and from lateral to medial (Fig. 3). This nerve is isolated with a rubber loop and retracted medially. The anterior scalene muscle is divided near its tendinous insertion on the first rib, taking care to avoid the branches of the thyrocervical trunk that lie beneath it. If branches of the thyrocervical trunk cross the anterior face of the scalene muscle, they can be ligated and divided, especially the transverse cervical and superior scapular arteries.

After section of the anterior scalene muscle, approximately 3-5 cm of the underlying subclavian artery can be seen and palpated. The artery is encircled in this area with a rubber vascular loop. The vertebral artery and internal mammary arteries are identified and may be controlled with vascular loops (Fig. 4).

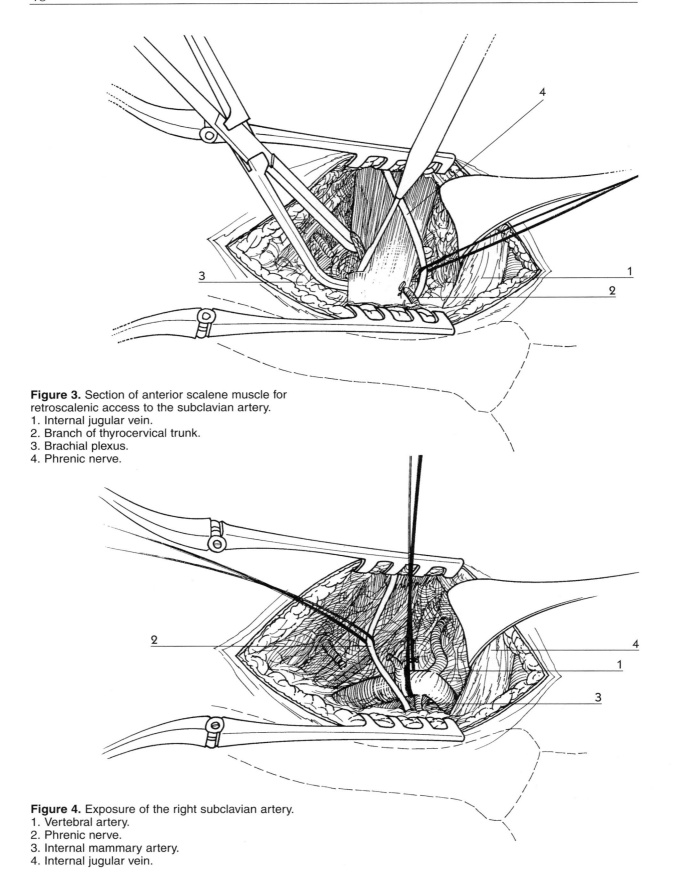

Figure 3. Section of anterior scalene muscle for
retroscalenic access to the subclavian artery.
1. Internal jugular vein.
2. Branch of thyrocervical trunk.
3. Brachial plexus.
4. Phrenic nerve.

Figure 4. Exposure of the right subclavian artery.
1. Vertebral artery.
2. Phrenic nerve.
3. Internal mammary artery.
4. Internal jugular vein.

Access to the Prescalene Subclavian Artery

This dissection requires lateral retraction of the internal jugular vein. The dissection is carried in a plane between the jugular and carotid artery. The sternal head of the SCM muscle and the subhyoid muscles are retracted medially. The proximal common carotid artery is encircled with a vascular loop and retracted medially. In the deeper recesses of the wound, the vertebral vein is identified and marks the adjacent location of the vertebral artery. In this area, one must look carefully for branches of the sympathetic chain (ansa subclavia) which surround the subclavian artery. These sympathetic fibers should be spared if possible. Their trauma can result in a Horner's syndrome. When dissection is completed in this area, the subclavian artery can be controlled proximal and distal to the vertebral artery. In the postvertebral portion, mobilization of the subclavian artery may be hindered by collateral branches of the thyrocervical trunk.

On the right side, the dissection is carried proximally to the junction of the subclavian artery with the common carotid artery. Depending on the morphology of the patient, one may be able to dissect this brachiocephalic branching through the cervical incision. One must be careful to avoid injury to any major lymphatic channels in this area. The recurrent laryngeal nerve must also be identified and preserved. The vagus crosses the anterior surface of the proximal subclavian artery with the recurrent nerve passing beneath and posterior to the surface of the artery.

On the left side, the subclavian artery can be deeper and less accessible. In its pre-vertebral portion, the artery is more posterior than on the right. The proximal subclavian artery can be encircled with a rubber vascular loop which can be used as a retractor as dissection is carried toward the mediastinum (Fig. 5). Occasionally, one can dissect the proximal subclavian artery with a fingertip gently advanced toward the aortic arch. However, such proximal dissection is generally difficult or impossible in large patients.

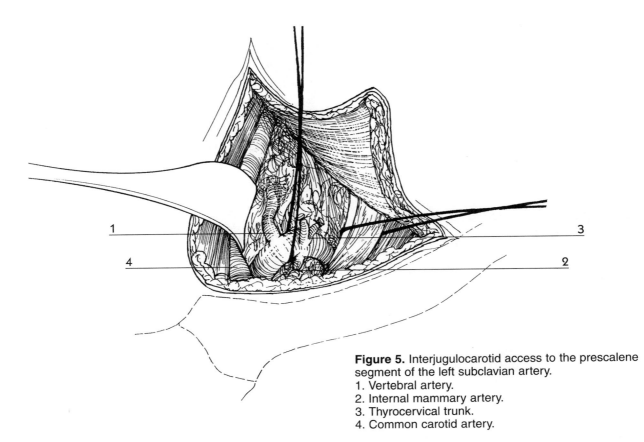

Figure 5. Interjugulocarotid access to the prescalene segment of the left subclavian artery.
1. Vertebral artery.
2. Internal mammary artery.
3. Thyrocervical trunk.
4. Common carotid artery.

Extensions of Previous Incisions

Because the proximal subclavian artery, particularly on the left, is in the mediastinum, the cervical incision may not provide adequate or safe exposure. The following options are often necessary.

Partial Medial Clavicular Resection

This approach is rarely used but may be helpful if one does not choose to perform a median sternotomy for proximal subclavian artery exposure (Fig. 1C). The supraclavicular incision is extended medially and then inferiorly over the clavicular head. The clavicular periosteum is incised with electrocautery, and the muscular attachments of the pectoralis major muscle are detached. The clavicle is sectioned at the union of the medial third and the lateral two-thirds with a Gigli saw or a small reciprocation saw. The sterno-clavicular and interclavicular ligaments, the costoclavicular ligament, and the tendon of the subclavius muscle are sectioned. The clavicle is disarticulated with care to avoid damage to the subclavian vein. This resection of the medial head of the clavicle gives a wider exposure to the subclavian artery in its intra-thoracic portion on the left and to the brachiocephalic arterial trunk on the right. As mentioned, this access is seldom utilized and would only be indicated in the case of a proximal venous hemorrhage which seemed inaccessible by the original incision.

Median Sternotomy (Fig. 6)

Whenever proximal subclavian artery exposure is needed on the right side, a median

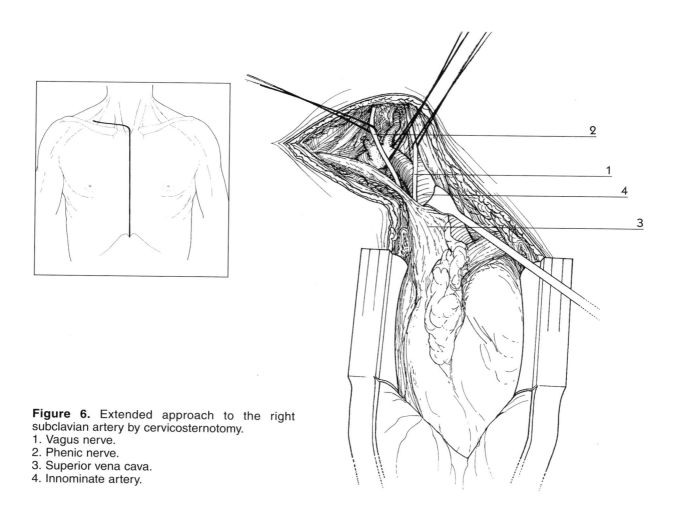

Figure 6. Extended approach to the right subclavian artery by cervicosternotomy.
1. Vagus nerve.
2. Phenic nerve.
3. Superior vena cava.
4. Innominate artery.

sternotomy should be performed. This approach is especially essential in penetrating trauma cases.

The patient is placed in the dorsal decubitus position with a soft towel roll slid beneath the shoulders. The head is extended slightly, and the neck is turned to the opposite side of the cervical exposure. The arms are generally placed along the side. The transverse supraclavicular incision is brought across and then taken inferiorly down the middle of the sternum. The sternotomy permits exposure of the brachiocephalic trunk for better control of the proximal subclavian and common carotid arteries. The innominate vein is mobilized and may be divided between ligatures to obtain adequate exposure. Generally, division of the brachiocephalic vein does not have any serious sequelae.

Left Anterior Lateral Thoracotomy

This approach is essential in cases of penetration trauma to the left neck, especially when one suspects that an injury of the proximal left subclavian artery has occurred. The patient is placed in a dorsal decubitus position with a soft block under the left shoulder. The left upper extremity is generally prepped into the operative field. An anterior lateral thoracotomy is performed in the third or fourth intercostal space. This approach permits control of the proximal left subclavian artery in the mediastinum. The distal subclavian artery is approached through a separate supraclavicular incision. In general, the so-called trap-door left upper thoracotomy for subclavian exposure is not easy to perform and can result in considerable postoperative pain.

Distal Subclavian Exposures

Occasionally, it is necessary to expose the distal subclavian artery beneath the clavicle. Such cases frequently occur when there has been complex trauma to the clavicle. Sometimes fractures of the clavicle or first rib are present.

When easy and rapid control of the subclavian artery is needed, the clavicle can be resected (Fig. 1D). This approach is especially helpful when the clavicle has been fractured or when a gunshot wound has fragmented the clavicle. Although clavicular resection may leave some chronic instability of the shoulder girdle, this disability has generally not been significant in our experience.

Surgical Access
to the Axillary Artery

Horizontal Infraclavicular Incision

The patient is placed in the dorsal decubitus position with a soft roll under the shoulder area. The entire upper extremity, supraclavicular area, and adjacent thorax are prepared.

The upper extremity can be placed in several positions. Although some prefer to place the arm along the body, more versatility is gained by preparing the arm so that it can move from the side to a position of abduction. This upper extremity mobility is especially useful in patients who are undergoing an axillofemoral bypass. By placing the upper extremity at approximately 45 degrees to the trunk, the surgeon has better access to the chest wall and axilla. In trauma cases, it is often necessary to move the upper extremity in several directions to obtain adequate exposure for complex wounds.

A horizontal incision is made approximately one fingerbreadth below the clavicle and carried from the medial third of the clavicle toward the deltopectoral groove. The coracoid process is also a good bony landmark for the lateral extent of the infraclavicular incision (Fig. 7A). The muscular aponeurosis is incised, and a dissection plane is developed between the fibers of the sternal and clavicular heads of the pectoralis major muscle. The separation of these fibers exposes the superficial surface of the clavipectoral fascia. This layer is opened to expose the underlying pectoralis minor muscle (Fig. 8). The acromiothoracic artery and vein cross the anterior surface of the pectoralis minor muscle and can

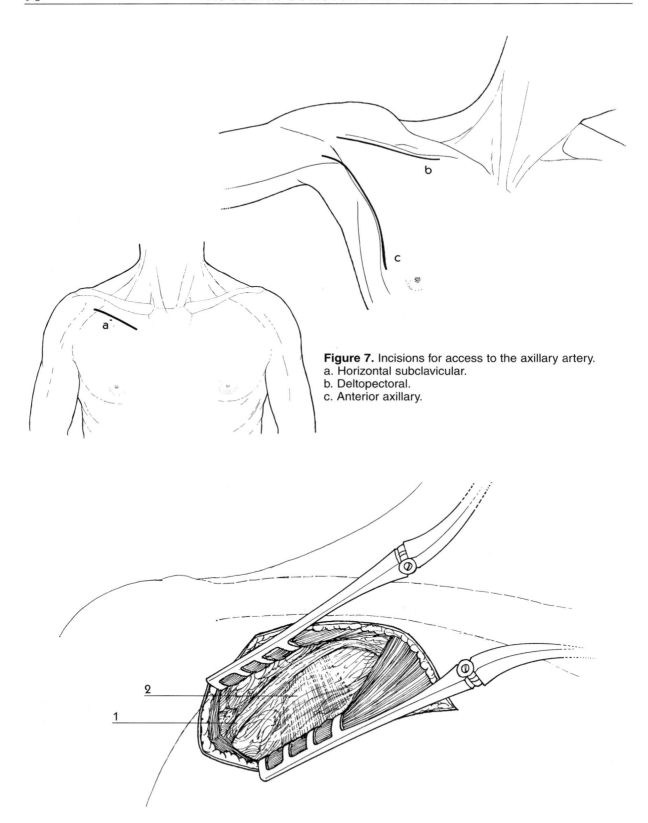

Figure 7. Incisions for access to the axillary artery.
a. Horizontal subclavicular.
b. Deltopectoral.
c. Anterior axillary.

Figure 8. Horizontal infraclavicular incision for approach to the axillary artery: superficial planes.
1. Cephalic vein.
2. Bulge of the pectoralis minor muscle under the clavipectoral fascia.

be traced medially to the axillary artery. Division of the pectoralis minor muscle near the coracoid process permits extensive exposure of the axillary artery. Division of the pectoralis minor muscle also avoids compression of any graft that may eventually pass in the subpectoral tunnel (Fig. 9). Although some surgeons choose not to divide the pectoralis minor muscle, we have seen no problems from its division and prefer the general exposure that is provided by its division.

Several structures in this area must be identified and preserved. The upper nerve to the pectoralis major muscle should be identified and can usually be preserved. The more anterior axillary vein is subsequently encountered and must be carefully dissected away from the artery. The axillary artery pulse is usually higher and deeper and can be easily palpated. The acromiothoracic arterial trunk guides one down to the axillary artery. This trunk can be conserved or ligated depending upon the need for more extensive axillary exposure. This portion of the axillary artery is generally suitable for implantation of an axillofemoral bypass (Fig. 10).

In this area, one must be careful to identify and preserve the branches of the brachial plexus. In general, regular electrocautery should not be used in this area. A bipolar cautery unit is preferable since it conducts a minimal current to any surrounding nerve.

Deltopectoral Incision

This exposure may be necessary for more distal lesions of the axillary artery and can be extended down onto the upper arm in cases of trauma. The arm is placed in slight abduction and internal rotation. The incision begins at the middle third of the clavicle and extends laterally into the deltopectoral groove. The lateral portion of the incision extends to the intersection of the anterior border of the

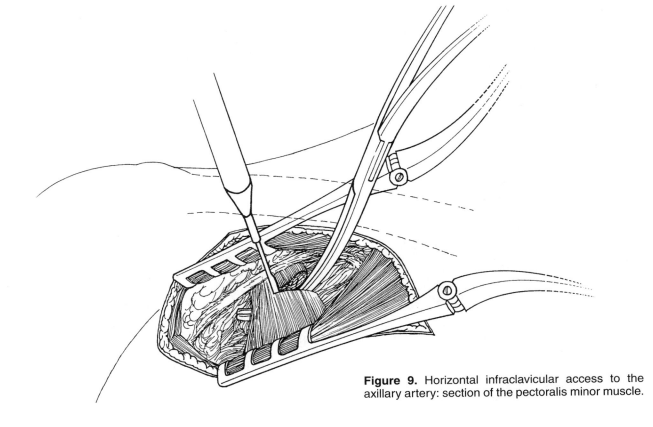

Figure 9. Horizontal infraclavicular access to the axillary artery: section of the pectoralis minor muscle.

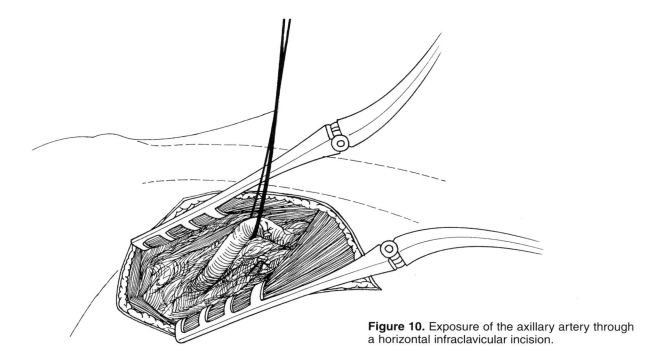

Figure 10. Exposure of the axillary artery through a horizontal infraclavicular incision.

deltoid muscle and the external border of the biceps muscle (Fig. 7B). The cephalic vein may be identified and left to the lateral aspect of the incision.

The pectoralis major muscle can be loosened or slackened by internal rotation of the arm. The clavipectoral fascia is identified and incised. The pectoralis minor muscle is detached from the coracoid process. The pectoralis major tendon is left intact and retracted. At the inferior portion of the incision, one can generally identify the cords of the brachial plexus where the median nerve and the musculocutaneous nerves form an "M" configuration on the anterior surface of the artery. Again, the nerves must be identified and protected from injury.

Transpectoral Incision

In occasional severe or complex penetration shoulder injury, it will be necessary to divide the pectoralis major muscle to obtain rapid and complete control of the underlying axillary artery. In general, we try to avoid

taking down the humeral head of the pectoralis major muscle. In many cases, it can be retracted or partially divided. However, one should not hesitate to take down the pectoralis major muscle if massive arterial or venous hemorrhage is occurring and control has not been adequately gained.

Anterior Axillary Incision

This incision is another method to expose the lower axillary artery in cases of localized trauma. The advantage of this incision is exposure of the lower axillary artery and brachial artery without dividing the pectoralis major tendon.

The patient is placed in the dorsal decubitus position with the arm in abduction (Fig. 7C). The lateral border of the pectoralis major muscle is identified, incised, and the median nerve is found and carefully retracted (Fig. 11). In some cases, section of the pectoralis minor tendon will facilitate proximal control of the axillary artery. Mobilization of the artery may require ligation and division of the lateral thoracic artery.

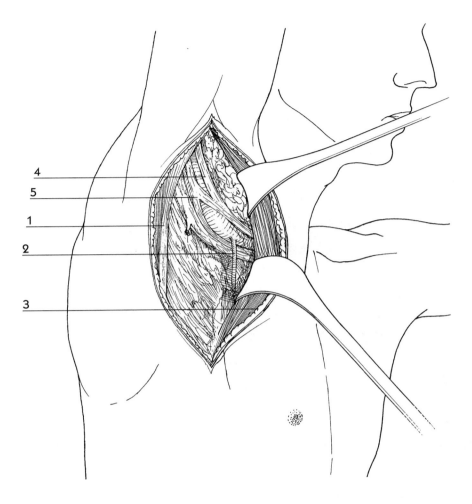

Figure 11. Exposure of the axillary artery through a subpectoral axillary incision.
1. Latissimus dorsi.
2. Lateral thoracic artery.
3. Pectoralis major.
4. Musculocutaneous nerve.
5. Median nerve.

Combined Infraclavicular and Deltopectoral Incisions

For more spacious exposure of the proximal and midaxillary arteries, one can extend the incision from the medial clavicle to the distal deltopectoral groove (Fig. 12). This exposure requires detachment of the clavicular head of the pectoralis major muscle at the anterior border of the clavicle, section of the pectoralis minor tendon from the coracoid process, and opening of the clavipectoral aponeurosis from the medial to lateral aspects of the incision. This wide exposure is especially useful in extensive trauma cases associated with voluminous hematoma. This incision allows total exposure of the first and second portions of the axillary artery and can be extended downstream to the level of the humeral head.

Extended Subclavian Axillary Exposure

This exposure involves the subclavian and axillary arteries (Fig. 13). Again, it is rarely necessary and may only be used in cases of extensive penetrating or blunt shoulder trauma. In general, it is used in cases where the clavicle has been fragmented by blunt or penetrating injury.

The fragmented clavicle is resected and debrided. Proximal distal control of injured

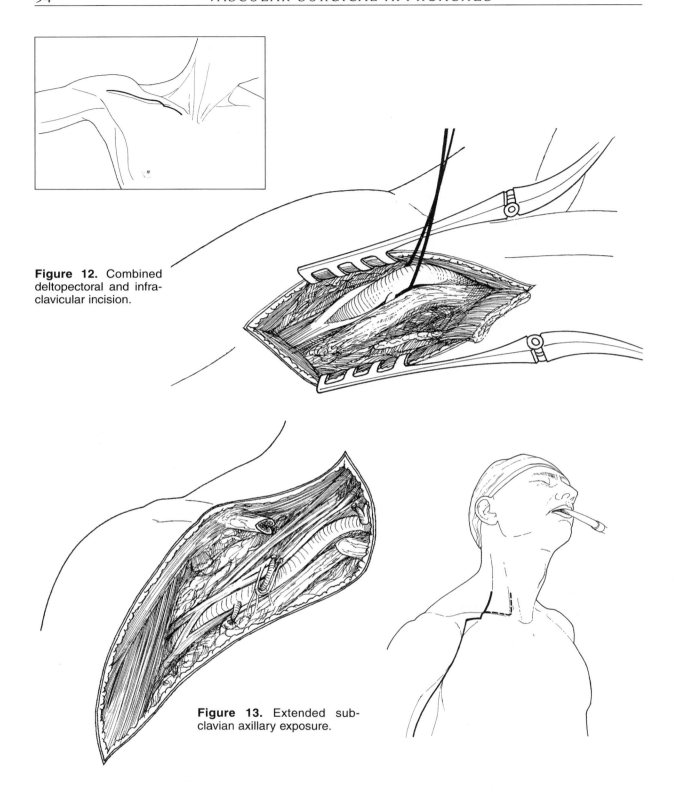

Figure 12. Combined deltopectoral and infra-clavicular incision.

Figure 13. Extended subclavian axillary exposure.

arteries and veins is obtained. Routes of the brachial plexus are identified. If they have been severed by trauma, they are generally marked with a fine suture for subsequent repair. Arterial and venous repair are performed. Nerve repairs will depend upon the extent of injury and the availability of surgeons with expertise in such repair.

8

Brachial Artery

Bertrand Ede

Present indications for brachial artery exposure fall into four main categories: arterial emboli, traumatic injury, chronic atherosclerosis of the upper extremity, and access for hemodialysis.

Anatomic Review

The brachial artery is the continuation of the axillary artery. It begins at the lower border of the pectoralis major muscle and runs from the armpit to the bend of the elbow in almost a straight line. It usually divides slightly below the elbow joint into the radial artery laterally and the ulnar artery medially. The brachial artery is located along with the other components of the neurovascular bundle in the triangular space that is formed by the biceps in front, the medial intermuscular septum covering the triceps in the back, the coracobrachial and brachial muscles laterally (Fig. 1). The artery can be easily palpated in the internal bicipital gutter. At the level of the elbow the brachial artery is in the medial bicipital space bound by the aponeurotic expansion of the biceps, the brachial muscle in the back, the pronator muscle medially, and the tendon of the biceps laterally. Throughout its course the brachial artery is accompanied by two venae comitantes. The median nerve crosses the brachial artery at

midcourse from lateral at the top to medial at the bottom. The radial nerve is in contact with the posterior side of the artery at the top but it quickly veers off to the inferior axillary space and to the back of the arm. The ulnar nerve which is first on the inner side of the brachial artery enters the back of the arm in the middle or lower third of the upper arm passing along the collateral upper ulnar artery behind the intermuscular septum. The deep brachial artery is the first large branch of the brachial artery. It arises shortly after the beginning of the brachial artery, enters the inferior axillary space along with the radial nerve and runs to the posterior side of the humerus. Other branches of the brachial artery are the deltoid artery, the artery of the humerus, the anterior ulnar artery, and the superior ulnar artery which accompanies the ulnar nerve to the back of the arm. The brachial artery contributes to the brachioaxillary network through its upper branches and to periarticular network of the elbow through its ulnar branches. An anatomic variant observed in one out of five patients is a

From Vascular Surgical Approaches, edited by Alain Branchereau and Ramon Berguer. ©1999, Futura Publishing Co., Inc., Armonk, NY.

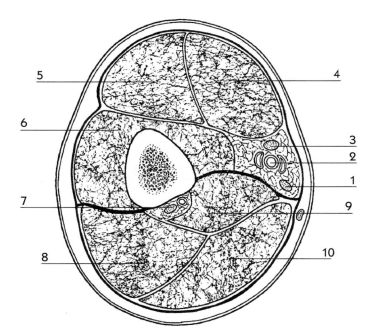

Figure 1. Cross-section at the middle third of the arm.
1. Ulnar nerve.
2. Brachial artery.
3. Median nerve.
4. Biceps, short belly.
5. Biceps, long belly.
6. Brachial muscle.
7. Radial nerve.
8. Triceps, lateral belly.
9. Triceps, medial belly.
10. Triceps, long belly.

superficial brachial artery[1] usually arising from the axillary artery and running subcutaneously in front of the median nerve in the bicipital gutter. This variant artery coexists with the brachial artery in 13% of cases and gives rise to the radial artery in 5% of these cases. In 9% of cases the superficial brachial artery is the only artery of the arm. The deep brachial artery can present several other variants: in 13% of cases it branches from the axillary artery and in 5% of cases from the posterior circumflex artery, a branch of the axillary artery.

Exposure in the Middle Third of the Arm

The following approach is traditionally used for ligature, thrombectomy or bypass.[2] The subject is lying supine with the upper arm at a 90 degree angle to the body and the forearm in extension-supination. The operator stands on the inner side of the arm and the assistant stands on the opposing side. The incision is made in the groove between the biceps and the triceps over a line that extends from the top of the armpit to the bend of the elbow (Fig. 2). An incision of about 6 cm to the junction between the upper third and middle third of the arm is usually sufficient. The incision can be slightly offset to the front to ensure preservation of the basilic vein posteriorly especially when the operation is being performed to create an angioaccess fistula. Opening the brachial aponeurosis allows mobilization and retraction of the internal border of the biceps. The neurovascular bundle can be seen under the medial border of the biceps. Incision of the thin aponeurotic membrane exposes the median nerve which usually crosses the anterior surface of the brachial artery. Once the nerve has been carefully released and protected, the artery can be separated from the two venae comitantes (Fig. 3). The main source of error is incision placement. Making the incision too far behind the biceps raises the risk of perforating the medial intermuscular septum and mistaking the ulnar nerve for the median nerve and the upper ulnar collateral artery for the brachial artery. The incision can be carried up to the armpit. It is also quick and easy to extend the incision down to the bend of the elbow.

Exposure at the Flexure

This approach allows exposure of the distal brachial artery as well as the origin of the radial and ulnar arteries. The arm is placed in exter-

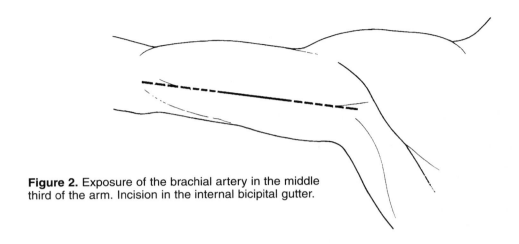

Figure 2. Exposure of the brachial artery in the middle third of the arm. Incision in the internal bicipital gutter.

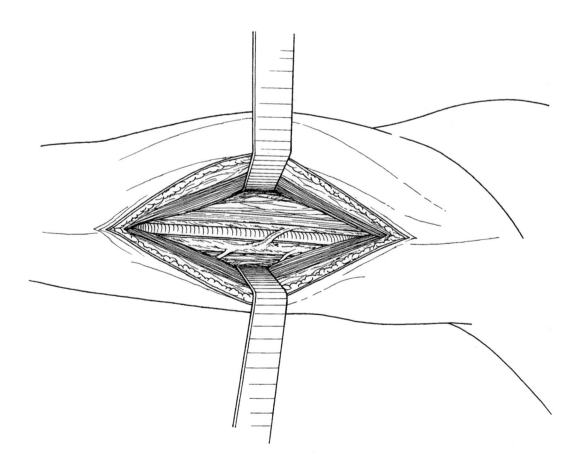

Figure 3. Exposure of the brachial artery in the middle third of the arm. The internal edge of the biceps and the median nerve are retracted to expose the artery.

nal rotation at a 90 degree angle to the body with the forearm in extension-supination. An S-shaped incision is made across the elbow. The superficial veins should be preserved especially when the operation is performed for hemodialysis. After opening the superficial aponeurosis, the tendon of the biceps can be seen at the bottom stretching obliquely to the outer side (Fig. 4). Pronating the arm slightly relaxes this tendon and facilitates its division. The brachial artery is exposed between the median nerve medially and the tendon of the biceps laterally. By carrying the incision downward it is possible to control the brachial bifurcation after retraction of the pronator muscle (Fig. 5). The radial artery appears as a continuation of the brachial artery, and the first centimeters of the ulnar artery can be seen just

before the vessel passes under the pronator and epitrochlear muscles.

Exposure of the Deep Brachial Artery

This approach was originally used to expose the radial nerve which accompanies the deep brachial artery on the posterior side of the arm.[3] The patient is placed in lateral decubitus on the unoperated side. The arm to be operated on is placed along the body with the forearm at a right angle in internal rotation. The operator stands behind the patient. The assistant stands in front of the operator holding the forearm in internal rotation. The incision is made along a

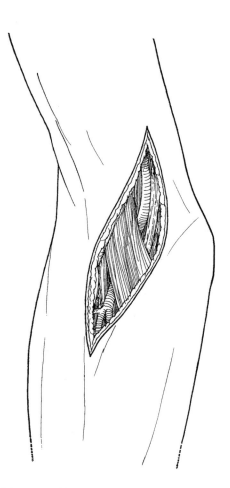

Figure 4. Exposure of the brachial artery at the elbow flexure. The aponeurotic expansion of the biceps crosses in front of the artery.

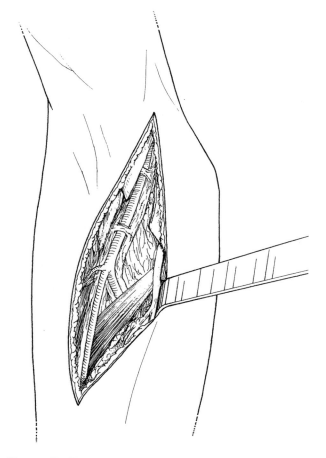

Figure 5. The brachial artery and its branches are exposed after division of the aponeurotic expansion of the biceps and retraction of the round pronator muscle.

line that extends from the acromial angle to the olecranon (Fig. 6). The incision should pass through the center of the posterior compartment of the arm in the space bounded on top by the long and the lateral bellies of the triceps. At the bottom of the incision the common tendon of the triceps must be sectioned and the fibers of the medial aspect of the triceps dissociated. The deep brachial artery and radial nerve run adjacent to the humerus.

Discussion

With a good knowledge of the anatomy of the arm, complications related to the surgical exposure of the brachial artery can be avoided. The features requiring special caution are the location of the median nerve and the possibility of a superficial brachial artery anatomic variant.

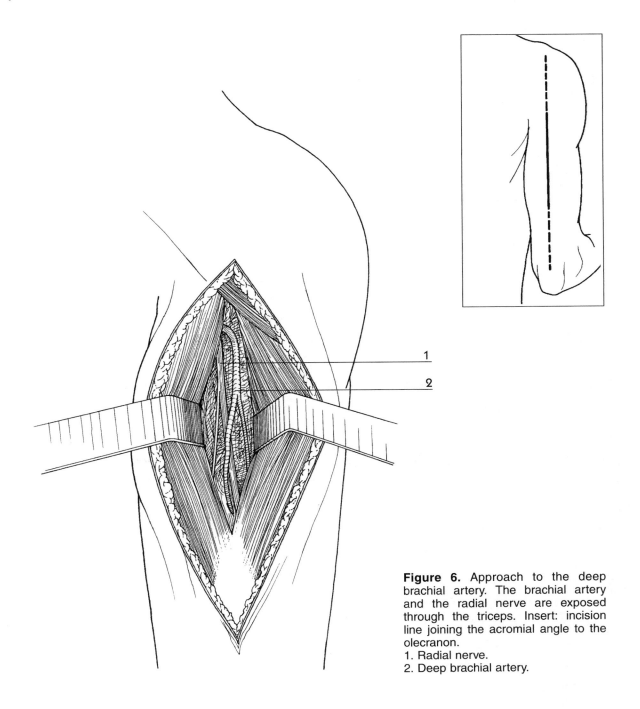

Figure 6. Approach to the deep brachial artery. The brachial artery and the radial nerve are exposed through the triceps. Insert: incision line joining the acromial angle to the olecranon.
1. Radial nerve.
2. Deep brachial artery.

Since it is in close contact with the humerus, the brachial artery may be injured in case of fracture or dislocation. Exposure of the brachial artery is done using the medial approach regardless of the type of injury or associated lesions; this exposure can be extended downward to allow control of the brachial bifurcation. In cases involving loss of tissue, especially on the anterior side of the bend of the elbow, it may be necessary to use a musculocutaneous flap to cover the artery.

Frequent use of the brachial artery for catheterization during cardiovascular examinations or endovascular procedures has led to an increase in the number of iatrogenic injuries. Thrombosis or false aneurysm usually requires surgical treatment.

In the rare cases of chronic ischemia of the upper extremity due to atherosclerotic disease or arteritis, there is often a need to expose the brachial artery. In the vast majority of cases the brachial artery is the recipient bypass site (carotido- or axillobrachial bypass) and only rarely is the donor site.

The brachial artery can be used for hemodialysis access when the veins of the forearm are inadequate. This can be achieved either by performing arteriovenous fistula at the elbow flexure or a brachial to basilic vein fistula. For brachial to basilic arteriovenous fistula the cutaneous incision is moved forward to avoid injury to the basilic vein.

References

1. Lippert H, Pabst R. *Arterial Variations in Man.* München, JF Bergmann Verlag, 1985, pp 69-70.
2. Cadenat FM. *Les voies de pénétrations des membres.* Paris, Doin, 1978, pp 84-98.
3. Fey B, Mocquot P, Oberlin S, Quenu J, Truffert P. *Traité de technique chirurgicale,* Tome 1 Paris, Masson, 1943 pp 381-400.

9

Arteries of the Forearm and Hand

Bernard Enon

Arterial blood is supplied to the forearm and hand by the two terminal branches of the brachial artery: the radial and the ulnar arteries. The superficial and deep arches of these arteries at the level of the hand constitute the limit for conventional vascular surgery. Microsurgery is required for more distal vessels.

Meticulous technique and use of magnifying glasses are crucial to the successful functional outcome of these operations which are often carried out after trauma involving bone fracture and tendon lacerations.

Anatomic Review

Brachial Artery at the Elbow Flexure

The brachial artery crosses the elbow in the medial bicipital gutter between the round pronator muscle medially, the tendon of the biceps laterally, and the tendon of the brachial muscle posteriorly. The brachial artery ends below the crease of the elbow about 2 cm after the midline of the joint where it divides into two terminal arteries: the radial artery and the ulnar artery. The common interosseous artery usually arises from the ulnar artery and sinks

deeply to reach the superior border of the interosseous ligament of the forearm, where it divides into an anterior and posterior branch.

Arteries of the Forearm

The radial artery has a straight course in the forearm. It runs in a fold of the antebrachial fascia where it is in relation posteriorly with the supinator muscles and the round pronator muscle, superficial flexor of the fingers, long flexor of the thumb, and the square pronator. Medially, it is in relation with the round pronator, superficial flexor of the fingers, and flexor carpi radialis. Laterally, the artery is

From Vascular Surgical Approaches, edited by Alain Branchereau and Ramon Berguer. ©1999, Futura Publishing Co., Inc., Armonk, NY.

contiguous to the brachioradialis. The upper half of the radial artery is covered by the brachioradialis muscle. In the middle third of the forearm the course of the radial artery is subfascial and superficial between the brachioradialis muscle laterally and the flexor carpi radialis medially.

The ulnar artery has an oblique and deeper course. Once it reaches the medial side of the forearm it runs vertically to the lower border of the pisiform bone. In the upper third of the forearm the ulnar artery is deep, located under the epitrochlear muscles. In the middle third of the forearm the ulnar artery is more accessible between the superficial and deep flexor muscles of the fingers. In the lower third of the forearm the ulnar artery is superficial between the tendons of the flexor carpi ulnaris medially and the superficial flexor of the fifth digit laterally, and is covered by the deep and superficial antebrachial fasciae. The ulnar nerve lies on its inner side during its course.

Arteries of the Wrist

The radial artery reaches the wrist gutter between the tendons of the brachioradialis muscle laterally and the flexor carpi radialis medially. At this point it is covered only by the superficial fascia. At the base of the radial styloid process, the radial artery describes a downward and outward curve and passes between the tendons of the long abductor of the thumb and the short extensor muscle of the thumb. It crosses the lower part of anatomic snuff box under the tendons of the short and long radial carpal extensors. It then passes between the bone and the tendon of the long extensor of the thumb to the dorsum of the hand crossing the upper part of the first interosseous space from the front to the back. The superficial palmar branch continues the vertical course of the radial artery before turning inward and anastomosing with the ulnar artery to form the superficial palmar arch.

The ulnar artery, accompanied by the ulnar nerve on its inner side and covered by two fasciae, runs along the lateral external border of the flexor carpi ulnaris in front of the square pronator muscle. It passes in front of the flexor

retinaculum of the carpus in a canal bounded medially by the pisiform bone and posteriorly by the flexor retinaculum. The ulnar artery then curves outward to give the palmar carpal branch that anastomoses with the radial artery (deep palmar arch).

Arteries of the Palm of the Hand

The radial artery crosses the upper part of the first interosseous space where it penetrates the first dorsal interosseous palmar muscle, and then passes between the first palmar interosseous muscle in front and the external part of the abductor of the thumb in the back. Upon reaching the underside of the deep palmar fascia, it anastomoses with the palmar carpal branch of the ulnar artery to form the deep palmar arch. The deep palmar arch lies on the bone under the deep palmar fascia and is accompanied by the deep branch of the ulnar nerve. It gives off ascending and descending branches. The descending branches include the palmar metacarpal arteries to the first, second, third, and fourth spaces.

After giving off the palmar carpal branch the ulnar artery curves, passes through the superficial palmar fascia, and runs in front of the superficial flexor tendons of the fingers and terminal branches of the median nerve. It anastomoses with the superficial palmar branch of the radial artery to form the superficial palmar arch.

Exposure
of the Brachial Artery
at the Elbow Flexure

The patient is supine with the upper extremity at a right angle to the body and the forearm in extension-supination. Since the artery is fairly superficial, a relatively short incision is sufficient. The incision should make an S-turn (Fig. 1). The first layer contains the superficial veins which should be left intact when the operation is performed for creation of a arteriovenous fistula for dialysis. Vein anatomy can present many variations. The perforating branch connecting with the deep veins should be preserved. The medial expansion of the tendon of the biceps is divided and the artery is encircled with tapes (Fig. 2). It is helpful to pronate the forearm to relax the tendinous expansion. This approach can easily be enlarged to allow exposure of the brachial artery above and the origins of the ulnar and radial arteries below. The artery is exposed between the tendon of the biceps on the

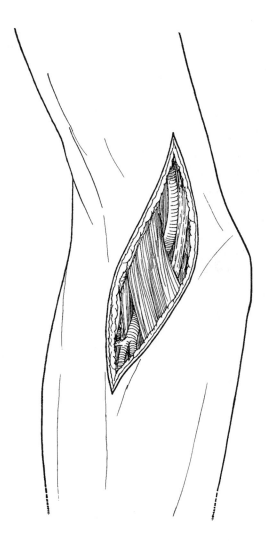

Figure 1. Exposure of the brachial artery at the elbow flexure before division of the aponeurotic expansion.

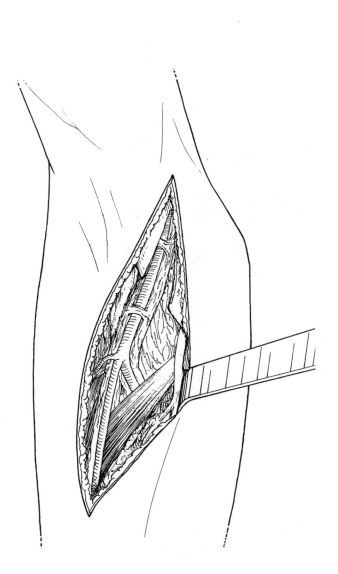

Figure 2. Exposure of the brachial artery at the elbow flexure after division of the aponeurotic expansion. A few centimeters of the brachial artery are exposed. By carrying the incision distally it is possible to expose the radial artery and the first centimeters of the ulnar artery.

outside and the median nerve on the inside: *The artery is between two white lines* (Fig. 3).

Exposure of the Arteries in the Forearm

Ulnar Artery and Common Interosseous Artery

The arm is placed in abduction and external rotation with the elbow raised. The forearm is placed in forced supination and slight flexion with the hand in hyperextension and abduction.

For exposure in the upper third of the forearm, the incision is a continuation of the one described in the previous section (Fig. 2). The median nerve, previously identified, disappears under the round pronator muscle. The latter is retracted inferomedially, now that it is relaxed by the pronation of the forearm. Using this approach, the bifurcation of the brachial artery and a long segment of the ulnar artery can be exposed. For lower access the arch of the superficial flexor muscle of the

fingers must be divided. The origin of the common interosseous artery is accessible using this approach (Fig. 4).

In the middle third of the forearm exposure is deeper and slightly more difficult. The incision is made along a line from the median epicondyle to the lateral edge of the pisiform bone. The space between the flexor carpi ulnaris medially and the superficial flexor of the fingers laterally is located. The major landmark is the ulnar nerve on the inner side. After incising the deep fascia the artery is exposed.

In the lower third of the forearm exposure of the ulnar artery is easy: lateral to the flexor carpi ulnaris. The ulnar nerve is medial to the artery (Figs. 5 and 6).

Radial Artery

The arm is placed in abduction with the forearm in extension-supination.

For exposure of the radial artery in the upper third of the forearm, the incision is made along a line from the middle of the elbow flexure to the point where the radial pulse is

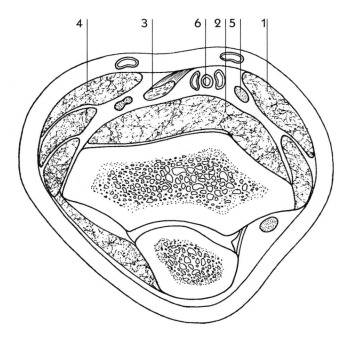

Figure 3. Cross-section of the right elbow: the brachial artery is between "the two white cords," the median nerve, and the tendon of the biceps.
1. Round pronator muscle.
2. Brachial muscle.
3. Tendon of biceps and its aponeurotic expansion.
4. Brachioradialis muscle.
5. Median nerve.
6. Brachial artery.

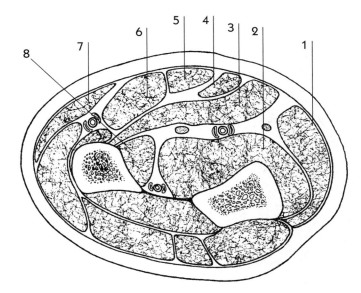

Figure 4. Cross-section of forearm between its upper and middle third.
1. Ulnar flexor of the carpus.
2. Deep flexor of the fingers.
3. Superficial flexor of the fingers.
4. Radial flexor of the carpus.
5. Long palmar muscle.
6. Round pronator muscle.
7. Brachioradialis muscle.
8. Flexor of the thumb.

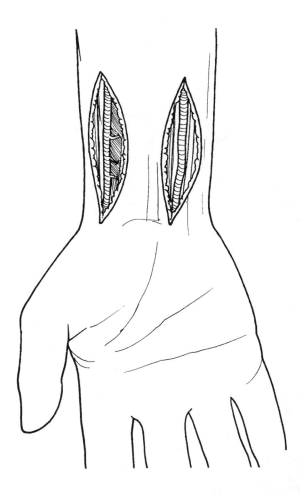

Figure 5. Exposure of radial and ulnar arteries in the lower third of the forearm.

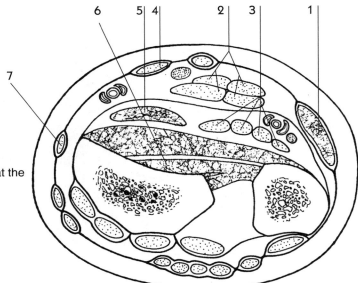

Figure 6. Cross-section of the right forearm at the junction between its middle and lower third.
1. Flexor carpi ulnaris.
2. Superficial flexor of fingers.
3. Tendons of the deep flexor of the fingers.
4. Flexor carpi radialis.
5. Long flexor of the thumb.
6. Square pronator muscle.
7. Brachioradialis muscle.

felt at the wrist. The brachioradialis muscle is retracted laterally (Fig. 4).

In the middle third of the forearm the incision line is the continuation of the one described above. A 6 cm incision in the upper third of the forearm allows identification of the round pronator muscle. The artery can easily be located resting on the anterior surface of the muscle (Fig. 4). It is not necessary to expose the nerve.

At the wrist the radial artery is superficial between the tendon of the brachioradialis muscle and the flexor carpi radialis. Access at this level is common for the creation of an arteriovenous fistula in which case special care is needed to protect the superficial vein network.

In the anatomic snuff box the artery is deeply situated. The major landmark is the cephalic vein which must be gently retracted to avoid injury especially when the purpose of the operation is to create an arteriovenous fistula. The radial artery can be found in the distal part of the incision near the bone structures as it sinks into the intermetacarpal space (Fig. 7).

Exposure of the Arteries in the Hand

Without mentioning the approaches used for plastic microsurgery which are beyond the scope of this book, there are numerous techniques for exposure of the arteries in the hand. All of these techniques require that the hand be placed in supination (Fig. 8).

Ulnar Artery

The ulnar artery gives rise to the superficial palmar arch. Injury can result from blunt or penetrating trauma but the most common cause of injury is repetitive trauma related to occupational (jack hammer) or sports (karate, barehanded jai alai) activities which can cause aneurysms that result in distal microembolization. The exposure is relatively simple. After incising the hypothenar eminence and the aponeurotic layer, the artery is exposed in the upper part of the palm at the origin of the superficial palmar arch. The length of the artery exposed is sufficient to allow construction of a distal bypass anastomosis or aneurysmal repair (Fig. 9).

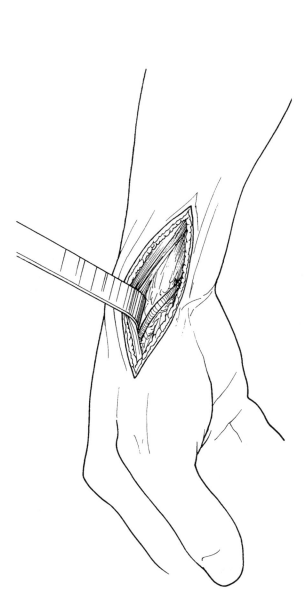

Figure 7. The radial artery can be exposed in the anatomic snuff box before it deepens into the intermetacarpal space.

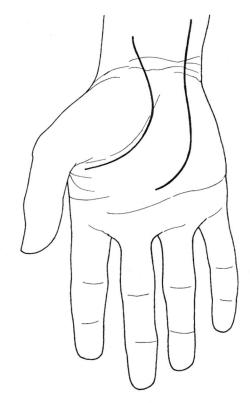

Figure 8. Incision for exposure of the arteries of the hand.

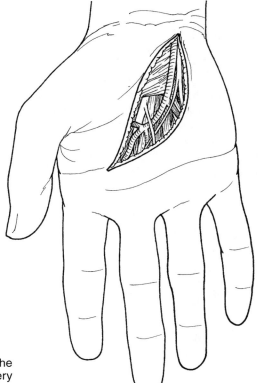

Figure 9. An arc-shaped incision passing through the hypothenar eminence allows exposure of the ulnar artery as well as the superficial palmar arch in the hand.

Radial Artery

Exposure of the deep palmar arch is a particularly difficult and disabling procedure that is rarely used. The approach through the medial border of the thenar eminence involves extensive dissection of the tendons and allows exposure of the origin of the deep palmar arch in the depth of the field.

Special Procedures

The previously described techniques are modified to suit the anatomic variations which may be encountered in this territory.

A high bifurcation of the brachial artery can occur as far up as the axilla. In these cases the standard approach to the brachial artery actually exposes the radial artery. The ulnar artery is located further posteriorly. In cases of agenesis of the radial artery the anterior interosseous artery may supply its territory and follow the same course throughout the forearm to the anatomic snuff box. The median artery (artery of the median nerve) is generally a small vessel but may be hypertrophic and even replace the radial and ulnar arteries in supplying blood to the hand. The radial artery can have a superficial course and wrap around the radius in the middle third of the forearm. In this case it can be palpated easily. The blood can be supplied to the hand exclusively by a radial or an ulnar artery. This latter arrangement is of special importance when the plan is to create an arteriovenous fistula at the wrist for hemodialysis or to cannulate the radial artery for blood pressure monitoring.

Discussion

A variety of causes can lead to pathology of the arteries in the area of the elbow. Emboli usually occur as emergencies. A transverse arteriotomy at the level of the bifurcation allows embolectomy. Open or closed trauma of the brachial artery at the level of the elbow is frequent (dislocation of the elbow, penetrating wounds, and iatrogenic trauma). The difficulty of treatment increases with the complexity of injury, such as with extensive subadventitial rupture or an open wound. By extending the exposure cranially and distally it is possible to use the conventional vascular reconstruction techniques of resection and reanastomosis, venous interposition, and bypass. The prognosis is usually determined by the extent of the associated nerve injuries.

When the operation is performed for angioaccess, care must be taken to preserve the superficial veins during exposure of the brachial artery. The use of the perforating vein of the venous "M" is especially effective to develop the superficial venous network. Axillobrachial, brachiobrachial, and brachioulnar bypass can be performed with conventional vascular surgical techniques. The main indication for surgery of the arteries of the forearm is open or closed trauma. The size of the vessels requires careful handling and use of magnifying glasses. Mechanical dilatation of arterial spasm using coronary dilators can be useful. The cephalic and basilic veins can be used for short radioradial or ulnoulnar bypasses.

Other than trauma, the main indication for exposure of the radial and ulnar arteries at the level of the wrist is creation of an arteriovenous fistula for hemodialysis. Mobilization of the superficial veins and arteries must be atraumatic and enable side-to-side or side-to-end anastomosis. The ulnar artery may be occluded at the wrist due to compression or aneurysm secondary to repeated injury. A number of procedures are feasible at the level of the wrist including segmental resection and reanastomosis for aneurysm, and radioradial or ulnoulnar bypass with venous interposition for thrombosis. At the level of the palm conventional vascular reconstruction requires exposure of the superficial palmar arch.

10

Superior Vena Cava

Pierre-Edouard Magnan

The superior vena cava (SVC) is exposed routinely by cardiac surgeons for extracorporeal circulation. Resection and/or bypass of the SVC are uncommon but may be required in patients with mediastinal or bronchopulmonary tumors. Since the SVC is located in the right part of the anterior mediastinum, it can be exposed by either a sternotomy or a right thoracotomy.

Anatomic Review

The SVC is formed by the junction of the right and left innominate (or brachiocephalic) veins behind the cartilage of the first rib. From its origin the SVC descends going slightly oblique posteriorly, and forming a gentle curve with a left concavity to conform itself to the right edge of the ascending aorta. Its intrapericardial termination is on the upper wall of the right atrium (Fig. 1). The mean diameter of the SVC is 2 cm and its mean length is 7 cm.[1] Anteriorly its relationships are the right pleura, the thymus, and the lymph nodes of the right anterior mediastinum. Posteriorly the SVC in its extrapericardial portion has a relationship with the right main stem bronchus and the termination of the right azygos vein, and in its intrapericardial portion with the right pulmonary artery. Its right wall is in contact with the mediastinal pleura and the right phrenic nerve, the left wall with the ascending aorta.

Exposure Via Sternotomy

The patient is placed in supine decubitus. The neck should be slightly extended by placing a roll under the shoulder blades. The arms are secured alongside the body. The surgical field extends from the lower part of the neck to the upper third of the abdomen vertically and laterally to the anterior axillary lines. When the procedure requires clamping of the SVC, central venous catheters are placed in the inferior vena cava. A vertical incision is made starting from the suprasternal notch to the abdomen below the xiphoid.

Superficial Layers

The subcutaneous tissue and presternal periosteum are divided with cautery. To completely mobilize the xiphoid process it is

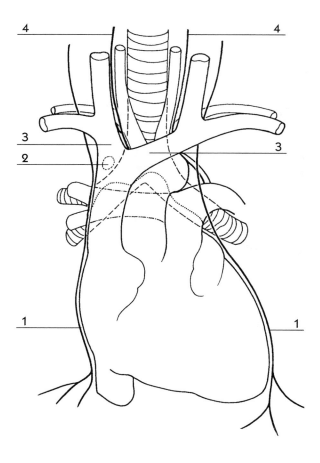

Figure 1. Anterior view showing the anatomic relations of the superior vena cava.
1. Phrenic nerve.
2. Azygos vein.
3. Innominate veins.
4. Vagus nerve.

necessary to incise the linea alba at the lower part of the incision. The sternum is divided using an alternating saw. Ventilation of the patient is momentarily discontinued during sawing of the sternum to reduce the risk of pleural injury. The sternum is spread apart gradually. As the ratchet retractor is opened, the interclavicular ligament is divided. The periosteum of the anterior and posterior sides of the sternum is coagulated with electrocautery. Bone wax can be used to obtain hemostasis of the divided bone but this method increases the risk of postoperative bone healing problems.

Deep Layers

Once the retractor has been fully opened, the anterior pleural folds are pushed to the sides using a stick sponge. The thymus gland is divided between ligatures. Dissection of the thymus begins at the lower border: a dissector is passed along the anterior aspect of the pericardium and brought out at the lower border of the left innominate vein. One may preserve the thymus gland by freeing its right border and flipping it on its left border to be used later to cover an eventual bypass. For full exposure of the intra- and extrapericardial SVC, the pericardium is opened with a vertical incision from the diaphragm to the aorta. The pericardium is held open using suture stays.

Vascular Layer

The dissection begins with the left innominate vein which is covered by the thyropericardial aponeurosis. Mobilization requires division of one or more thymic veins along its lower border and inferior thyroid veins along the upper border at the junction between the two innominate veins. The posterior wall is then freed from the innominate artery. The termination of the right innominate vein is located behind the cartilage of the first rib. It is dissected by mobilizing its medial wall from the areolar tissue that contains the lymphatic network of the anterior mediastinum and by ligating and dividing the right internal mammary vein which retains the anterior wall of the innominate vein against the bone. The right phrenic nerve and the covering mediastinal pleura must be detached from the external border of the right innominate vein using a swab stick or scissors. It may be helpful to open the pleura. The posterior wall of the vein is dissected by pulling the vein anteriorly. This technique separates the vein from the vagus nerve that stays behind.

The anterior wall of the extrapericardial SVC is free. Its left border can be easily separated from the ascending aorta. The right border on the outer side can be released from the pleura and the phrenic nerve using the same technique that was used to free the proximal end of the right innominate vein. On the posterior aspect it is necessary to locate the arch of the azygos vein which crosses the upper border of the right main stem bronchus before inserting the dissector between the bronchus and the SVC (Fig. 2). Control of the intrapericardial SVC is more straightforward. After incising the left border of the serous layer of the pericardium, a dissector is introduced from right to left behind the SVC and brought out between the ascending aorta and vena cava. Care must be taken to avoid injuring the right pulmonary artery which is in direct contact with the posterior caval wall (Fig. 3).

Extensions

The sternotomy can be carried up into the neck to allow exposure of the internal jugular or subclavian veins. To expose the internal jugular vein the skin incision is made along the anterior border of the sternocleidomastoid muscle in continuity with the sternotomy incision. The platysma is cut using cautery and the sternocleidomastoid muscle is retracted laterally. The anterior jugular vein is divided between two ligatures and the sternocleidomastoid muscle and the intermediary tendon of

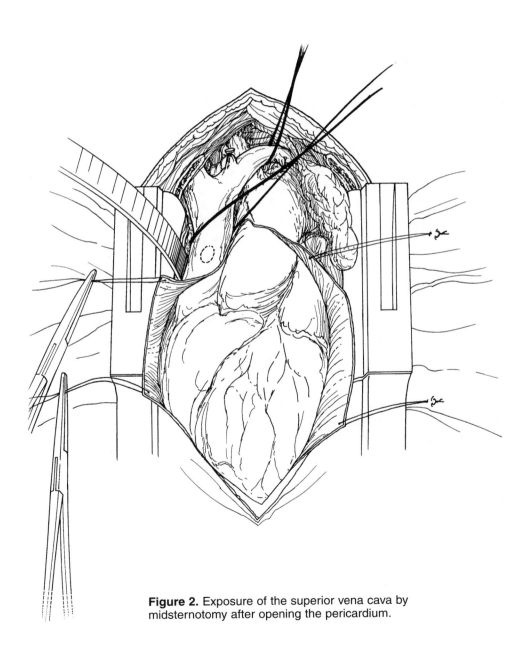

Figure 2. Exposure of the superior vena cava by midsternotomy after opening the pericardium.

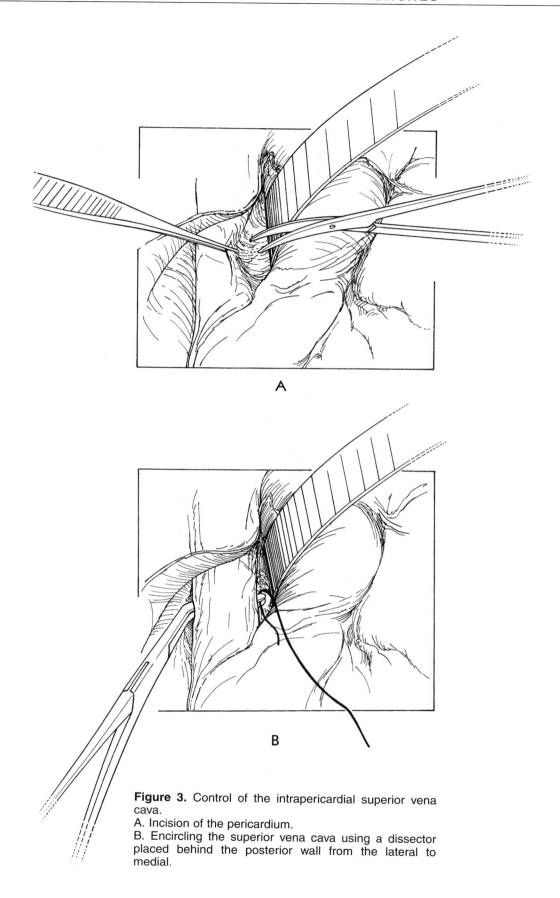

Figure 3. Control of the intrapericardial superior vena cava.
A. Incision of the pericardium.
B. Encircling the superior vena cava using a dissector placed behind the posterior wall from the lateral to medial.

the omohyoid muscle are divided using cautery. The internal jugular vein can then be exposed and dissected by separating it from the common carotid artery and the vagus nerve.

To expose the subclavian vein the skin incision is made parallel to the clavicle. The sternal head of the sternocleidomastoid muscle and the omohyoid and sternocleidohyoid muscles are divided using cautery. Because the subclavian vein is located behind the clavicle, its exposure is more difficult than that of the internal jugular vein. Opening the sternum facilitates exposure by allowing dissection to be continued beyond the innominate vein in the groove formed by the sternum and clavicle. The subclavian vein is mobilized by ligating and dividing the anterior and external jugular veins in its upper border. In the back, care is exercised to preserve the phrenic and vagus nerves on the right and the phrenic nerve on the left. These nerves cross the posterior border of the subclavian vein in front of the artery. Bilateral cervical exposure can be done by *T-ing* the median sternotomy with a transverse cervical incision. In all cases the sternocleidohyoid and omohyoid muscles are divided to achieve exposure of all the large venous attachments (right and left internal jugular and subclavian veins).

Exposure Via Right Thoracotomy

The patient is placed in the left lateral decubitus using a bean bag to immobilize the shoulder and buttocks. An axillary roll is placed to facilitate spread of the ribs and to take some weight off of the left axilla. Allowing the right arm to hang freely across the top of the left arm helps to move the scapula from the field after muscle section. The patient must be ventilated using a double lumen endotracheal tube to allow exclusion of the right lung.

Opening the Rib Cage

The incision begins in the back two fingerbreadths from the spine in the angle formed by the spine and scapula. It follows parallel to the spinal border of the scapula and passes 2 cm below the tip of the scapula. At that point it curves and follows the ribs to the front stopping at the anterior axillary line. The latissimus dorsi muscle is divided from one end to the other perpendicular to the fibers using cautery. The lower part of the muscle is detached from the serratus. The triangular aponeurosis at the lower edge of the rhomboid muscle and over the posterior border of the serratus is divided along the border of these muscles in order to leave an attachment posteroinferiorly. This opens the virtual space on the inner side of the scapula. By introducing his hand into this space the operator can locate the fourth intercostal space which provides the best exposure of the SVC. The serratus muscle is then divided using an electric scalpel along the costal insertions so that its pedicle is sectioned as low as possible.

The fourth intercostal space is opened after exclusion of the right lung. The rib edges are protected with drapes and a Finiochietto thoracic retractor is placed. As soon as the retractor has been opened, division of the intercostal muscles is completed to the spine in the back, and to the costal cartilages in front.

Deep Layer

The excluded lung is pushed down to the back using a malleable retractor. When the intrapericardial portion of the SVC is to be exposed, the pericardium is opened by a vertical incision behind the phrenic nerve (Fig. 4). In some cases the nerve is located near the lung pedicle and must be dissected before opening the pericardium. Mobilization of the phrenic nerve is begun by incising the mediastinal pleura on both sides of the nerve leaving enough pleural margin to allow mobilization of the nerve without directly grabbing it. The pericardial aspect of the nerve is mobilized using scissors or a peanut dissector after the nerve has been encircled with a loop. Mobilization is continued upward along the external border of the SVC. Control of the vein itself is achieved by incising the reflexion of the pericardium in front of the right pulmonary artery. This allows insertion of a dissector between the pulmonary artery and the medial side of the vena cava. The tip of the

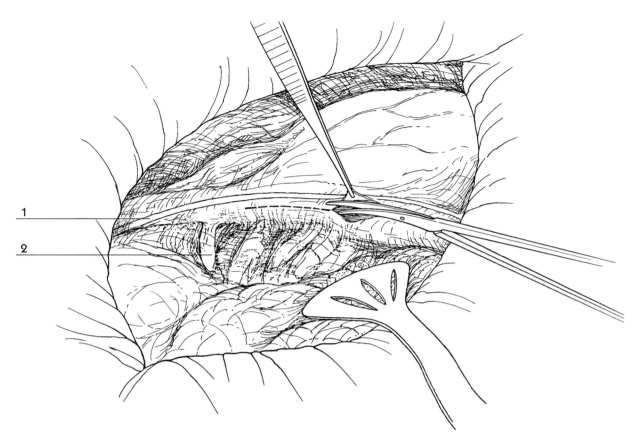

Figure 4. Exposure of the superior vena cava by right thoracotomy. The broken line behind the phrenic nerve indicates the direction of the pericardial incision.
1. Phrenic nerve.
2. Azygos vein.

dissector should exit in the aortocaval window between the ascending aorta and the medial wall of the vena cava. The termination of the azygos vein is controlled on the upper border of the right main stem bronchus by incising the parietal pleura along each border. In this way the azygous vein can be encircled with a dissector and looped.

Dissection of the extrapericardial portion of the SVC begins with mobilization of the phrenic nerve from its lateral wall. Near its termination the posterior aspect of the SVC is detached from the origin of the left main stem bronchus. It can be helpful to divide the azygos between two ligatures. Using scissors the

posterior and medial walls of the SVC are freed from the lymphatic rich areolar tissue on the right side of the trachea.

Control of the junction between the two innominate veins is more difficult than when using the anterior approach. In this region the areolar tissue lining the pleura is denser and may bleed and require electrocoagulation. The right innominate vein is controlled after locating the phrenic nerve which crosses its posterior aspect and after freeing its medial wall from the anterior mediastinal lymphatic network which separates it from the vagus nerve and from the innominate artery. Control of the left innominate vein is more difficult. A long incision of the mediastinal pleura is made perpendicular to the SVC in front of its origin. The main danger for dissection is the innominate artery which crosses the back of the left innominate vein. Using this approach it is preferable to use tourniquets rather than clamps to occlude the innominate vein.

the vein itself is often obstructed and it may be easier to perform bypass without direct exposure. The proximal anastomosis can be made to one or more of its tributaries and the distal anastomosis to the right atrium or its appendix.

Discussion

There are a variety of reasons to expose the SVC. The most common is cannula placement for cardiopulmonary bypass. In this case only the intrapericardial segment of the SVC needs to be exposed. Circumferential dissection is necessary to allow clamping around the cannula to cut off blood flow to the right heart. Resection of the SVC may be necessary for surgical treatment of primary tumors[2] or after invasion by mediastinal or pulmonary tumors.[3-5] Obstructive indications for bypass of the SVC are uncommon but the procedure may be necessary in cases that result in disability and do not respond to treatment.[6-10] Thrombectomy of the SVC is rarely indicated in cases of septic thrombophlebitis.[11]

For resection the choice of approach depends on the type and location of the tumor. Although sternotomy is feasible for bronchopulmonary tumors invading the SVC,[10] a right thoracotomy is generally used.[3,5] Sternotomy is better suited for treatment of primary tumors of the SVC and mediastinal tumors.[4] For bypass or thrombectomy a sternotomy is the most frequent approach[6-10] since it is well-tolerated and can be carried upward by means of left and/or right cervical incisions to allow access to the subclavian and/or jugular veins. In patients with superior vena cava syndrome

References

1. Rouvière H. Anatomie humaine. Tome 2. Tronc. Onzième édition. Paris, Masson, 1974.
2. Abrat RP, Williams M, Raff M, et al. Angiosarcoma of the superior vena cava. *Cancer* 1983; 52: 740-743.
3. Dartevelle P, Chapelier A, Navajas M, et al. Replacement of the superior vena cava with polytetrafluoroethylene grafts combined with resection of mediastinal pulmonary malignant tumors: Report of thirteen cases. *J Thorac Cardiovasc Surg* 1987; 94: 361-366.
4. Dartevelle PG, Chapelier AR, Pastorino U, et al. Long-term follow-up after prosthetic replacement of the superior vena cava combined with resection of mediastinal pulmonary malignant tumors. *J Thorac Cardiovasc Surg* 1991; 102: 259-265.
5. Thomas P, Magnan PE, Moulin G, et al. Extended operation for lung cancer invading the superior vena cava. *Eur J Cardiothorac Surg* 1994; 8: 177-182.
6. Doty DB, Baker WH. Bypass of superior vena cava with spiral vein graft. *Ann Thorac Surg* 1976; 22: 490-493.
7. Doty DB, Doty JR, Jones KW. Bypass of superior vena cava. Fifteen years' experience with spiral vein graft for obstruction of superior vena cava caused by benign disease. *J Thorac Cardiovasc Surg* 1990; 99: 889-896.
8. Gloviczki P, Pairolero PC, Cherry KJ, Hallett JW Jr. Reconstruction of the vena cava and of its primary tributaries: A preliminary report. *J Vasc Surg* 1990; 11: 373-381.
9. Moore WM, Hollier LH, Pickett TK. Superior vena cava and central venous reconstruction. *Surgery* 1991; 110: 35-41.
10. Magnan PE, Thomas P, Giudicelli R, et al. Surgical reconstruction of the superior vena cava. *Cardiovasc Surg* 1994; 2: 598-604.
11. De Marie S, Hagenouw-Taal J, Schultze Kool LJ, et al. Suppurative thrombophlebitis of the superior vena cava. *Scand J Infect Dis* 1988; 21: 107-111.

11

Pulmonary Vessels

Pascal Thomas, Pierre Fuentes, Pascal Di Mauro

Direct access to the pulmonary vessels was first performed by Trendelenburg in 1907[1] for treatment of pulmonary embolism. Today direct access to the pulmonary vessels is done for a variety of indications, the most common being lung resection. Management of thoracic trauma, especially penetrating wounds of the thorax, requires familiarity with the dissection of the pulmonary vessels to achieve hemostasis and optimal preservation of lung parenchyma.

Anatomic Review

The pulmonary artery is 4-5 cm long and is in close contact with the ascending aorta. Under the aortic arch it divides into the right and left pulmonary arteries. The bifurcation into these two arteries is located against the anteroinferior wall of the left main stem bronchus and is covered by the fibrous pericardium that attaches it to the aortic arch.

The origin of the right pulmonary artery is covered by the aorta and fibrous pericardium except at its lower border which remains covered by serous pericardium and forms the transverse sinus. The vessel exits the pericardium behind the superior vena cava about 2 cm above the junction between the superior vena cava and the right atrium. After passing under the carina, the vessel runs under the medial border and then along the anterior side of the right main stem bronchus. In the lung pedicle the right pulmonary artery is positioned above the pulmonary veins. The superior pulmonary vein is located in front and its upper border partially covers the right pulmonary artery. At this level the first branch arises, i.e. the anterior trunk which is a large vessel ascending in front of the upper lobe bronchus. The right pulmonary artery, covered in front by the veins that form the upper component of the superior pulmonary vein, penetrates the small fissure at the root of the upper lobe bronchus and runs to the superolateral border of the intermediate bronchus. Herein a second branch is given off, i.e. the posterior ascending artery of the upper lobe or retrobronchial artery. Almost at the same point anteriorly is the origin of one or two middle lobar arteries along the lateral border of the middle lobe bronchus. The right pulmonary

From Vascular Surgical Approaches, edited by Alain Branchereau and Ramon Berguer. ©1999, Futura Publishing Co., Inc., Armonk, NY.

artery then penetrates into the large fissure and gives off a branch to the superior segment of the lower lobe and then divides into two main branches for the rest of the lower lobe.

After exiting the pericardium the left pulmonary artery ascends leftward leaving the superior pulmonary vein below and anteriorly. At its origin the upper border of the left pulmonary artery is connected to the lower border of the aortic arch by the ligamentum arteriosum. The subaortic loop of the left recurrent nerve is located lateral to the arterial ligament and is in contact with the upper border of the left pulmonary artery. The artery crosses the upper and lateral wall of the left main stem bronchus and gives off one or two anterior branches to the apex. At the point where it wraps around the posterior aspect of the upper lobe bronchus, before the left pulmonary artery enters the large fissure, it gives off an apical branch. In the fissure there are two to three medial branches to the upper lobe and a lateral branch to the superior segment of the left lower lobe. The artery terminally bifurcates just distally to the lingular artery. The relationship between the segmental arteries of the lower and upper lobe is highly variable. The hilus of the lung projects at the level of the fifth intercostal space on the midaxillary line. A thoracotomy along the upper border of the sixth rib allows direct access to the pulmonary vessels.[2] Intubation should be performed with a double-lumen catheter to enable selective ventilation and exclusion of the lung on the operated side. This exclusion, which is necessary to avoid lung injury, should start as soon as the ribs are open and be maintained throughout the intrathoracic dissection.

Thoracotomy Techniques

Posterolateral Thoracotomy

A posterolateral thoracotomy is the *gold standard* technique allowing direct exposure of the hilus of the lung. The main drawback of this route is that it requires extensive muscle cutting. Various alternatives have been described to counter this problem.[3]

Patient Position

The patient is placed in the lateral decubitus resting on the contralateral side. A roll may be placed under the tip of the scapula. The ipsilateral arm is positioned on an arm rest that forms a 90 degree angle with the shoulder of the patient. The scapula is displaced above, forward, and upward out of the operating field after dividing the muscles. The pelvis is positioned perpendicular to the table by turning the patient's trunk slightly to the front. The contralateral lower extremity is flexed in order to stabilize the position of the body on the table. For further stability, supportive devices are also placed under the sacrum and sternum.

Skin Incision

In the back the incision begins midway between the angle of the scapula and the spinous processes. It continues parallel to and at 2 cm from the border of the scapula. At the bottom of the scapula the incision follows the ribs. The resulting incision is slightly S-shaped (Fig. 1).

Superficial Layer

The subcutaneous tissue is cut with cautery to expose the muscle layer at the back of the incision. The muscle layer consists of the trapezius and rhomboid posteriorly and latissimus dorsi and serratus anterior in the anterior two-thirds. The latissimus dorsi and the serratus anterior that lies underneath are divided with cautery, from back to front, taking care to coagulate any blood vessels that appear as the muscle fibers retract (Fig. 2). Posteriorly the trapezius and the underlying rhomboid muscles are also divided all in the line of the skin incision.

Opening of the Intercostal Space

The rib cage is explored behind the scapula by inserting the hand in the space between the serratus muscle and the thorax. The intercostal spaces are counted from the first rib, the neck of which can be felt slightly lateral to the

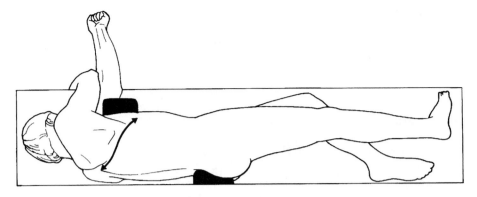

Figure 1. Posterolateral thoracotomy.

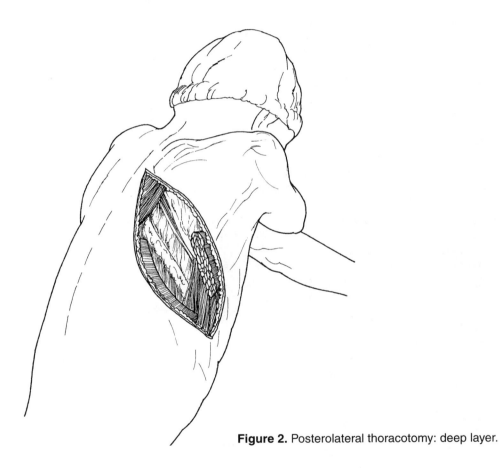

Figure 2. Posterolateral thoracotomy: deep layer.

spinous processes at the apex of the thorax. After discontinuing ventilation of the lung ipsilateral to the thoracotomy, the fifth intercostal space is opened up close to the upper border of the sixth rib using a cautery. Retraction of the lung can be assisted with a swab or small malleable retractor. A Tuffier-type spreader retractor is placed and opened moderately. Using this method the intercostal opening can be enlarged and the fifth space can be opened from the sympathetic chain in the back to the chondrocostal junction in the front. The Finochietto spreader is placed on the posterior axillary line with the ratchet in the front. The ribs should be spread slowly in order to avoid rib fracture. In the elderly, in order to avoid fracturing the ribs while spreading the wound edges, the fifth rib should be resected subperiosteally or divided posteriorly.

Lateral Thoracotomy

The main advantage of a lateral thoracotomy is to allow adequate exposure of the root of the lung without cutting of the large muscles of the chest wall. Other advantages are less postoperative pain, better shoulder movement, and improved function of the rib cage in the immediate postoperative period. However, a lateral thoracotomy is time-consuming, provides only limited access to the posterior mediastinum, and increases the risk of postoperative hematoma due to the need for extensive dissection.[4]

Patient Position

The position of the patient is exactly the same as that described in the previous section except that the torso is rotated more to the back. The trunk is thus twisted in the opposite direction from that used for posterolateral thoracotomy. The ipsilateral arm is raised suspended above the head. Excessive tension should not be applied to the upper extremity to avoid stretching the brachial plexus.

Skin Incision

The fifth intercostal space is located by counting the ribs from the bottom to the top.

Reference landmarks are the seventh rib, which is the first not connected directly to the sternum, or the tenth rib which is immediately above the floating ribs. The skin incision follows the outline of the sixth rib beginning in the back two fingerbreadths below the tip of the scapula and passes under the outline of the latissimus dorsi muscle. In men the incision ends below the nipple. In women the end of the incision is in the crease under the breast (Fig. 3).

Superficial Layer

The subcutaneous layer is divided with cautery. The dissection frees extensively the anterior border of the latissimus dorsi muscle preserving the periaponeurotic areolar tissue. The posterior aspect of the latissimus dorsi muscle is then separated from the serratus. In the back this dissection should be sufficient to allow ample retraction of the muscle later on. Prior to closure it is important to place drains in the dissected muscles to avoid postoperative hematomas.

Deep Layer

The latissimus dorsi muscle is retracted backward using a short retractor. The neurovascular pedicle of the serratus anterior muscle can then be fully exposed. The serratus muscle is divided from front to back following the direction of its digitations on the fifth and sixth ribs and stopping in front of its motor nerve. The space between the serratus muscle and the thorax is opened along the whole posterior

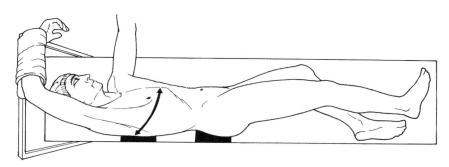

Figure 3. Lateral thoracotomy.

aspect of the muscle using a finger. A long retractor placed in the space and resting on the edge of the rib and scapula can be used to fully expose the ribs.

Opening of the Intercostal Space

The lung on the side of the thoracotomy is excluded from ventilation. The fifth intercostal space is opened along the upper border of the sixth rib using cautery. In front the residual insertions of the anterior serratus muscle must be detached. A Tuffier retractor is placed and opened gently. As in the posterolateral thoracotomy, this technique allows enlargement of the intercostal incision towards the back and to the front by extending the incision as the rib retractor is gradually opened.

Exposure of Vessels

Extrapericardial Approach

The dissection begins with complete mobilization of the lung followed by division of the inferior pulmonary ligament that attaches the inferior lobe to the esophagus and diaphragm. The mediastinal pleura is then incised circumferentially around the hilus. The vessels are located within the areolar lymphatic tissue the thickness of which varies according to the patient's body fat. The vessels can be exposed using a swab to push back the parenchymal margins of the hilum.

Right Side

The vessels are exposed on the anterior aspect of the hilum. The superior pulmonary vein is the element closest to the surface (Fig. 4). It covers the posterior ascending artery, an inferior branch of the right pulmonary artery. Above the pulmonary vein is the anterior trunk, the first branch of the right pulmonary artery, concealed by areolar and lymphatic tissue. The inferior pulmonary vein, the lowest component of the pedicle, can be

easily isolated from the posterior aspect after division of the inferior pulmonary triangular ligament. The right pulmonary artery is located behind the superior vena cava. It is important to expose the subadventitial layers of this artery by liberating gradually its inferior, anterior, and superior walls. Extra-adventitial exposure is hazardous because of the risk of injuring this low-pressure vessel which is particularly fragile. Passage of the angle-clamp behind the artery must not be done blindly and should be preceded by encircling the artery with the index and thumb. If the bifurcation is located close to the hilus it is possible that the anterior trunk of the right pulmonary artery will need to be exposed separately. In this case a tape should be placed around the superior pulmonary vein to pull it down in order to expose the occasionally present second anterior branch and the posterior ascending branch. The dissection of the vein should be carried out from the top to the bottom to minimize the risk of injuring the artery.

Left Side

The vessels are exposed in the upper part of the pulmonary pedicle (Fig. 5). The left pulmonary artery is located above the superior pulmonary vein in front. The main stem bronchus is found further back covered by the subaortic lymph nodes of the recurrent chain (Fig. 6). The surgeon must not pull excessively on the lung to avoid injury to the apical branches, the posterior apical and the anterior arteries that are short and broad. Isolation of the pulmonary veins is usually easy.

Intrapericardial Approach

The pericardium is opened along its full vertical length behind and parallel to the phrenic nerve. The incision is best made from the bottom up. Using a scalpel, a small slit is first made in the pericardium which is held with small-jawed forceps. The opening is then enlarged sufficiently to insert the fingers so that the pericardium can be separated from the heart surface. The pericardium is then opened up to its reflection line on the pulmonary artery.

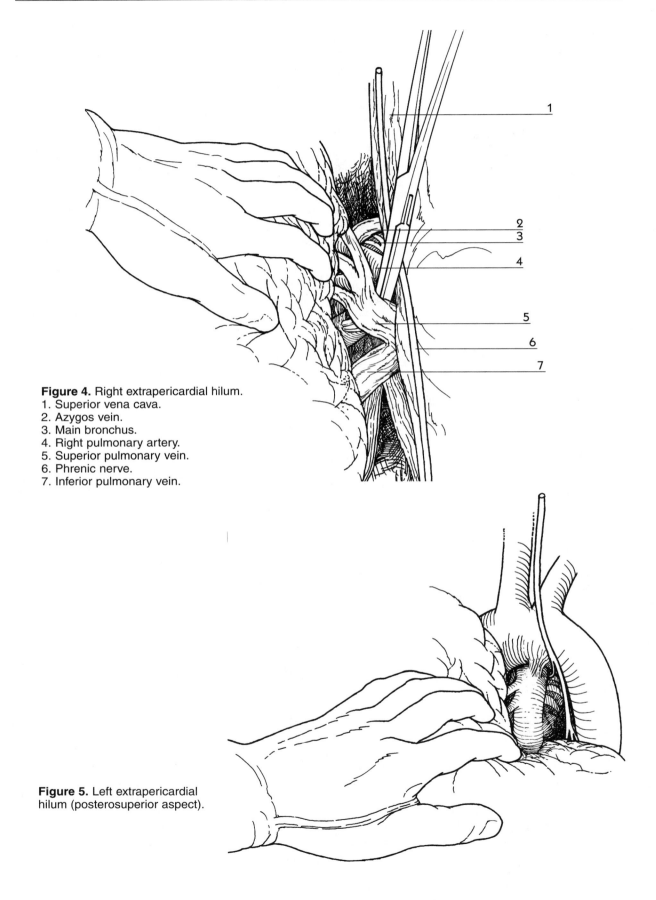

Figure 4. Right extrapericardial hilum.
1. Superior vena cava.
2. Azygos vein.
3. Main bronchus.
4. Right pulmonary artery.
5. Superior pulmonary vein.
6. Phrenic nerve.
7. Inferior pulmonary vein.

Figure 5. Left extrapericardial hilum (posterosuperior aspect).

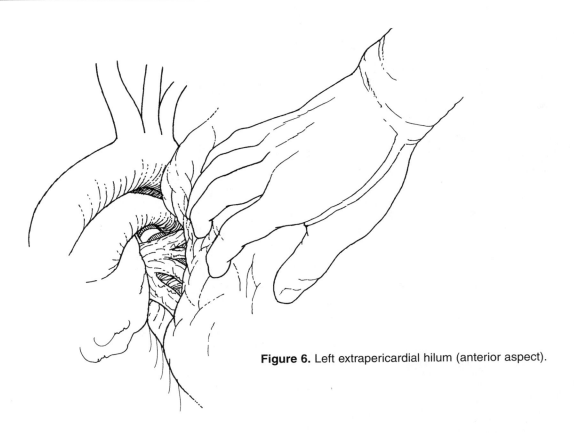

Figure 6. Left extrapericardial hilum (anterior aspect).

Right Side

After collapsing the posterior leaf of the pericardial reflection, it is possible to locate both pulmonary veins either separately or at their junction. In some cases it may be necessary to mobilize the right infundibulum of the left atrial appendage. The epicardial layer should be incised in the groove that runs behind the junction of the superior vena cava with the right atrium and then continues down to the inferior vena cava. Further dissection in this groove (Söndergaard procedure) (Fig. 7) should be performed carefully using a swab. The inferior wall of the right pulmonary artery is exposed above the superior pulmonary vein and behind the superior vena cava (Fig. 8). Prior mobilization of the superior vena cava using a tape may facilitate this dissection. The artery can also be exposed in the transverse sinus between the superior vena cava and ascending aorta (Fig. 9). Encircling and retracting the superior vena cava with a tape is indispensable to expose the artery. After incision of the overlying pericardium, the anterior and inferior walls of the artery are dissected. The main problem is the dissection of the posterior side of the artery since repair of a tear in this location requires cardiopulmonary bypass. Using a blunt dissector the posterior wall of the artery is progressively detached from the pericardium starting at the bottom and working up to the upper margin of the artery. The left index finger is used to guide the dissecting instrument. If any difficulty is encountered, the arch of the azygos vein can be divided to allow ample forward retraction of the superior vena cava and access to the upper part of the transverse sinus. This technique allows safer exposure of the superior wall of the pulmonary artery.

Left Side

Dissection of the pulmonary veins is not difficult unless the intrapericardial segment of

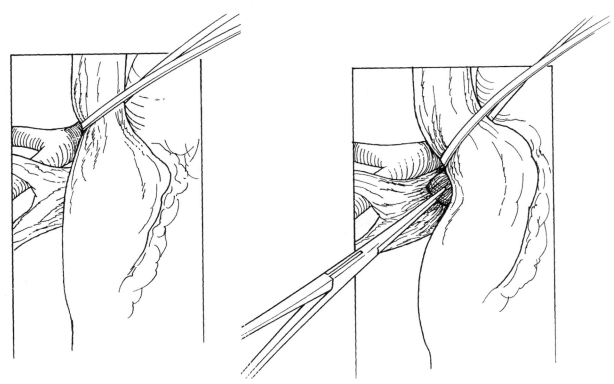

Figure 7. Söndergaard maneuver.

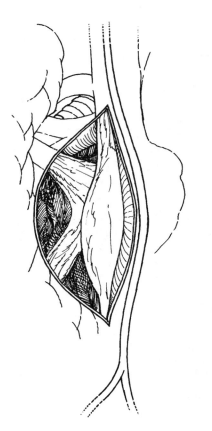

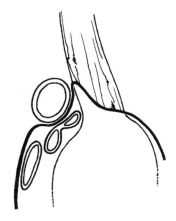

Figure 8. Anterior view of the right intrapericardial hilum. The drawing on the right shows a parasagittal section immediately behind the superior vena cava. It shows the position of the intrapericardial veins and the groove of the pulmonary artery on the posterior membrane of the pericardium.

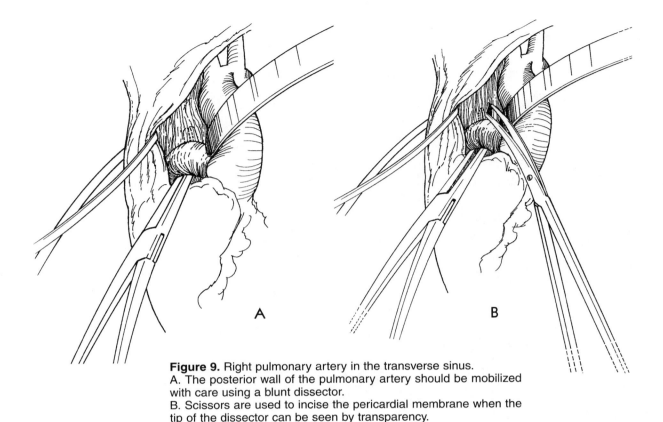

Figure 9. Right pulmonary artery in the transverse sinus.
A. The posterior wall of the pulmonary artery should be mobilized with care using a blunt dissector.
B. Scissors are used to incise the pericardial membrane when the tip of the dissector can be seen by transparency.

the inferior pulmonary vein is short (Fig. 10). The left pulmonary artery can be isolated medial or lateral to the arterial ligament. For isolation medial to the ligament, the incision should be made parallel to the artery along the pericardium attached to its anterior wall. The artery is mobilized from the top down using a blunt dissector placed between the superior pulmonary vein and artery. Extending control of the artery more proximally requires section of the arterial ligament between two ligatures after identifying the recurrent nerve as it loops under the aorta. Section of the arterial ligament allows good exposure of the origin of the left pulmonary artery and of the main pulmonary artery. The roof of the pericardium is incised parallel to the artery and the dissector is inserted above and behind the artery staying in contact with the main stem bronchus which serves as the buttress point. The emergence of the tip of the dissector below the lower margin of the artery is controlled by palpation using the left index finger.

Intrafissural Approach

The difficulty with exposure of the pulmonary artery in the fissure is different in both sides. On the left there is only one fissure, i.e. the oblique fissure or large fissure, in which the entire pulmonary artery can be exposed. On the right there is also the horizontal or small fissure in which the pulmonary artery (intermediary vessel) is covered by vessels ensuring venous run-off from the posterior segment of the right upper lobe. Complete exposure of the right pulmonary artery can only be achieved after division of the upper lobe venous drainage. The difficulty of fissural mobilization depends on how complete the fissure is, and there can be considerable variation. The large fissure can be a mere superficial groove and the small fissure is rarely complete. On the right, exposure of the pulmonary artery in the fissure begins with careful exposure of the artery at the site where the oblique fissure meets the horizontal fissure.

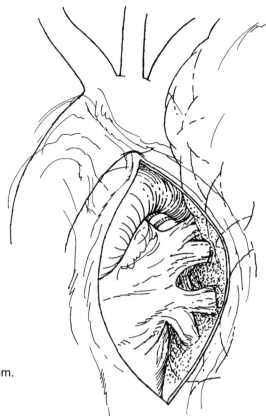

Figure 10. Left intrapericardial hilum.

On the left, we start by visualizing the pulmonary artery below the arch of the aorta and dissecting towards the fissure and dividing the tissue from the visualized artery to the periphery of the lung.

Right Side

After the initial approach the oblique and horizontal fissures are opened. It is often necessary to resect a group of lymph nodes in order to expose the pulmonary artery. One or two segmental branches supplying the middle are encountered anteriorly. One or occasionally two branches supply the superior segment of the lower lobe commencing opposite the middle lobe artery. Dissecting the artery distally it terminates in three or four segmental arteries supplying the rest of the lower lobe (Fig. 11). The superior segmental artery has to be ligated separately when resecting the right lower lobe.

Left Side

As mentioned above, the left pulmonary artery is visualized below the arch of the aorta and dissected towards the fissure and the fissure is dissected from the visualized artery towards the periphery. The segmental branches of the lobes are dissected while making headway in dissecting the main left pulmonary artery (Fig. 12). Occasionally the dissection is easier retrograde if the fissure is developed and the artery is seen between the lingula and the lower lobe. The anterior trunk to the upper lobe is dissected last. It is the most difficult one for obtaining length. Retracting the apical venous branch of the superior pulmonary vein helps in the exposure.

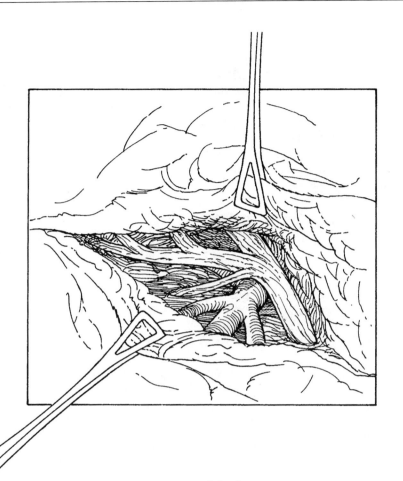

Figure 11. Right pulmonary artery in the fissure.

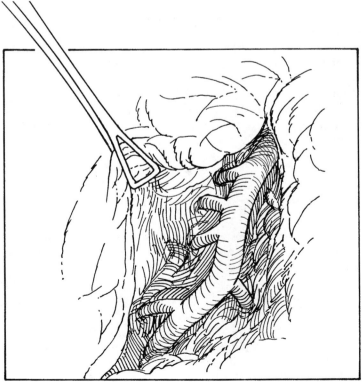

Figure 12. Left pulmonary artery in the fissure.

Median Approaches

Complete Median Sternotomy

This is the method of choice for exposure of the pulmonary artery and bifurcation.[5] However, it does not allow easy access to the intrapericardial pulmonary veins which are covered by the heart particularly on the left side. The advantage of a complete median sternotomy is that extracorporeal circulation can be set up easily if necessary.

Patient Position

The patient is placed in supine decubitus with the arms alongside the body and a roll under the scapula to facilitate spreading of the sternum.

Incision

The incision begins at the upper border of the manubrium and is carried down to 2 cm below the xiphoid. The subcutaneous areolar tissue, periosteum layer and sometimes the insertion fibers of the pectoralis major muscle that reach the midline are incised using cautery. Below, the linea alba is incised to free the posterior surface of the xiphoid from the peritoneum. Above, the transverse interclavicular ligament is divided at the upper border of the manubrium. Using the finger, it is then possible to expose the posterior side of the sternum by pushing the pleura back laterally away from the median line.

Section of the Sternum

The midline of the sternum is marked with cautery. Opening the sternum is performed using an alternating saw from the top down following the marks. Ventilation is halted for the time the saw is used so as not to open the mediastinal pleura if this is not needed for the operation. Use of a small Tuffier sternal retractor allows spreading of the sternal edges. At the top of the incision, section of the remaining elements of the interclavicular

ligament and of the sternothyroid muscles allows maximal exposure. For the same reason the lower part of the incision and the anterior sternal insertions of the diaphragm should be detached. After hemostasis of the margins of the sternum, the latter is spread using a large ratchet retractor. The spreading should be cautious to avoid tearing the left innominate vein.

Opening of the Pericardium

Fat and residual thymus tissue is removed from the anterior side of the pericardial sac. Dissection is performed from the bottom up and continued to the left innominate vein which is exposed on the anterior side after ligating off one of the two thymic veins. The pericardial sac is grasped in the median line using small jaw forceps and tented up before making a slit in it. This incision is then completed up to the reflection line on the ascending aorta and down to the diaphragm. On the left side, dissection of the aorta at the level of the pulmonary artery facilitates exposure. The borders of the pericardium are suspended using suture threads and forceps attached to the drapes on both sides.

Transverse Bithoracotomy

This approach is routinely used for double lung and heart-lung transplantation.[6] It allows simultaneous exposure of the mediastinum and both pleural cavities. The pulmonary vessels can be controlled not only at the origin in the pericardium but also laterally as via conventional thoracotomy. Using this approach, extracorporeal circulation can be set up without difficulty.

Patient Position

The patient is placed in supine decubitus position with the arms attached to the operating table above the head. A roll is placed transversally under the shoulders in order to raise the thorax. A support is placed laterally on each side of the hips and the lower extremities are secured to the operating table.

In this way the table can be tilted to one side or the other to obtain exposure comparable to that obtained by lateral thoracotomy.

Skin Incision

Since bithoracotomy provides anterior access to the thorax, it is preferable to approach the two pleural cavities in the fourth intercostal space. The fourth space is located by counting the ribs from the bottom up. The skin incision follows the outline of the fifth rib on both sides. It begins behind the posterior axillary line covering the bulge of the latissimus dorsi muscle. In front the two incisions join horizontally on the midline of the sternum (Fig. 13).

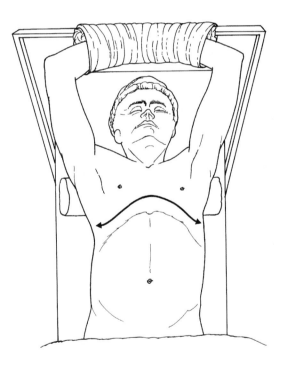

Figure 13. Bithoracotomy.

Opening of the Thorax

The steps to open the thorax are the same as those described for the lateral thoracotomy.

The internal mammary arterial pedicles on the anterior part of the thoracic incisions must be divided between ligatures before transverse division of the sternum. Once the sternum has been sawed across, the assistant raises the upper part of the thorax while exposing the deep side of the sternum, taking care to avoid injuring the phrenic nerves which are located at the top of the incision. A ratchet retractor is inserted on either side with the ratchet to the outside. The pericardium is opened using the same technique as described for sternotomy.

Exposure of the Pulmonary Vessels

Exposure of the pulmonary artery can be improved by passing a tape in the transverse sinus underlying both the posterior side of the aorta and pulmonary artery. The left branch of the tape is grasped using a dissector introduced from the left side behind the aorta. This tape is used to control the pulmonary artery without the need to dissect and expose it with its attendant risk of injury. On the right, the two branches can be controlled separately in the transverse sinus between the superior vena cava and the ascending thoracic aorta. On the left, they can be controlled on the inner side of the ligament arteriosum. Isolation of the pulmonary veins is difficult by sternotomy, particularly on the left side, since it requires handling of the heart and this can have adverse consequences unless performed under cardiopulmonary bypass. Conversely, bithoracotomy and alternative tilting of the operating table allow performance of any of the procedures described by thoracotomy in both sides.

Discussion

The choice of approach depends on the procedure that is to be performed as well as the location of the vessel involved. The indications for lateral and posterolateral thoracotomy are the same. However, exposure of pulmonary vessels on the right is easier by lateral thoracotomy since they can be exposed on the anterior surface of the hilum. On the left a posterolateral thoracotomy offers more direct access to the posterosuperior part of the hilum where one encounters the main difficulties for dissection of the pulmonary artery. These details are of practical importance only for surgical treatment of cancer. Problems related to isolation of pulmonary vessels are mainly due to their fragility. In this regard the necessity for subadvential dissection of the pulmonary artery and its branches should be emphasized (Fig. 14). For arterial clamping it is better to use a Rummel-type device than a conventional clamp. Penetrating wounds are better treated via a posterolateral thoracotomy which is quicker to perform and offers wider exposure. This approach allows access by the same incision to several intercostal spaces (from the third to the seventh). Clamping of the hilus is not advisable due to the risk of injuring the artery against the hard surface of the main stem bronchus. It is preferable to control

bleeding with the finger and to expose the vessels inside the pericardium. Control of bleeding from a lesion of the pulmonary artery in the fissure is also hardly feasible without controlling the hilus. Using these guidelines it is possible to minimize the amount of lung tissue resected.

Sternotomy is the approach of choice for exposure of the pulmonary artery and the proximal part of its branches for surgical treatment of acute pulmonary embolism with or without circulatory assistance. Although rarely indicated, retrograde embolectomy can be performed by the left thoracic route.[7] The left pulmonary artery is controlled intrapericardially, medial to the ligamentum arteriosum. The arteriotomy is performed astride the origin of a large lobar artery and of the pulmonary

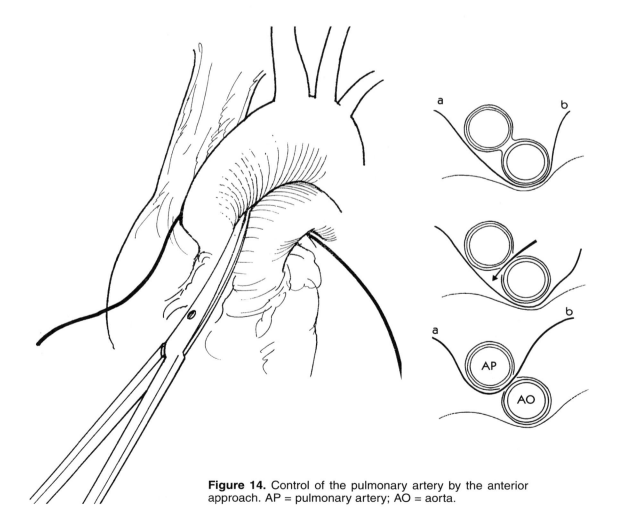

Figure 14. Control of the pulmonary artery by the anterior approach. AP = pulmonary artery; AO = aorta.

artery itself. The embolectomy is done in two steps. After proximal clamping of the artery to limit blood loss, disobstruction of the distal left pulmonary artery is performed first. The pulmonary artery and its right branch are then explored in retrograde fashion.

Surgery of the aorta by the left thoracic approach may require circulatory assistance. Despite recent technical advances, canulation of the femoral vein often leads to poor venous return and insufficient flow rate. Left heart bypass can be set up by canulating the left atrial appendage through its posterior wall at the level of the junction of the inferior pulmonary vein. This method of canulation is not completely risk free since tears of the left atrial appendage are difficult to repair using this approach. Undoubtedly, the safest solution is right-to-left bypass canulating the pulmonary artery.[8] This method is performed either by a direct intrapericardial approach to the main pulmonary artery or via the left pulmonary artery. The direct intrapericardial approach requires enlarging the exposure by extending the thoracotomy up to the sternum anteriorly. The transverse bithoracotomy approach should be used only for double- or single-lung transplantation. This technique allows placement of circulatory assistance at any point and doing the anastomosis required for transplantation.[9] Vascular complications involving anastomoses are not uncommon and may have serious consequences since they can lead to bronchial complications and jeopardize the immediate and long-term outcome of transplantation. This type of complication can occur on the pulmonary artery as well as veins. While stenosis can result from poor construc-

tion of the anastomosis, the most frequent cause is excessive length of the native pulmonary artery or of the left atrial patch and both may require reoperation.

References

1. Trendelenburg F. Zur Operation der Embolie der Lungarterie. *Deutsch Med Wschr* 1908; 34: 1173.
2. Griffith BP, Magee MJ, Gonzalez IF, et al. Anastomotic pitfalls in lung transplantation. *J Thorac Cardiovasc Surg* 1994; 107: 743-754.
3. Noirclerc M, Chauvin G, Fuentes P, et al. Les thoracotomies. *Encycl Méd Chir Paris,* Techniques chirurgicales, Thorax, 42205, 4.5.11, 16 p.
4. Massard G, Wihlm JM, Lion R, et al. Thoracotomie postérolatérale avec conservation partielle du muscle grand dorsal. Possibilités de myoplastie immédiate ou différée. *Encycl Méd Chir Paris, Techniques chirurgicales,* Thorax, F.r. 42205, 1991, 3 p.
5. Hazelrigg SR, Landreneau RJ, Boley TM, et al. The effect of muscle-sparing versus standard posterolateral thoracotomy on pulmonary function, muscle strength and postoperative pain. *J Thorac Cardiovasc Surg* 1991; 101: 394-401.
6. Tran Viet T, Grunenwald D, Neveux JY. Sternotomies verticales et horizontales. *Encycl Méd Chir Paris,* Techniques chirurgicales, Thorax, 42210, 4.11.03, 12 p.
7. Pasque MK, Cooper JD, Kaiser LR, et al. Improved technique for bilateral lung transplantation: Rationale and initial clinical experience. *Ann Thorac Surg* 1990; 49: 785-791.
8. Grunenwald D, Tran Viet T, Neveux JY. Traitement chirurgical de l'embolie pulmonaire aiguë. *Encycl Méd Chir Paris,* Techniques chirurgicales, Thorax, 42745, 11-1987, 14 p.
9. Bouchard F, Bessou JP, Tabley A, et al. Ruptures traumatiques isthmiques de l'aorte au stade aigu: Réévaluation du traitement chirurgical. *Ann Chir Thor Cardiovasc* 1992; 46: 116-124.

12

Supraaortic Trunks

Ramon Berguer

Reconstruction of the supraaortic trunks comprises 6% of the extracranial operations performed by our group. The most common etiology for the lesions found in these patients is atherosclerosis. Takayasu's disease, traumatic injury, and traumatic dissection are rare. In a patient with symptomatic and severe lesions of the supraaortic trunks, the first question is whether it should be reconstructed by a direct transthoracic operation or via a cervical approach. In some patients, especially those with an embolizing innominate artery lesion, the best choice is a transthoracic approach. In those patients who have symptomatic and severe lesions of either common carotid (CCA) or subclavian (SA) arteries, the best choice is a cervical operation which is less morbid than the transthoracic approach and has an excellent long-term patency rate. The transthoracic approach is often needed in patients with atherosclerotic involvement of all branches of the aortic arch because of the lack of an appropriate donor vessel upon which to base the reconstruction. In this chapter we will review the surgical access for transthoracic and cervical reconstructions of the supraaortic trunks.

Anatomic Review

The aortic arch gives off three branches to supply the head and the upper extremities. The most common anatomic distribution is an innominate artery supplying the right CCA and the right SA, a left CCA and a left SA. A common anatomic variation is an ostium shared in part by the left CCA and innominate arteries that occurs in 16% of the patients. In 8% of the patients the left CCA and innominate arteries arise from a common trunk and the left SA is the only other branch of the arch. A shared origin or a common trunk presents specific problems for the technique of endarterectomy. In 6% of the patients, the left vertebral arises directly from the arch between the left CCA and left SA. In 0.5% of the cases the right subclavian arises as the last branch of the arch at the beginning of the descending aorta and crosses the midline behind the esophagus before reaching the right supraclavicular area. This is called a retroesophageal right subclavian artery. Patients with this latter

From Vascular Surgical Approaches, edited by Alain Branchereau and Ramon Berguer. ©1999, Futura Publishing Co., Inc., Armonk, NY.

anomaly have a nonrecurrent inferior laryngeal nerve on the right side and their main thoracic duct empties in the right rather than the left subclavian vein. In addition, the right vertebral artery takes origin from the right CCA rather than from the retroesophageal subclavian.

The origin of the innominate artery and, rarely, the origin of the left CCA may be at the pericardial reflection line. Beyond its origin the innominate artery is immediately behind the innominate or brachiocephalic vein which crosses over the artery transversely. At this level the vein has one or two venous branches inferiorly that drain the thymus and usually a thyroid ima vein in its superior wall that drains the thyroid. The innominate artery bifurcates above the level of the brachiocephalic vein behind the head of the clavicle into the right CCA and right SA. The vagus nerve is situated lateral to the CCA and crosses over the first portion of the subclavian before sending a recurrent loop below the subclavian (the right recurrent laryngeal nerve) that ascends behind and medial to the origin of the right CCA. The right SA gives off the right vertebral artery at its first branch. At the point where it gives off the vertebral artery, the right SA is crossed by the right vertebral vein that empties into the right subclavian vein after crossing the artery. The right internal mammary artery arises from the inferior border of the subclavian artery shortly after the vertebral artery take-off. The thyrocervical trunk arises further laterally from the superior wall of the SA.

The right CCA ascends in the neck behind the sternomastoid muscle partially covered by the internal jugular vein. The vagus nerve lies between it and the jugular vein in a posterior plane. Above its origin the left CCA is crossed by the prethyroid muscles: the sternothyroid and the sternohyoid muscles. The left CCA ascends in the left neck in a position identical to the right carotid. The carotid arteries bifurcate at the C3-C4 level into the internal and external carotid arteries.

The left SA is a posterior mediastinal structure, retropleural in location. It gives off the left vertebral artery as it ascends through the posterior mediastinum. The internal mammary artery originates in its inferior border slightly beyond the level of take-off of the left vertebral artery. The left vertebral artery is also covered by the left vertebral vein which crosses the artery before emptying into the left subclavian vein.

Transthoracic Approach

The patient is supine with the arms placed at the side of the body. Central venous lines on the left side of the neck are avoided in those patients in whom the left CCA or left SA are to be part of the reconstruction since the brachiocephalic vein may need to be divided to achieve adequate exposure. A small longitudinal roll is placed along the spine between the scapulae. The head rests on a doughnut roll. If the operation is going to be limited to the innominate and its branches, the head is slightly rotated to the left and fixed in this position. If both sides of the neck will need to be accessed a nasotracheal tube is used and is taped to the forehead so the neck can be moved by the anesthesiologist from one side to the other as required. The entire neck is prepped on one or both sides as needed. The anterior chest and upper third of the abdomen are included in the operative field.

Operation

The basic incision is midline from the suprasternal notch to beyond the xiphoid (Fig. 1). The incision has a small cervical (supraclavicular) extension for access to the proximal right SA and CCA. The cervical extension may also be made following the general line of a carotid incision anterior to the sternomastoid, if the distal CCA and the carotid bifurcation components are to be part of the distal anastomosis of the graft. If both the innominate artery and the right carotid bifurcation need to be repaired, the latter is generally exposed through a separate incision. In these cases we prefer a separate incision for the carotid and we do the sternotomy with a small supraclavicular component to have access to the proximal portion of the branches of the innominate. Whichever of the two cranial extensions is used, the sternomastoid muscle is retracted laterally. The interjugular anastomotic vein is divided between ligatures and the prethyroid muscles are cut. When the carotid cranial extension is used, the dissection of the carotid sheath and carotid bifurcation is the same as when doing a carotid endarterectomy (as described in Chapter 1).

Over the sternum the incision is midline. Once the subcutaneous tissue is divided the periostium is incised along the midline which is determined by palpating the anterior border of the intercostal spaces. The incision is outlined with cautery to decrease bleeding from the sternal periostium. The supraclavicular notch is entered and an oscillating saw is used to open the sternum of its entire length.

At the top of the incision, the interclavicular ligament is divided. Both halves of the sternum are alternatively lifted so that their anterior and posterior periostial cover can be cauterized. Field towels are placed over sternal edges and a sternal retractor is inserted and partially opened. The opening of the sternum is done gradually to avoid bone or ligamentous injury to the costovertebral junctions posteriorly. The thymus is split along its midline using cautery and a few bridging vessels are cauterized (Fig. 2). The inferior thymic vein is divided between ligatures near its origin from the brachiocephalic vein. The latter is isolated and slung with a small rubber drain to be retracted first cranially and then distally as the innominate artery is dissected (Fig. 3). An additional length of brachiocephalic vein is freed on both sides to decrease the tension on it when the sternal retractor is further opened later on. The retractor is further opened a few notches at this point. The pericardium is tented up and opened. It is opened from the ventricular surface to its reflection line, usually below the origin of the innominate artery. The

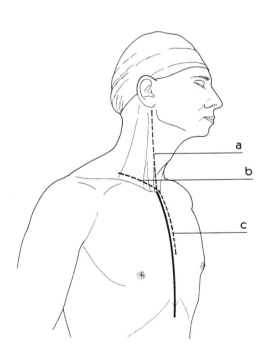

Figure 1. Different incisions for approaching the supraaortic trunks through a transternal route. (a) Cervical extension along the internal edge of the sternomastoid muscle. (b) Short supraclavicular extension. (c) Hemisternotomy.

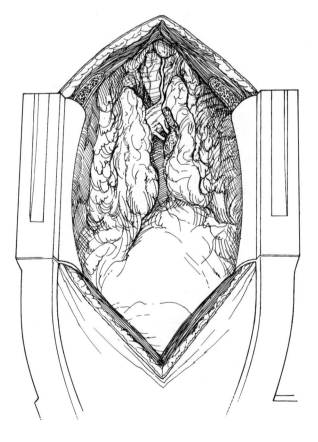

Figure 2. View of the anterior mediastinum after midsternotomy. The two lobes of the thymus have been separated and the thymic veins draining into the inferior wall of the brachiocephalic venous trunk are seen.

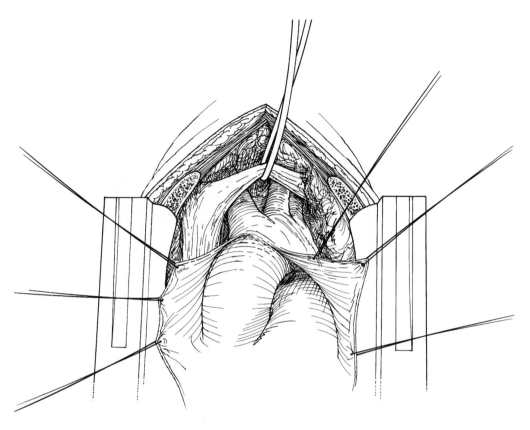

Figure 3. The brachiocephalic venous trunk is mobilized after ligature of the small veins that drain into it.

edges of the pericardium are held with stay sutures and placed under minimal tension on the frame of the retractor. Care should be taken not to put too much tension on the right-sided pericardial sutures since this can compromise venous inflow through the superior vena cava. The ascending aorta is exposed. Enough of its anterior and lateral walls are freed of visceral pericardium and fat for placement of the partial exclusion clamp later on. The dissection proceeds along the distal innominate artery retracting now the brachiocephalic vein caudally and exposing the origins of two branches of the former (Fig. 4). The right CCA dissection is pursued close to the vessel taking care not to injure the recurrent nerve that crosses obliquely the posterior aspect of the origin of the common carotid artery at some distance from it. The origin of the SA is dissected. The vagus nerve and its recurrent branch are identified and the artery is looped

close to its origin, bearing in mind the location of the recurrent nerve that should be visible at this point. Both the right CCA and the right SA are encircled with silastic loops.

The origin of the left CCA can be exposed through this incision by continuing the dissection on top of the aortic arch. Only the first two inches of left CCA are easily accessible. Any further cranial exposure requires division of the subhyoid muscles on the left side. The artery is slung with a loop that can serve as a gentle traction device for further dissection.

At this point any necessary dissection at the level of either carotid bifurcation is completed. This can be done as a continuation of the sternotomy or as a separate incision. If the limb of the graft is to go to a left carotid bifurcation, the graft will be tunneled under the prethyroid muscles on the left.

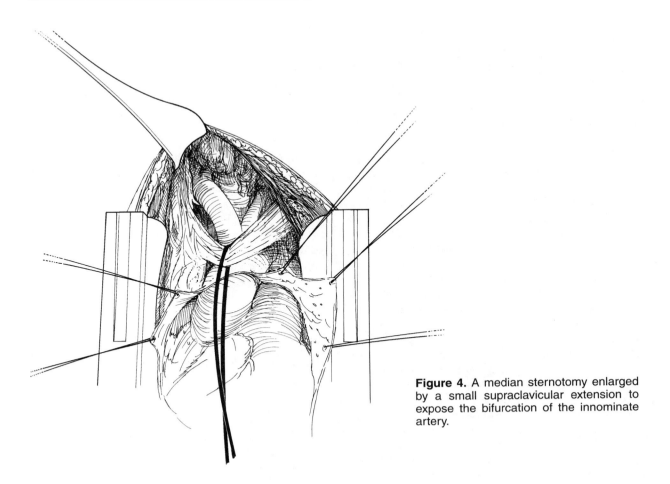

Figure 4. A median sternotomy enlarged by a small supraclavicular extension to expose the bifurcation of the innominate artery.

In preparation for its partial occlusion clamping, the aorta has been stripped of some of the visceral precardium that occasionally covers it with fat deposits. This is done in a small area that corresponds to the clamping site. The systolic pressure is then lowered to 100-110 mmHg so that the partial exclusion clamp will not be dislodged by the expanding pulsation of the ascending aorta. The construction or the bypass is end-to-side proximally and generally end-to-end distally but is not part of this description.

If access is needed to the left subclavian artery, which is a posterior mediastinal structure, the sternal borders need to be separated further and this cannot be accomplished safely without dividing the stretched out brachiocephalic vein. After dividing the vein we tag it with some heavy sutures in order to reconstruct it at the end of the procedure. We used to divide it without reconstructing it but we experienced a substantial incidence of left jugular and left subclavian vein thrombosis. When isolating the left subclavian artery care must be taken not to injure the left phrenic and left vagus nerves that cross in front of the subclavian as they enter the chest cavity. The subclavian artery is isolated in its first portion exposing the origin of the vertebral artery which in this projection is clearly visible to the operator.

Partial Midsternotomy (Fig. 1)

In cases where access is needed to the innominate artery alone for a direct endarterectomy, an upper midsternotomy provides a more economical and functional approach. We use this approach for lesions that occupy the distal half of the innominate artery and for those that will require clamping limited to the anterior wall of the ascending aorta. The advantage of the upper midsternotomy is that the lower half of the sternum remains intact providing chest stability and decreasing postoperative pain.

When the upper midsternotomy is used for distal innominate lesions there will be a need to isolate the origin of the innominate branches, the right SA, and the right CCA. The incision therefore starts with a short supraclavicular component which is then continued along the midline over the first three segments of the sternum. The preparation of the sternum is identical to that of the full midsternotomy except that it stops at the level between the third and fourth segments of the sternum. We use an alternating saw which is brought through the midline until the level of the third sternal segment at which point the cut is brought to the right margin of the sternum. The upper half of the sternum has now been divided and a small Tuffier retractor can be inserted and slowly opened to proceed with dissection of the upper mediastinum as was done for the full sternotomy. Preconclusion of the reconstruction, the sternum is closed using three loops of wire inserted in the same manner as for a full sternotomy. The anterior mediastinum is drained superiorly to the supraclavicular area.

Cervical Approach to Supraaortic Trunks

The approach to the proximal subclavian arteries has been described in Chapter 7 and the approach to the common carotid artery is part of the standard exposure for carotid endarterectomy (Chapter 1). In addition to the standard description provided in those chapters, the following remarks apply specifically to cervical reconstructions of the supraaortic trunks.

For a reconstruction based ipsilaterally, that is a carotid-subclavian bypass, a subclavian-carotid bypass, or a transposition of one of the above vessels into the other, the incision is supraclavicular. It is drawn out from the clavicular head to permit access to the subclavian and carotid arteries. Ipsilateral subclavian-carotid bypasses are done between the midcervical portion of the common carotid artery and the retroscalene segment of the subclavian. Occasionally when exposing the SA and particularly in thin individuals, we prefer to divide the lateral half of the scalenus anticus and place the bypass in the segment of SA between the latter and the brachial plexus. This avoids the dissection of the entire prescalene fat pad and of the phrenic nerve.

In subclavian-carotid transpositions on either side, it is the first segment of the SA that must be isolated. On the right side this is an easier maneuver than on the left where the subclavian is deeper and more posterior. On the right side the isolation of the SA must avoid injury to the recurrent or vagus nerves; on the left side injury to the thoracic duct is to be avoided, ligating it when needed. Control of the proximal stump of the SA is obtained by clamping. Closure of the stump must be done in two layers sometimes using pledgeted sutures. The long end of the suture is not cut until the clamp is released and there is no evidence of any suture line bleeding under normotensive conditions.

Cervical reconstruction of the supraaortic trunks often requires going from one side of the neck to the other. To cross the neck we have advocated the use of the retropharyngeal tunnel (Fig. 5) as opposed to the pretracheal route which was traditionally used. This tunnel may be used to cross the midline with a graft between carotids or/and subclavian arteries on opposite sides of the neck. The plane for the retropharyngeal tunnel is defined first by palpating the transverse process of the cervical vertebrae and sliding the finger over the lamina prevertebralis as the finger feels the anterior lips of the vertebral bodies. The tunnel enters the space between the carotid anteriorly and the sympathetic chain posteriorly, slides over the lamina prevertebralis in the midline, and emerges at the same level on the opposite side. A bypass graft can be tended through this tunnel which is enlarged with two fingers so that there is no pressure on it.

In some patients in whom a transthoracic approach is not advisable and who have a

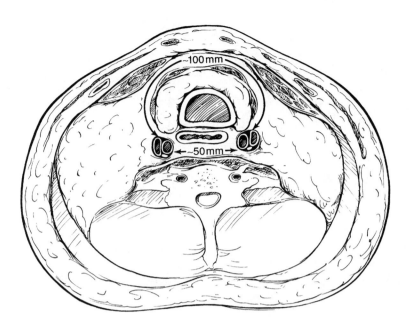

Figure 5. Pathway of the retropharyngeal tunnel.

lesion at the bifurcation of the innominate artery, this artery may be approached by a cervical incision by resecting the middle third of the clavicle. The resection of the middle third of the clavicle is necessary in most patients. In some anatomic circumstances in patients with long thin necks and with a high bifurcation of the innominate artery, one may gain control of the latter without resecting the clavicle.

In order to resect the middle third of the clavicle an incision is made with a cautery onto the periostium of the clavicle. Using cautery and a periostium elevator the clavicle is denuded of soft tissue from its middle third to the sternoclavicular junction which is entered. Laterally at the junction of the middle and inner thirds, the clavicle is encircled, hugging the bone closely to avoid injury of the underlying vein. A Gigli saw is used to divide the clavicle. The stump of the clavicle is held with a Kocher clamp and, using periostium elevators, the subclavian muscle and the remainder of the soft tissue is separated from the clavicular head. The latter is then removed from its sternoclavicular joint. This provides additional exposure in the upper mediastinum to dissect the distal most portion of the innominate artery and to obtain control of it. The medial claviculectomy results in a cosmetic deformity and occasionally in displacement and pain in the acromioclavicular joint.

13

Coronary Arteries

Xavier Barral, Jean-Pierre Favre, Jean-Paul Gournier

Expanded use of percutaneous coronary angioplasty has not reduced the number of coronary bypasses. Today bypass procedures are performed electively and the morbidity-mortality rate is only slightly higher than that of percutaneous revascularization. A number of technological advances have been made including better perioperative myocardial protection, refinement in microsurgical technique, better surveillance, and more sophisticated critical care. However, the first prerequisite for successful outcome of coronary bypass is mastery of the surgical technique. In this regard proper identification and exposure of the coronary arteries to be bypassed is of primary importance.

Anatomic Review

The two arteries supplying blood to the heart are named coronaries because they encircle the surface of the epicardium like a crown (corona in Latin). Both vessels arise from the ascending aorta slightly above the free margin of the semilunar valves at the level of the sinus of Valsalva.

Right Coronary Artery

The right coronary artery arises from the anterior side of the sinus of Valsalva about 1.5 cm above and inside the insertion of the semilunar aortic valve. It quickly describes a rightward curve toward the right atrium. In some cases the first branch of the right coronary, i.e. the infundibular artery which supplies the pulmonary infundibulum, originates from the aorta. The second branch supplying the right atrial appendix is for the sinoatrial nodal artery. At the level of the right atrium, the right coronary artery which is covered by fat and in rare cases may be concealed under a myocardial bridge, courses down the sulcus between the atrium and ventricle (Fig. 1). It gives off one or two marginal branches to the right ventricle. The longest marginal branch runs along the lower edge of the right ventricle. After reaching the diaphragmatic edge of the heart, the right coronary artery runs in the sulcus between the left atrium and ventricle to the crux cordis at

From Vascular Surgical Approaches, edited by Alain Branchereau and Ramon Berguer. ©1999, Futura Publishing Co., Inc., Armonk, NY.

the intersection of the interatrial and interventricular sulci (Fig. 2). At this point the artery generally divides into two terminal branches, one of which (the descending branch) courses along the posterior interventricular sulcus towards the tip of the heart and supplies blood to the septum and lower wall of the two ventricles, and the other (the transverse branch) gives off the diaphragmatic branches that supply the lateral wall of the left ventricle.

Left Coronary Artery

The left coronary artery arises from the anterolateral or left aortic sinus. It is a short artery about 5-25 mm in length that curves around the back side of the pulmonary artery then passes forward and leftward between the pulmonary artery and the left atrial appendage. At this point it divides into two branches: the anterior descending artery and the circumflex artery (Fig. 3).

Anterior Descending Artery

The anterior descending artery (ADA) courses in the anterior interventricular sulcus parallel to the great cardiac vein. In some cases it ends before reaching the apex and in others it continues into the posterior interventricular sulcus. The ADA gives off three types of branches. The largest branches are the diagonal arteries which supply the anterolateral wall of the left ventricle. There are two or three diagonal arteries (Figs. 1 and 3). The septal branches of the ADA are located more deeply and supply the anterior two thirds of the interventricular septum. The first and largest septal branch arises immediately below the origin of the ADA. The first septal branch divides into two or three fairly large branches and is an important anatomic landmark for the angiographic description of the ADA (Fig. 4).

Circumflex Artery

In contrast with the ADA, which is the continuation of the left coronary artery, the circumflex artery is a perpendicular branch arising in the fat tissue between the pulmonary artery and the left atrium. It runs in the sulcus between the left atrium and ventricle along the left border of the heart and ends on the diaphragmatic surface of the left ventricle (Fig. 2). It reaches the cross of the heart in only 10% of cases. The circumflex artery is in contact with the coronary sinus and this relationship greatly hinders surgical exposure. The number and size of the branches of the circumflex artery are inversely proportional to the development of the right coronary artery and its branches. When the right coronary artery is dominant, the circumflex artery is not highly developed. The circumflex artery vascularizes the left atrium and the lateral wall of the left ventricle.

The largest collateral branch of the circumflex artery is called the first or left marginal artery. It is the continuation of the circumflex artery located midway between the anterior and posterior borders of the left ventricle. There is frequently a second marginal artery parallel to the first (Fig. 3). When the right coronary artery is hypoplastic, the circumflex artery also gives off diaphragmatic or posterolateral branches to the lateral wall of the left ventricle.

In some cases a large descending artery is observed in the middle part of the lateral wall of the left ventricle arising in the angle formed by the origin of the ADA and the circumflex artery. This artery, which is called the bisecting artery or ramus intermedius, gives the appearance of a trifurcated left coronary artery. The bisecting artery can reach the apical region (Figs. 1 and 3).

Hemodynamically Significant Anomalies

Several congenital heart malformations give rise to hemodyamically significant anomalies of myocardial blood supply. These anomalies, which can become symptomatic even without embolic or inflammatory atherosclerotic lesions, can be divided into four main groups.[1]

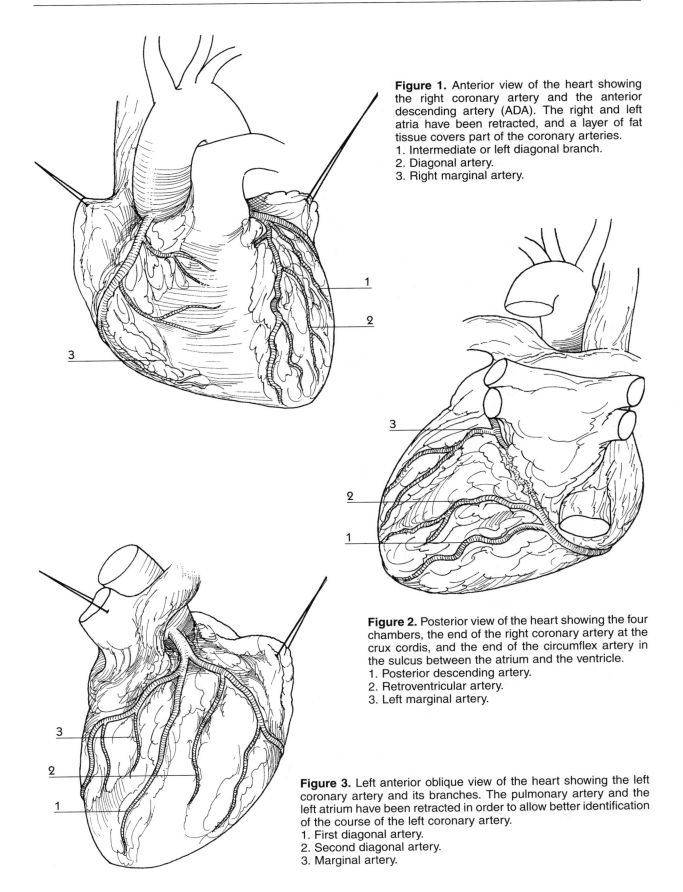

Figure 1. Anterior view of the heart showing the right coronary artery and the anterior descending artery (ADA). The right and left atria have been retracted, and a layer of fat tissue covers part of the coronary arteries.
1. Intermediate or left diagonal branch.
2. Diagonal artery.
3. Right marginal artery.

Figure 2. Posterior view of the heart showing the four chambers, the end of the right coronary artery at the crux cordis, and the end of the circumflex artery in the sulcus between the atrium and the ventricle.
1. Posterior descending artery.
2. Retroventricular artery.
3. Left marginal artery.

Figure 3. Left anterior oblique view of the heart showing the left coronary artery and its branches. The pulmonary artery and the left atrium have been retracted in order to allow better identification of the course of the left coronary artery.
1. First diagonal artery.
2. Second diagonal artery.
3. Marginal artery.

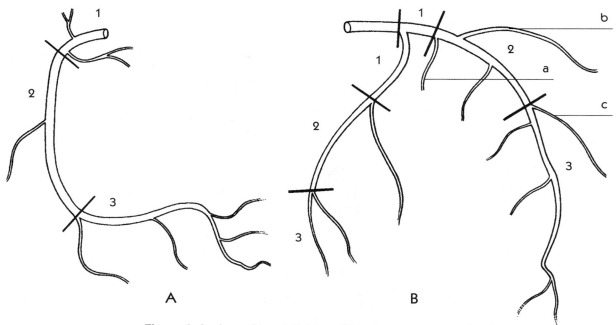

Figure 4. Angiographic subdivision of the coronary artery network.

A. Illustration of an anterior oblique view of the three segments of the right coronary artery:
1. From the origin to the superior genu.
2. From the superior genu to the inferior genu.
3. From the inferior genu to the cross of the heart.

B. Illustration of an anterior oblique view of the left coronary artery network with subdivisions of the ADA and circumflex arteries.

ADA
1. From the origin to the first septal artery.
2. From the first septal artery to the second diagonal artery.
3. From the second diagonal artery to its termination.

Circumflex Artery
1. From its origin to the first marginal artery.
2. From the first to the second marginal artery.
3. Distal to the second marginal artery.

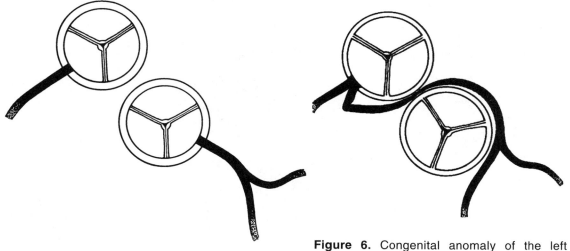

Figure 5. Left coronary artery arising from the pulmonary artery.

Figure 6. Congenital anomaly of the left coronary artery arising from the same orifice as the right coronary artery. Compression of the artery results in diminished flow.

Intracardiac Fistula and Arteriovenous Fistula

Fistulas can occur between a coronary artery and a heart chamber or between a coronary artery and the superior vena cava, pulmonary artery, or coronary sinus. Depending on the size of the orifice, fistulas can range from minimal to massive. Approximately 50% of patients with coronary fistulas develop cardiac failure. Ischemia can be compounded by arteriovenous steal, rupture, or bacterial contamination.

Abnormal Origin from the Pulmonary Artery

Abnormal origin of the coronary artery from the pulmonary artery is the second most common congenital anomaly of the coronary system. In most cases the left coronary artery is involved (Fig. 5) but involvement of the right coronary artery, the ADA, and even both coronary arteries has been observed. Coronary insufficiency usually develops in early childhood due to perfusion of the myocardium by hypoxic blood. Without treatment this anomaly generally leads to death within 2 years.

Coronary Atresia

Atresia of a coronary artery is an uncommon congenital anomaly. It can be an isolated or associated with other anomalies such as supravalvular aortic stenosis, homocystinuria, Friedrich's ataxia, or Hurler's syndrome.

Abnormal Origin of the Left Coronary Artery on the Right Sinus

Abnormal origin of the left coronary artery from the right sinus is an uncommon anomaly. The left coronary artery arises either from the same orifice as the right coronary artery or directly from the right coronary artery. In this case the artery runs obliquely backward between the pulmonary infundibulum and the aorta and then behind the pulmonary artery before assuming its normal course and dividing into the ADA and circumflex artery (Fig. 6). Flow rate in the proximal segment is reduced due to plication and compression of the left coronary artery between the aorta and pulmonary artery proximally. Sudden death after strenuous physical activity is observed in young adults.

Nonhemodynamically Significant Anatomic Variations

Unlike the previous four anomalies which have dramatic hemodynamic effects, several nonhemodynamically significant anatomic anomalies can be observed. These lesions can pose problems for catheterization and identification.

The origin of the coronary arteries can occur higher or more laterally near a commissure in the sinus of Valsalva. The left coronary artery may be absent with the ADA and circumflex arteries arising directly from the left sinus. The right coronary artery can arise from the left sinus, with the circumflex artery arising from the right coronary artery and winding around the right and back side of the aorta. The ADA can arise from the right sinus or from the right coronary artery. The most frequent variation is the presence of an isolated single coronary artery arising from the right or left sinus. Single coronary arteries can display several courses which Lipton classified into nine subgroups.[2] Other more uncommon variations include duplication of the ADA or of the posterior descending artery. Intramyocardial courses constitute a particularly interesting variation due to the presence of an intermuscular bridge of variable thickness and length over a segment of a coronary artery. Diagnosis can be achieved on the basis of cineangiocardiography showing narrowing of the vessel during systole and normal diameter during diastole. This variation is uncommon in arteries located in the sulcus between the atria and ventricles (right coronary artery and circumflex artery). In contrast, it is frequent in the first and second diagonal arteries and in the marginal arteries.

Interpreting Coronary Arteriographs

Unlike peripheral bypass procedures which can be undertaken without angiography, coronary bypass requires preoperative coronary angiography to determine the number of vessels to be bypassed and select the site of anastomoses. Ventriculography is also necessary to determine myocardial status and to ascertain the viability of the muscle in the zones to be revascularized. Several imaging angles are necessary to allow complete visualization of the right and left coronary arterial networks.[3]

The right coronary artery can be easily and reliably visualized using a 60 degree left anterior oblique angle and 30 degree right anterior oblique angle. Using these two angles, the three segments of the right coronary artery (Fig. 4) can be studied from the origin to the end of its division branches to determine the presence and degree of stenosis and the quality of collateral circulation. One of the few mistakes that can be made consists of pushing the catheter tip too far into the artery and overlooking a stenosis near its orifice.

The left coronary arterial network is more complicated and requires more imaging angles to accurately assess subdivisions, plications, and overlapping branches. In addition to the 30 degree and 60 degree left and right anterior oblique angles, lateral, craniocaudal, and caudocranial images are necessary to unfold the circumflex and proximal ADA. The right anterior oblique cranial angle is needed to eliminate any superimposition that may exist and to rule out possible overlapping between the circumflex and diagonal arteries, and the ADA. In practice, the relative value of each imaging angle varies from case to case depending on anatomic features. Branching of the left coronary network (Fig. 4B) is more difficult to interpret.

Standard Exposure Technique

Patient Position

The patient is placed in dorsal decubitus with a roll under the shoulders in order to extend the neck slightly. The arms are positioned at the side of the body. Pressure points should be protected to avoid postoperative neurologic deficits. The operative field should include the lower neck below central lines, puncture sites, the anterior thorax and abdomen, and both lower extremities. The thighs should be placed in external rotation with the knees slightly bent. This precaution is necessary to allow additional graft harvesting if necessary. The surgeon stands on the right side of the patient with the assistant(s) on the opposite side. The instrument nurse stands to the right of the surgeon. The table should be raised higher than for conventional vascular surgery to facilitate venous return to the extracorporeal circulation (ECC) system. Surgical drapes should be placed so that the anesthesiologist is able to access the patient's head and also monitor myocardial contraction.

Exposure of the Heart

The skin incision begins in the middle of the upper end of the manubrium and continues four fingerbreadths below the xiphoid process. After hemostasis of the subcutaneous tissue, a longitudinal sulcus is made in the sternum using an electric scalpel and then the sternum is opened using a sternotomy saw. Careful hemostasis of the internal and external table of the sternum is performed. Since the use of bone wax to stop bleeding from the spongy bone can lead to pseudarthrosis, we resort to this technique only in cases of massive bleeding. Residual thymic tissue below the innominate vein is removed between two ligatures. The right and left pleural cul-de-sacs are retracted. The pericardium is incised longitudinally from its aortic reflection line at the top down to the diaphragm at the bottom. The pericardium is suspended with sutures placed over the sternal retractor.

The ascending aorta and the heart should be inspected with minimal handling. Attention should be paid to detect parietal calcifications and to identify zones of myocardial dyskinesia and akinesia suggested by ventriculography. In general, only the right coronary arteries, ADA, and diagonal arteries can be inspected without risking a hypotensive reaction. Inspection of the circumflex and marginal arteries requires rotation of the heart and thus cannot be done until cardiopulmonary bypass (CPB) is initiated.

Before starting CPB the graft material is harvested. The internal mammary, radial or gastro-omental arteries or the saphenous vein can be used. After harvesting graft material CPB is initiated. It is only after starting CPB and immobilizing the heart that the coronary arteries are actually exposed. The anastomotic sites selected on the basis of coronary angiographic findings are confirmed by careful examination of the vessels to be bypassed. Operating loupes are especially useful for this purpose.

Right Coronary Artery

For surgical purposes the right coronary artery can be divided into three segments (Fig. 4A): the proximal segment from the origin to half the distance to the right border, the middle segment extending to the right border, and the distal segment which goes from the marginal branch to the origin of the posterior descending artery. In most cases the distal segment of the artery is exposed. Using a moist lap, the assistant raises the right ventricle upward and leftward (Fig. 7) thus bringing the lower border of the heart, which separates the anterior and diaphragmatic surfaces of the right ventricle, into the middle of the operating field. In this way the right coronary artery can be easily identified in the sulcus between the atrium and the ventricle. If the periventricular fat layer is thick, suture threads can be passed and used for traction to expose the coronary artery. The extent of dissection of the artery depends on the amount of calcification. In most cases a few centimeters is sufficient. Exposure of its branches is not necessary. However, in some cases dissection may be extended toward the terminal branches of the

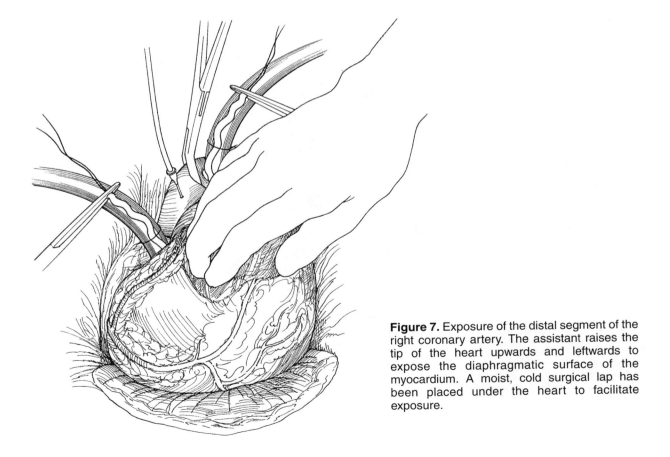

Figure 7. Exposure of the distal segment of the right coronary artery. The assistant raises the tip of the heart upwards and leftwards to expose the diaphragmatic surface of the myocardium. A moist, cold surgical lap has been placed under the heart to facilitate exposure.

right coronary artery on the posterior side of the heart. The first vessel that is encountered is the posterior descending artery. The retroventricular artery is located more posteriorly on the diaphragmatic side and exposure requires further rotation of the heart. To facilitate exposure, a damp compress can be placed under the heart so that the tip of the organ points toward the patient's shoulder.

Sometimes the coronary artery is exposed in the sulcus between the atrium and the ventricle immediately above the origin of the right marginal branch. The advantage of this approach is that it does not require rotation of the heart, but the disadvantage is that it can be hindered by the presence of fat tissue or a myocardial bridge (Fig. 8).

Circumflex Artery

Surgically, the circumflex artery is described as having two segments: the proximal segment from the origin to the first marginal artery and the distal segment which includes the terminal circumflex artery with the marginal arteries. Surgical treatment of the proximal segment is difficult due to the presence of the left atrium and the great cardiac vein. The bypass is usually anastomosed to the distal segment. Depending on the size of the heart and the depth of the artery in the organ, the surgeon may remain on the patient's right side or temporarily move to the left side. Tilting the operating table to the right is often useful to roll the heart over.

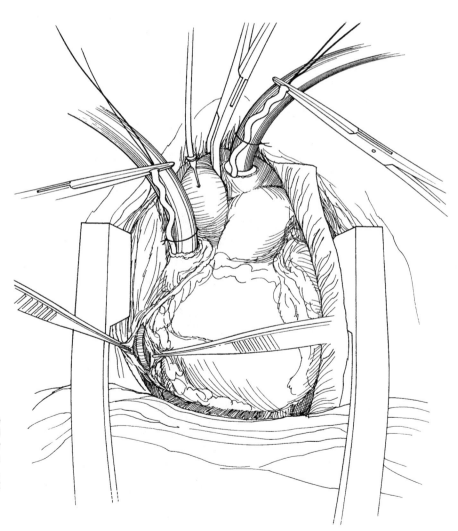

Figure 8. Exposure of the distal end of the second segment of the right coronary artery in the sulcus between the atrium and the ventricle. Rotation of the heart is not necessary for this exposure.

The heart is rotated upward and held by the assistant so that the tip points toward the apex of the lung (Fig. 9). One or two compresses soaked in ice-cold saline can be placed in the pericardial cavity to raise the heart and place the posterior surface of the left ventricle on a horizontal plane. Another refinement consists of using a gauze strip passed behind the superior vena cava towards the origin of the aorta. It is then attached using two Kocher forceps on the right border of the sternotomy. This allows the heart to be held in rotation with the raised tip pointing toward the top right side of the operative field. This maneuver frees up the assistant's hand who can then use a swab to flatten out the posterior convexity of the left ventricle and facilitate exposure of the marginal artery. Anastomoses to marginal arteries should be made as close to the origin as possible to obtain the largest possible lumen diameter. The optimal site for anastomosis is located by palpating the circumflex artery at its exit from the sulcus between the atrium and the ventricle just above the marginal branches. Careful incision of the epicardium enhances visualization of the arteries to assess the existing lesions. If a sequential bypass is to be performed, it is better to expose all the vessels to be bypassed and choose the optimal anastomotic sites before starting any revascularization.

Anterior Descending and Diagonal Arteries

Surgically, the ADA can be divided into three segments (Fig. 4B): the proximal segment

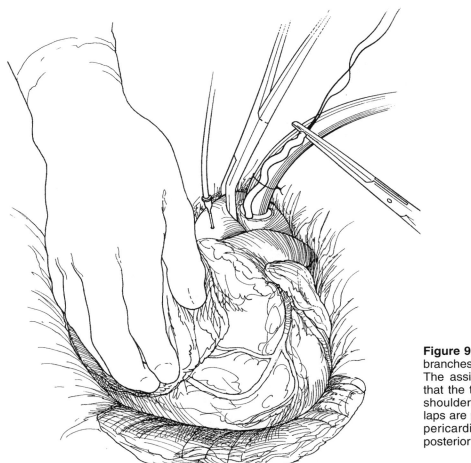

Figure 9. Exposure of the marginal branches of the circumflex artery. The assistant rotates the heart so that the tip points towards the right shoulder. Ice cold saline-soaked laps are placed in the bottom of the pericardial cavity to raise the posterior surface of the left ventricle.

running from its origin on the left coronary artery to the first septal artery slightly below the left atrium; the middle segment between the first septal artery and the second diagonal artery; and the distal segment which corresponds to the distal ADA beginning at the second diagonal artery and ending with the artery behind the apex. In most bypasses the anastomosis is performed to the second or third segments.

A compress soaked in ice-cold saline can be placed in the bottom of the pericardial cavity in order to raise the left ventricle. The ADA can be easily located running in the interventricular sulcus to the tip of the heart. It is superficial and easy to expose in the middle of the operating field. The middle segment of the vessel is usually exposed on either side of

the second diagonal artery. The artery is usually visible immediately under the epicardium and sometimes covered by a layer of fat tissue and criss-crossed by a few small veins. After palpation of the sulcus to locate the artery and careful incision of the epicardium, a few centimeters of the artery should be exposed (Fig. 10).

The same approach can be used for exposure of the diagonal arteries. The main axes of these vessels form an angle of about 45 degrees with the ADA. In most cases the diagonal arteries can be easily located on the anterolateral surface of the left ventricle. The first proximal diagonal artery is below the right side of the left atrium, 1 cm or 2 cm under the sulcus between the atrium and the ventricle. Pushing the ventricle down with a swab

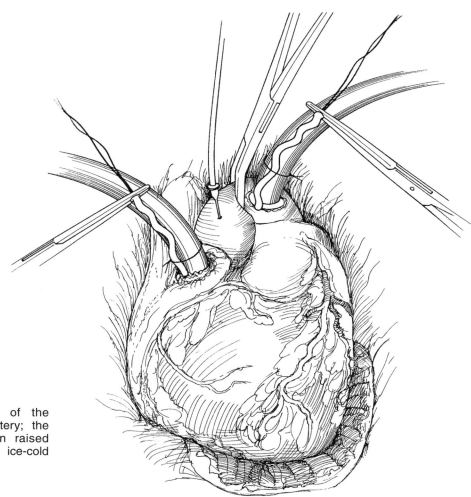

Figure 10. Exposure of the anterior descending artery; the left ventricle has been raised using a lap soaked in ice-cold saline.

flattens the convexity of the heart and facilitates exposure of the diagonal artery.

Left Coronary Artery

In some cases isolated noncalcified lesions of the left coronary can be treated by endarterectomy and venous angioplasty.[4] After opening and dissecting amply the aortopulmonary window, two techniques can be used to expose the left coronary artery. The anterior approach is achieved by incising the anterior surface of the aortic sinus. The incision should be performed in a leftward direction from the front and back to the orifice of the left coronary artery. The left coronary artery is then incised on the anterior side distal to the stenosis. Leftward retraction of the pulmonary artery allows exposure of a healthy zone of the left coronary artery. If exposure is not sufficient, it may be necessary to divide the pulmonary artery above the sinus of Valsalva (Fig. 11A). The posterior approach is achieved via an incision in the front of the aortic sinus extending rightward and backward toward the ostium of the left coronary artery and passing above the commissure between the noncoronary and the left coronary valve leaflets. After opening the posterior three quarters, the aortic sinus can be retracted to the front and leftward in order to expose the posterior side of the aorta and the origin of the left coronary artery, which can then be opened distal to the stenosis (Fig. 11B).

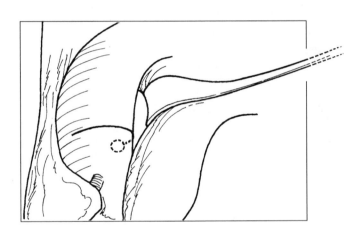

A

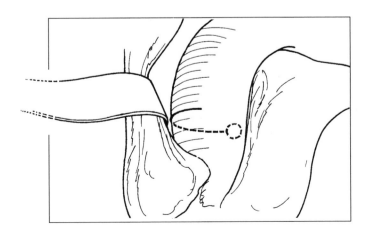

B

Figure 11. Direct exposure of the left coronary artery.
A. Anterior exposure. The pulmonary artery is retracted.
B. Posterior exposure. The superior vena cava is retracted to the right and the root of the aorta to the left.

First Septal Artery

Bypass of the first septal artery can be beneficial for patients in whom that vessel is well developed. The proximal segment of the ADA is exposed in the longitudinal sulcus opposite the left atrium. Exposure of the ADA leads directly to the first septal artery. To avoid injury to the right ventricle, the surgeon must stay close to the first septal artery.[5]

Intramyocardial Segments

Intramyocardial segments are uncommon. In cases involving myocardial bridges over the ADA, the usual technique consists of exposing the second diagonal artery near the sulcus and using it as a guide for careful retrograde dissection. An alternative technique is to use the anterior surface of the distal ADA as a guide for careful retrograde dissection. Overlying fat tissue and muscle fibers are progressively divided and the veins crossing the surface of the myocardium are ligated. The main risk of dissection is perforation of the right ventricle. This complication must be avoided since repair often requires inserting wide suture which can lead to occlusion of the vessel to be bypassed.

Reoperation

Great care is necessary when reopening the sternum especially if the pericardium was not closed during the first procedure or if no mention was made of this in the surgical report. To reduce the risk of injuring the heart, the suture wires should not be removed after they are cut. The internal surface of the sternum should be detached from the underlying tissue with particular care. The retractor should be spread very progressively. The ascending aorta and right atrium are dissected first to allow cannulation for CPB before complete mobilization of the heart. In the case of massive bleeding early in the procedure, immediate femoral cannulation is the safest response. If adherences are not extensive, mobilization can be achieved without stopping the heart. If adherences are extensive or if dissection requires handling of the heart which can result in decreased output, it may be advisable to finish the mobilization after initiating CPB. Identification and palpation of the sulci is particularly important during reoperations. Similarly, location of the previous bypass and suture lines is needed in order to choose the new anastomotic sites.

Conclusion

Identification and exposure of the coronary arteries is not difficult especially in patients undergoing a first procedure. However, much skill and care are required since the quality of the anastomosis and outcome are dependent on the quality of exposure. In cases involving reoperation, myocardial bridges, or anatomic variations, dissection may be more difficult. Good exposure is necessary even if it entails prolonging the pump time.

References

1. Levin D, Fellows JE, Abrams HL. Hemodynamically signifiant primary anomalies of the coronary arteries: Angiographic aspects. *Circulation* 1978; 58: 25-32.
2. Lipton M J, Barry WH, Obrez I, et al. Isolated single coronary artery: Diagnosis, angiogaphic classification and clinical signifiance. *Radiology* 1979; 130: 39-45.
3. Abrams HL. *Coronary arteriography: A Practical Approach* Boston, Little Brown and Cie, 1983.
4. Dion R, Verhelst R, Schoevaerdts JC, et al. La plastie chirurgicale du tronc commun de l'artère coronaire gauche. *Ann Chir* 1989; 43: 85-89.
5. Thevenet A, Du Cailar CI, Wintrebert P. Chirurgie des artères coronaires: *Encycl Med Chir*, Paris, Techniques chirurgicales, Thorax 42700, 4-9-04.

14

Exposure for Harvesting Coronary Bypass Grafts

Dominique Blin, Olivier Chavannon

The quality of autogenous grafts is a crucial factor for the outcome of coronary artery bypass. The internal mammary artery is now the most frequently used graft in coronary surgery. In addition to the internal mammary artery, which is almost routinely utilized during bypass procedures, graft material of various quality can be obtained from other donor sites.

Internal Mammary Artery

The internal mammary artery (IMA) or internal thoracic artery was first used for the Vineberg procedure in 1946.[1] It was not used for coronary bypass until 1968.[2] After initial reluctance on the part of many surgeons, the IMA has now become the graft of choice for myocardial revascularization because of better patency rates.[3,4]

Anatomic Review

The IMA arises from the subclavian artery as a single vessel in 80% of cases and as part of a trunk in 20% of cases (more often on the left).[5,6] It enters the thorax between the subclavian artery and vein and descends behind the rib cage 1-1.5 cm outside the edge of the sternum. The IMA is covered by the pleura, the endothoracic fascia and the internal intercostal muscles on the lower two thirds[7] of its trajectory.

The phrenic nerve crosses the ventral surface of the IMA from top to bottom and from lateral to medial at a mean distance of 1.8 cm from the origin of the IMA at the level of the subclavian vein[6,8,9] (Fig. 1). The IMA gives off a number of collaterals (Fig. 2): anterior pericardiac arteries (superior and inferior), the superior phrenic artery (accompanying the phrenic nerve) which arises at a mean distance of 3.9 cm from the origin of the IMA,[6] anterior intercostal arteries, perforating arteries, and sternal arteries. In 16.6% of cases there may be

From *Vascular Surgical Approaches*, edited by Alain Branchereau and Ramon Berguer. ©1999, Futura Publishing Co., Inc., Armonk, NY.

Figure 1. Origin of the internal mammary artery (IMA) and its relation with the phrenic nerve.
1. Phrenic nerve.
2. Accessory IMA.
3. IMA.
4. Pericardiophrenic artery.

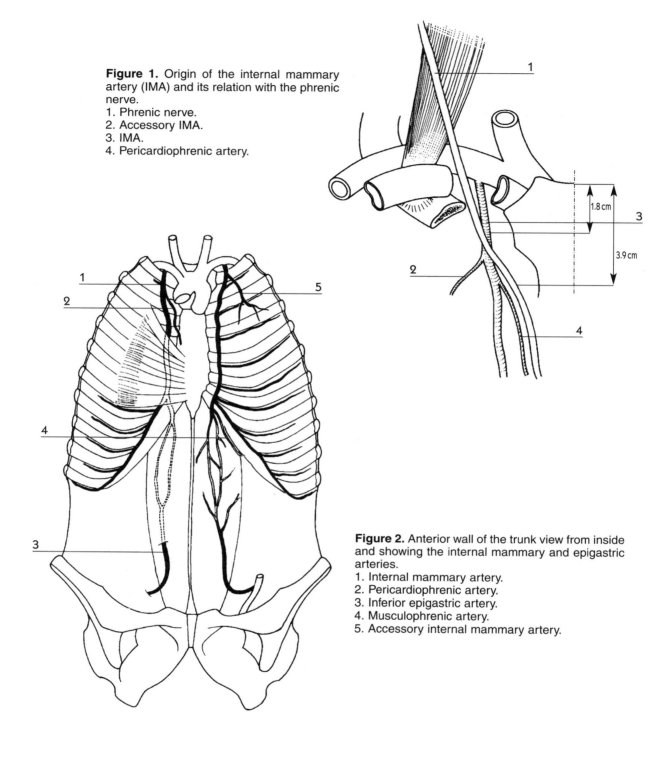

Figure 2. Anterior wall of the trunk view from inside and showing the internal mammary and epigastric arteries.
1. Internal mammary artery.
2. Pericardiophrenic artery.
3. Inferior epigastric artery.
4. Musculophrenic artery.
5. Accessory internal mammary artery.

a lateral costal branch of the IMA[10] arising at a mean distance of 2.5 cm from the origin of the IMA, then running obliquely behind and on the outer side of the internal surface of the wall of the thorax. Awareness of this variation is necessary since failure to divide this vessel can lead to significant steal syndrome.[10] Recently, using the lateral costal branch as a graft has been proposed,[11] based on histologic findings showing features similar to those of the IMA and on its mean diameter of 1.7 mm.[10] The IMA ends in the sixth intercostal space where it divides into a musculophrenic branch which descends obliquely behind the cartilages of the false ribs and an abdominal branch (superior epigastric artery) which joins the inferior epigastric artery behind the rectus.

The IMA is an elastic artery[12] that has some useful features for coronary bypass: low susceptibility to atherosclerosis and a diameter similar to that of coronary arteries. It can be used without proximal implantation and has the possibility of sequential anastomosis. The main problem is harvesting, which is difficult because of the fragility of its wall.

General Considerations

Preoperative work-up should include Doppler ultrasound of the supraaortic vessels to rule out the presence of subclavian artery stenosis which is a contraindication for harvesting of the IMA. Some authors have proposed its outlining by angiography during preoperative coronary studies[13] but this additional examination is not necessary in all cases.

Technique

The patient is placed in dorsal decubitus with the arms down by the body. If necessary a transverse roll can be placed under the shoulder blades. After standard median sternotomy, an IMA retractor is placed in position. The surgeon sits on the patient's right. The table is raised and tilted to the opposite side. Magnifying glasses should be used for greater safety. The pleura is retracted and each section of the artery is freed from its fibrous attachments and from its pericardial collaterals using an electric knife. This allows progressive opening of the retractor and exposure of the posterior surface of the sternum (Fig. 3).

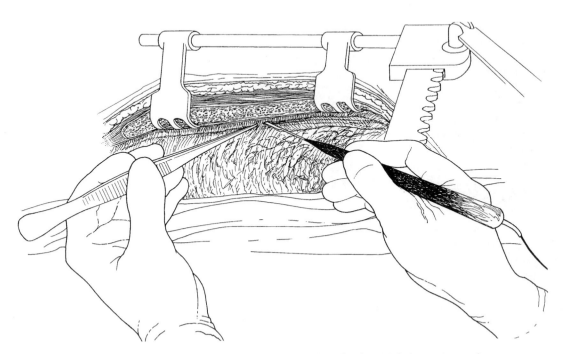

Figure 3. Harvesting the internal mammary artery. The dissection begins by dividing the fibers that connect the pleura to the chest wall. The retractor is opened gradually as the dissection progresses.

Harvesting of the Internal Mammary Artery

The technique consists of harvesting the IMA as part of a pedicle that includes the artery, veins, connective tissue, fat, muscle, and endothoracic fascia. The internal intercostal muscles nearly always cover the lower portion of the artery. Dissection is performed using a cautery at a low power setting[14] and never by grasping the artery directly with an instrument. Dissection should begin at the level of the sixth costal cartilage by an incision one centimeter medial to the IMA and continue until contact is made with the periosteum. The internal branch which is adherent to the sternum at this point is then dissected (Fig. 4). After initiating dissection, saline with papaverine should be injected into the cleavage plane to facilitate separation[15] and diminish spasm. Dissection is pursued from bottom to top so as to create a groove on the medial side of the vessels which are then progressively detached from the sternum.

Once a sufficient length has been dissected, the lateral border of the pedicle can be mobilized. In this way a strip of tissue is obtained which can be pushed down with the left hand so that dissection can be continued upwards (Fig. 5). Since the vessels are often poorly visualized and/or reenter the intercostal space, dissection must be performed with the electric scalpel as far forward as possible in contact with the lower edge of the ribs. Some authors[9] have recommended carrying the dissection upwards, identifying the phrenic nerve and dividing the mammary vein. The advantages of this technique are to achieve a pedicle that lies easily in the mediastinum and to allow division of the proximal collateral branches which could otherwise generate a steal syndrome. The disadvantage is an enhanced risk of injury or devascularization of the phrenic nerve. Distally the bifurcation and origin of the two terminal branches of the IMA can be preserved for use as a segmental bypass. If necessary the distal dissection can be carried down to the first few centimeters of the superior epigastric artery. Some authors[16] have recommended either preservation of the distal bifurcation of the IMA to ensure optimal blood

supply to the lower part of the sternum or, if the bifurcation cannot be preserved, resection of the xiphoid process. The artery is divided distally after systematic heparinization. The distal branches are ligated and temporary hemostasis of the pedicle is achieved by placing a small bulldog Fogarty clamp.

Variant Techniques

Opening of the pleura gives good exposure quickly, allows more direct access, and provides a longer pedicle. This is useful to perform distal and sequential bypasses and makes it possible to let the lung pass in front of the bypass. The disadvantage of opening the pleura is to create a free space in which blood can collect. The mechanism has been implicated in numerous pleuropulmonary complications.[17,18] Only 9% of patients in whom the pleura is opened have normal postoperative lung x-ray images compared to 42% in whom the pleura is left intact.[18] The stripped mammary artery can be isolated by dissecting close to the artery and ligating all collaterals. This technique is lower but provides a longer pedicle, and results in less devascularization of the thoracic wall.[19] While long-term patency does not seem to be better,[20-23] there is a higher risk of intraoperative injury to the IMA. When a sequential bypass is planned it is better to clear the myocardial surface of the IMA pedicle for the full length of the potential implantation sites.

Intraoperative Complications

Injury during harvesting of the IMA usually occurs when a branch is torn off resulting in a subadventitial hematoma.[9] Other causes of injury include undue traction and the use of excessively high cautery settings which can cause endothelial damage and impair graft patency.[14] The free graft technique must be resorted to if there is a frank injury to the pedicle. Twisting of the pedicle which is difficult to identify, also requires use of the free graft technique implanting the IMA on the ascending aorta, in a vein graft, or in another mammary graft.

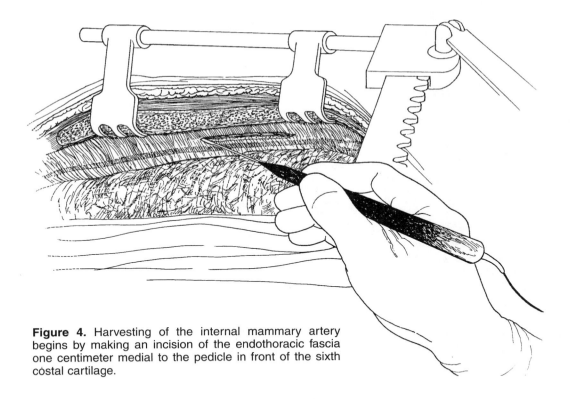

Figure 4. Harvesting of the internal mammary artery begins by making an incision of the endothoracic fascia one centimeter medial to the pedicle in front of the sixth costal cartilage.

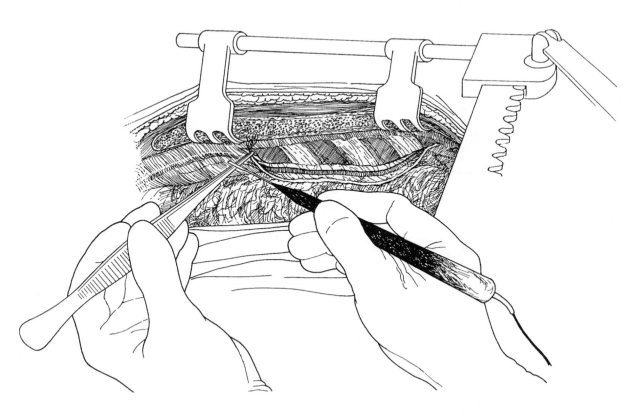

Figure 5. Harvesting of the internal mammary artery. The intercostal arterial branches are coagulated against the lower edge of the ribs.

Postoperative Complications

Impaired sternal blood supply increases the incidence of sternal nonunion and mediastinitis.[24] These complications are frequent when both internal mammary arteries are harvested. Bilateral harvesting is contraindicated in patients with diabetes and respiratory insufficiency and in obese women. Limiting the width of the pedicle greatly reduces the risk of devascularization of the sternum.[19] Postoperative bleeding is greater following IMA grafts than after vein grafts, particularly following bilateral IMA harvesting.[25] Pleuropulmonary complications are more likely if the pleura is opened.[9] Phrenic nerve paralysis is a common complication of coronary surgery and may follow mammary artery harvesting but may also be due to other factors. Pain and paresthesia of the thoracic wall due to division of anterior intercostal nerve branches usually regresses[9] but can lead to permanent disability.[26] Paresthesia of ulnar distribution secondary to stretching of the brachial plexus is common after sternotomy and has also been attributed to the harvesting of the IMA. Because of this, it is recommended that the opening of the mammary retractor be kept at a moderate setting. Mammary artery harvesting has been implicated in impaired postoperative pulmonary mechanics probably due to devascularization of the intercostal muscles.[27]

Subclavian artery steal syndrome is uncommon[13] but stenosis of the subclavian artery is observed in 0.3% of patients.[28] Steal syndrome caused by large collateral branches of the IMA, by the accessory mammary artery, or the superior phrenic artery has been reported[29] and is treated by embolization.

Gastroepiploic Artery

The gastroepiploic artery was first used for indirect myocardial revascularization with the Vineberg technique in the 1960s. The first reported use for coronary bypass was in 1987.[30,31] Early cases of gastroepiploic artery grafting involved young hyperlipidemic patients without a saphenous vein or with a calcified ascending aorta, but its indications have been expanded in view of the superiority of arterial grafts.

Anatomic Review

The right gastroepiploic artery (RGE) is the main branch of the gastroduodenal artery. It runs along the greater curvature of the stomach between the layers of the greater omentum. In 5% of cases the artery does not reach the midpoint. In 34% of cases the artery reaches beyond the proximal two thirds of the greater curvature.[31] It anastomoses directly with the left gastroepiploic artery in 35% of cases.[32] Removal of the RGE does not affect the blood supply of the gastric mucosa.[33] The RGE, with a diameter comparable to that of the coronary arteries, is a muscular artery that goes easily into spasm after handling. Like the IMA the RGE has histologic features that makes it less susceptible to atherosclerosis.[12,34]

Technique

The position of the patient is the same as for the harvesting of the IMA. Placement of a nasogastric tube facilitates handling of the stomach. Gastroepiploic grafts are harvested last, after mammary artery grafts, although simultaneous harvesting is feasible.[35] The sternal retractor is placed with the ratchet to the top. The midline incision is prolonged downwards towards the abdomen. Before beginning its harvest, the quality of the vascular pedicle is assessed. The omentum is opened and the arterial pedicle is isolated; its branches are divided flush with the stomach and occluded with ligatures or with a stapling device. Mobilization of the greater curvature is continued slightly to the left and then to the level of the pylorus on the right. Traction on the superior border of the gastrocolic ligament allows exposure of the lower branches without exposing the transverse colon. The lower edge of the arterial pedicle is then mobilized using the same technique (Fig. 6) to obtain a band sufficiently wide to limit the risk of axial twisting.

After systemic heparinization the pedicle is divided on the left side and this generally

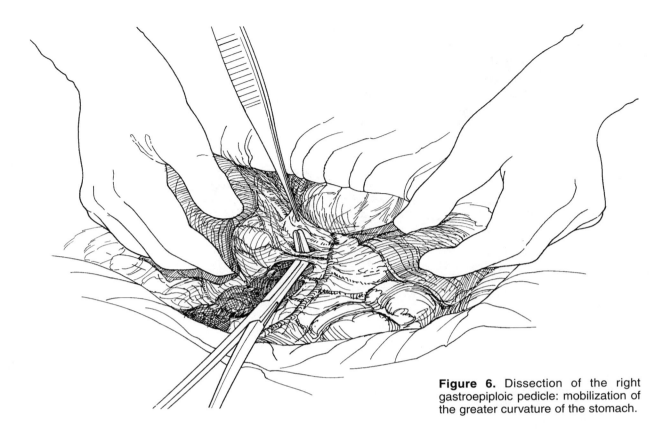

Figure 6. Dissection of the right gastroepiploic pedicle: mobilization of the greater curvature of the stomach.

allows bringing the free end of the graft to the ascending aorta. Some authors advise injection of papaverine solution into the distal end of the graft to control spasm[36] but this maneuver has been implicated in injury of the intima and in detrimental effects on the elasticity of the vessel.[23] After determining the implantation site, the length of the pedicle is trimmed accordingly. Once cardiopulmonary bypass is started, an opening is made in the diaphragm to bring the pedicle to its site of implantation. Hemostasis of the diaphragmatic opening is ensured and care is taken to protect the inferior phrenic vein from injury. If the left lobe of the liver hinders the pathway of the arterial graft, it can be mobilized by dividing the triangular ligament.

Contraindications and Complications

The only absolute contraindications for use of the gastroepiploic artery are prior gastric surgery and stenosis of the celiac artery.

Mesenteric angiography should be considered in elderly patients with multiple atherosclerotic lesions[36] and in patients in whom mesenteric ischemia is suspected. Prior gallbladder or submesocolic surgery does not preclude the harvesting of the gastroepiploic artery but may make it more difficult. Previous gastroduodenal ulcer, inguinal hernia, older age, and obesity are only relative contraindications. Complications are usually minor, mostly postoperative ileus. The incidence of postoperative ventral hernia is higher than after simple sternotomy.

Inferior Epigastric Artery

The inferior epigastric artery was first used for coronary bypass by Puig in 1988.[37] Since then several studies have reported controversial results. In our opinion this technique should be used only if other grafts are unavailable. The inferior epigastric artery is a muscular artery arising from the anterior wall of the external iliac artery immediately below the inguinal ligament (Fig. 2). It first ascends behind the right rectus muscle between the transversalis fascia and the peritoneum and then crosses the fascia and continues between the muscle and posterior sheath. It ends either by anastomosing with the superior epigastric artery or by dividing into branches that supply the rectus muscle.

The hockey-stick like incision (Fig. 7) begins lateral to the umbilicus approximately

in the middle of the anterior surface of the right rectus muscle. It descends vertically and ends with an outside turn 2 cm above the inguinal ligament.[38] After opening the anterior rectus sheath, the muscle is retracted to expose the arterial pedicle (Fig. 8). After ligating its branches, the origin of the artery is exposed on the outside of the right rectus muscle, ligated, and divided (Fig. 9). Contraindications are previous transverse laparotomy of any kind and eventration. Complications are the same as those of any procedure involving the abdominal wall: hematoma, suppuration, and dehiscence.

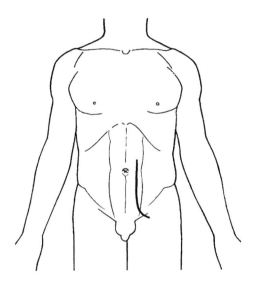

Figure 7. Incision for harvesting of the inferior epigastric artery (Reproduced with permission from Mill-Everson[38]).

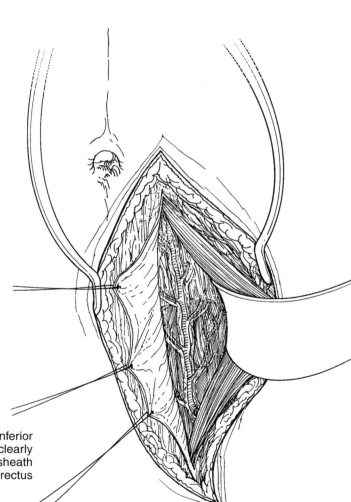

Figure 8. Harvesting of the right inferior epigastric artery: the pedicle is clearly visualized after opening the rectus sheath and retracting the belly of the right rectus muscle.

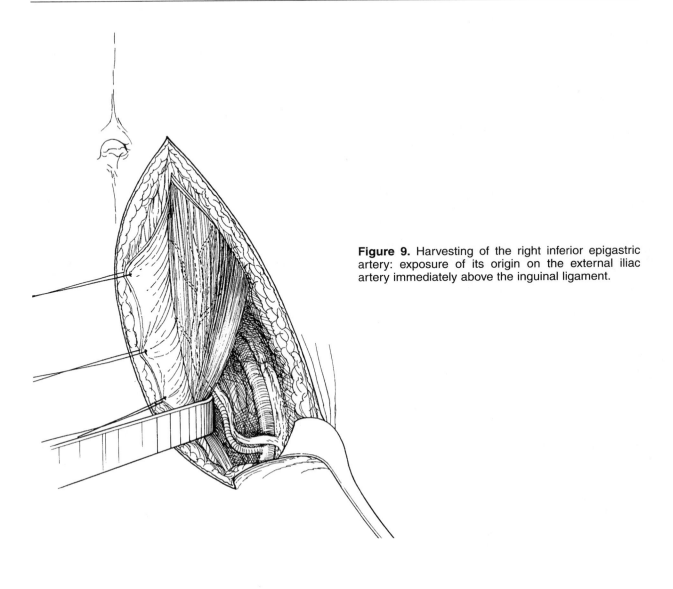

Figure 9. Harvesting of the right inferior epigastric artery: exposure of its origin on the external iliac artery immediately above the inguinal ligament.

Other Grafts

Techniques for exposure of other arteries that may be used as arterial grafts for coronary bypass are described elsewhere in this book. The use of the radial branch was first proposed by Carpentier in 1973[39] and then abandoned due to poor results. Its use has recently been rehabilitated by Acar.[40] The artery must not be stripped or mechanically dilated and is harvested *en bloc* with its accompanying veins and surrounding fat tissue. During dissection, care must be taken to preserve intact the neighboring anterior branch of the radial nerve since its injury can lead to paresthesias of the thumb.

The use of the splenic artery as a free or pediculated graft is discouraged because of the serious disadvantages it presents.

References

1. Vineberg AM. Development of anastomosis between coronary vessels and transplanted internal mammary artery. *Can Med Assoc J* 1946; 55: 117-119.
2. Green GE. Internal mammary artery to coronary artery anastomosis: Three year experience with 165 patients. *Ann Thorac Surg* 1972; 14: 260-271.

3. Loop FD, Lytle BW, Cosgrove DM, et al. Influence of the internal-mammary-artery graft on 10 year survival and other cardiac events. *N Engl J Med* 1986, 314, 1-6.

4. Grondin CM, Campeau L, Lesperance J, et al. Comparison of late changes in internal mammary artery and saphenous vein grafts in two consecutive series of patients 10 years after operation. *Circulation* 1984, 70 (suppl. I), 208-212.

5. Lippert H, Pabst R. *Arterial variations in man.* Classification and frequency. München, Bergman Verlag, 1985.

6. Henriquez-Pino J, Mandiola-Lagunas E, Prates JC. Origin of the internal thoracic artery and its relationship to the phrenic nerves. *Surg Radiol Anat* 1993; 15: 31-34.

7. Paturet G. *Traité d'anatomie humaine, tome III, Appareil Circulatoire.* Paris, Masson, 1958, 663 pages.

8. Locicero J, Hoyne WP, Locicero MA, et al. Anatomic variations of the phrenic nerve at the superior thoracic aperture (thoracic inlet): Implications for the cardiothoracic surgeon. *Clin Anat* 1988; 1: 125-129.

9. Green GE. Use of internal thoracic artery for coronary artery grafting. *Circulation* 1989; 79 (suppl. I): 30-33.

10. Henriquez JA, Mandiola EA, Prates JC. Lateral costal branch of the internal thoracic artery. *Clin Anat* 1993; 6: 295-299.

11. Hartman AR, Mawulawde KI, Dervan JP, Anagnostopoulos CE. Myocardial revascularization with the lateral costal artery. *Ann Thorac Surg* 1990; 49: 816-818.

12. Van Son JA, Smedts F, Vincent JG, et al. Comparative anatomic studies of various arterial conduits for myocardial revascularization. *J Thorac Cardiovasc Surg* 1990; 99: 703-707.

13. Tonz M, Von Segesser L, Carrel T, et al. Steal syndrome after internal mammary artery bypass grafting an entity with increasing significance. *Thorac Cardiovasc Surg* 1993; 41: 112-117.

14. Lehtola A, Verkkala K, Jarvinen A. Is electrocautery safe for internal mammary artery (IMA) mobilization? A study using scanning electron microscopy (SEM). *Thorac Cardiovasc Surg* 1989; 37: 55-57.

15. John LCH, Edmondson SJ, Rees GM. Modified technique of internal mammary artery harvest. *Ann Thorac Surg* 1991; 52: 157-158.

16. Francel TJ, Dufresne CR, Baumgartner WA, O'Kelley J. Anatomic and clinical considerations of an internal mammary artery harvest. *Arch Surg* 1992; 127: 1107-1111.

17. Noera G, Pensa PM, Guelfi P, et al. Extrapleural takedown of the internal mammary artery as a pedicle. *Ann Thorac Surg* 1991; 52: 1292-1294.

18. Landymore RW, Howell F. Pulmonary complications following myocardial revascularization with the internal mammary artery graft. *Eur J Cardiothorac Surg* 1990; 4: 156-162.

19. Parish MA, Asai T, Grossi EA, et al. The effects of different techniques of internal mammary artery harvesting on sternal blood flow. *J Thorac Cardiovasc Surg* 1992; 104: 1303-1307.

20. Huddleston CB, Stoney WS, Alford WC, et al. Internal mammary artery grafts: Technical factors influencing patency. *Ann Thorac Surg* 1986; 42: 543-549.

21. Noera G, Pensa P, Lodi R, et al. Influence of different harvesting techniques on the arterial wall of the internal mammary artery graft: Microscopic analysis. *Thorac Cardiovasc Surg* 1993; 41: 16-20.

22. Mills NL, Bringaze WL. Preparation of the internal mammary artery graft: Which is the best method? *J Thorac Cardiovasc Surg* 1989; 98: 73-79.

23. Van Son JA, Smedts F. Comparative study between the gastroepiploic and the internal thoracic artery as a coronary bypass graft. *Eur J Cardiothorac Surg* 1991; 5: 505-507.

24. Seyfer AE, Shriver CD, Miller TR, Graeber GM. Sternal blood flow after median sternotomy and mobilization of the internal mammary arteries. *Surgery* 1988; 104: 899-904.

25. Aarnio P, Kettunen S, Harjula A. Pleural and pulmonary complications after bilateral internal mammary artery grafting. *Scand J Thorac Cardiovasc Surg* 1991; 25: 175-178.

26. Mailis A, Chan J, Basinski A, et al. Chest wall pain after aortocoronary bypass surgery using internal mammary artery graft: A new pain syndrome? *Heart Lung* 1989; 18: 553-558.

27. Berrizbeitia LD., Tessler S, Jacobowitz IJ, et al. Effect of sternotomy and coronary bypass surgery on postoperative pulmonary mechanics: Comparison of internal mammary and saphenous vein bypass grafts. *Chest* 1989; 96: 873-876.

28. Carrier M, Perrault LP, Hudon G, et al. Résultats de la dilatation percutanée de sténoses de l'artère sous-clavière chez des malades porteurs de greffons mammaires internes. *Ann Chir* 1993; 47: 855-859.

29. Habbab MA, Amro AA. Nonsurgical (embolization) treatment of the coronary internal mammary flow diversion phenomenon. *Am Heart J,* 1993; 126: 456-458.

30. Pym J, Brown PM, Charrette EJP, et al. Gastroepiploic-coronary anastomosis: A viable alternative bypass graft. *J Thorac Cardiovasc Surg* 1987; 94: 256-259.

31. Suma H, Fukumoto H, Takeuchi A. Coronary artery bypass grafting by utilizing in situ right gastroepiploic artery: Basic study and clinical application. *Ann Thorac Surg* 1987; 44: 394-397.

32. Yamato T, Hamanaka Y, Hirata S, Sakai K. Esophagoplasty with an autogenous tubed gastric flap. *Am J Surg* 1979; 137: 597-602.

33. Suma H, Wanibuchi Y, Furuta S, Takeuchi A. Does use of gastroepiploic artery graft increase surgical risk? *J Thorac Cardiovasc Surg* 1991; 101: 121-125.

34. Suma H, Takanashi R. Arteriosclerosis of the gastroepiploic and internal thoracic arteries. *Ann Thorac Surg* 1990; 50: 413-416.

35. Mills NL, Everson CT. Right gastroepiploic artery: A third arterial conduit for coronary bypass. *Ann Thorac Surg* 1989; 47: 706-711.

36. Suma H, Wanibuchi Y, Terada Y, et al. The right gastroepiploic artery graft. *J Thorac Cardiovasc Surg* 1993; 105: 615-623.

37. Puig LB, Ciongoli W, Cividanes GV, et al. Artéria epigastrica inferior como enxerto livre. Uma nova alternativa na revascularizaçao direta do miocardio. *Arq Brad Cardiol* 1988; 50: 259-261.

38. Mills NL, Everson CT. Technique for use of the inferior epigastric artery as a coronary bypass graft. *Ann Thorac Surg* 1991; 51: 208-214.

39. Carpentier A, Guermonprez JL, Deloche A, et al. The aortocoronary radial artery bypass graft: A technique avoiding pathological changes in grafts. *Ann Thorac Surg* 1973; 16: 111-121.

40. Acar C, Farge A, Chardigny C, et al. Utilisation de l'artère radiale pour les pontages coronaires. Nouvelle expérience 20 ans après. *Arch Mal Cœur Vaiss* 1993; 86: 1683-1689.

15

The Aortic Arch

Marie-Nadine Laborde, Eugène Baudet

Surgery of the aortic arch has developed slowly because of the complexity of the techniques involved. First introduced in 1955 by D.A. Cooley, the surgical treatment of lesions of the aortic arch has always come up against the enormous difficulties related, on one hand, to the severity and extent of the lesions and, on the other, to the necessity of ensuring brain perfusion during the period when the branches of the aortic arch are clamped. The choice of approach depends on the lesion to be treated. The surgeon should choose the approach that will result in the best exposure and least trauma. The majority of patients requiring cardiopulmonary bypass require a standard midsternotomy. Rarely, a transverse submammary incision is used. Other approaches, such as the posterolateral thoracotomy, are rarely used in limited lesions that do not require cardiopulmonary bypass. In practice, all types of approaches to the aortic arch should be considered in light of the need for:

- *best exposure for the lesion to be treated;*
- *access to other areas than those harboring the main lesion;*
- *minimum derangement of the respiratory function; and*
- *cardiopulmonary bypass.*

Anatomic Review[1,2]

The aortic arch is the arch-shaped part of the aorta that crosses over the main left bronchus. It follows the ascending aorta and continues into the descending thoracic aorta. Almost horizontal, it lies at the level of the fourth thoracic vertebra and heads obliquely backwards and to the left. It is shaped like a double concavity, one open inferiorly and the other facing the right (Fig. 1).

The inferior surface relates to the left pulmonary artery, to the left main bronchus, and to the cardiac ganglia. It is linked to the left pulmonary artery by the ligamentum arteriosum and is surrounded by the recurrent (inferior) left laryngeal nerve. Three large

From Vascular Surgical Approaches, edited by Alain Branchereau and Ramon Berguer. ©1999, Futura Publishing Co., Inc., Armonk, NY.

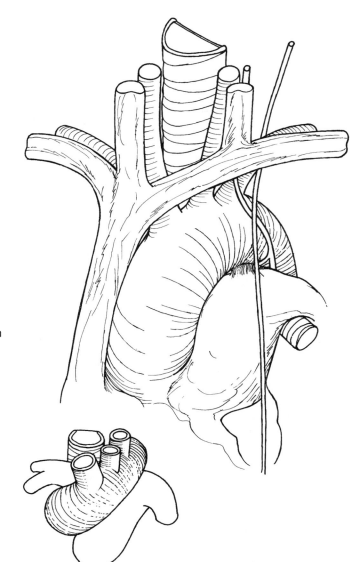

Figure 1. The aortic arch and its relationships in left anterior oblique views.

arterial trunks arise from its superior wall: the brachiocephalic arterial trunk (innominate artery), the left common carotid artery, and the left subclavian artery. There are a number of anatomic variations of the origin of these vessels. The left wall of the aortic arch is crossed by the left vagus nerve, the cervical cardiac rami, and the left phrenic nerve. It is surrounded by the left mediastinal pleura. The right posterolateral wall crosses, from front to back, the trachea, the esophagus, the thoracic duct, and a number of lymphatic vessels.

General Considerations[3]

The lesions which generally require surgery may extend to the ascending aorta and to the upper part of the descending aorta and thus call for an extensive exposure (Fig. 2). A median sternotomy involving the entire length of the sternum provides adequate exposure for the treatment of lesions of the aortic arch. This incision can be enlarged by a left anterolateral thoracotomy entering the fourth or fifth intercostal space for further exposure of the

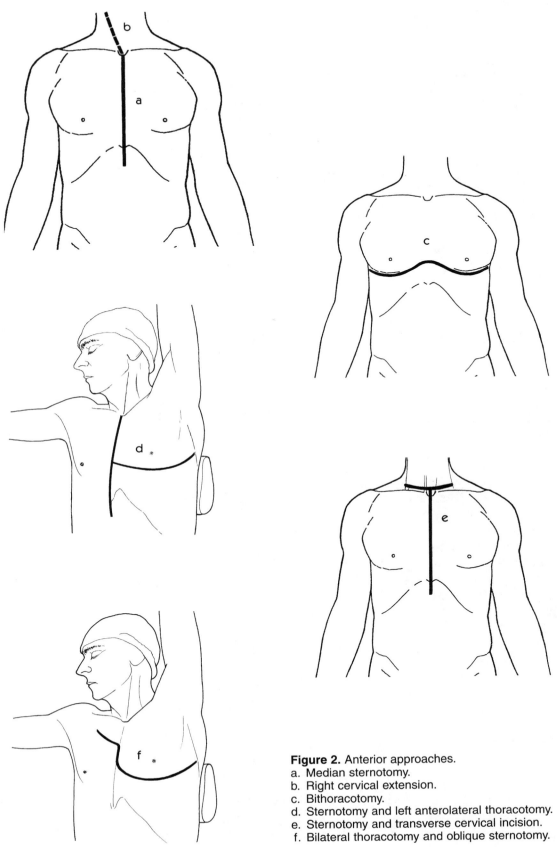

Figure 2. Anterior approaches.
a. Median sternotomy.
b. Right cervical extension.
c. Bithoracotomy.
d. Sternotomy and left anterolateral thoracotomy.
e. Sternotomy and transverse cervical incision.
f. Bilateral thoracotomy and oblique sternotomy.

distal aortic arch and descending thoracic aorta. It can also be prolonged upwards by a right cervical incision allowing access to the innominate artery and its branches or augmented by a transverse cervical incision. The submammary bilateral thoracotomy, though no longer in use, gives the widest exposure. This was the traditional approach used for cardiac surgery before being superseded by the median sternotomy. It allows treatment of the lesions of the arch which have spread to the ascending and descending aorta as far as the diaphragm. A left posterolateral thoracotomy should only be used for limited lesions of the aortic isthmus and descending aorta that do not reach the left common carotid artery.

Median Sternotomy[4]

Patient Position

The patient is placed in supine decubitus, the thorax raised either by a break in the operating room table or by a roll under the shoulders. The arms are secured alongside the body at the elbow level using a sheet, which should not be too tight, to avoid pressure over the nerves (ulnar) or vessels (radial arterial line, venous catheters). The central venous catheter should not be inserted through the left upper extremity or the left jugular vein because it may be necessary to divide the brachiocephalic venous trunks. The surgeon is to the right of the patient with the two assistants on the opposite side. The nurse is at the foot of the patient to the right of the surgeon. The anesthesiologist should have access to the patient's head. Due to the usual need for cardiopulmonary bypass, the left groin should be in the field for cannulation.

Superficial Planes

The skin incision begins 1 cm above the manubrium and ends 4 cm below the xiphoid process. The subcutaneous tissue is cut with an electric cautery. The skin over the upper edge of the manubrium is raised with a retractor. At

this level in front of the subhyoid muscles, there is a transverse vein that joins the two anterior jugular veins and is divided and ligated. The interclavicular ligament, which is thick and fibrous, is cut until an index finger can be slid behind the sternum. The mediastinum behind the xiphoid process is cleared with a finger. To avoid opening the pleura, the anesthesiologist stops ventilation for a few seconds while the sternum is cut from top to bottom along the median line, with an alternating saw. Hemostasis of the sternal edges is achieved with cautery. In a redo operation an oscillating saw is employed. It has the advantage of sparing soft tissue which is particularly important if the pericardium was not closed after the previous sternotomy. In the case of a voluminous aneurysm of the ascending aorta and in certain redos when there is a risk of aortic rupture during the sternotomy, the reopening can be performed with the assistance of a femorofemoral cardiopulmonary bypass or, in extreme cases, with hypothermic arrest.

At the upper end of the incision, the subhyoid muscles, which insert behind the sternum, are separated in the midline using scissors in order to have better access to the supraaortic trunks. If further exposure is required for the supraaortic trunks, the sternotomy should be enlarged by making a T-shaped transverse incision (Fig. 2) and dividing the subhyoid muscles, but keeping the sternal insertions of the sternomastoid muscles. If this is still not sufficient, it is also possible to section these latter muscles and reconstruct them at the end of the operation.

Medium Layer

The pericardium is opened vertically along the midline, from the diaphragm at the lower end as far as its upper reflection on the aorta, the pulmonary artery, and the superior cava. This opening should be completed by horizontal incisions, taking care not to open the pleura at the level of the diaphragm. The pericardial edges are suspended from the sternal borders (Fig. 3).

The brachiocephalic venous trunk, which crosses the supraaortic trunks transversally, is

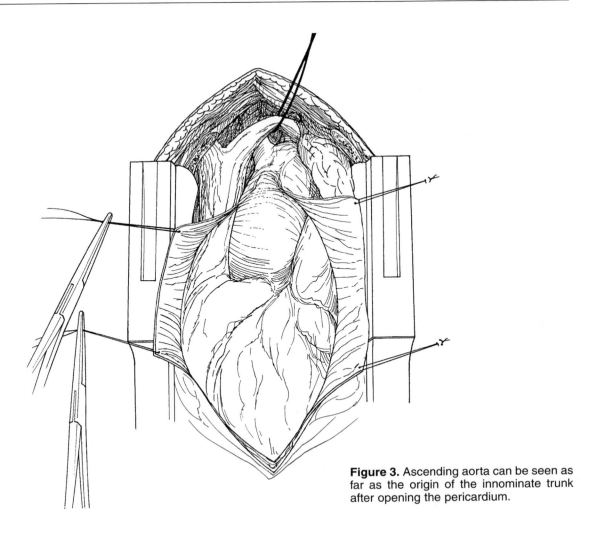

Figure 3. Ascending aorta can be seen as far as the origin of the innominate trunk after opening the pericardium.

isolated on a loop and pulled upwards. This mobilization is needed to obtain easy access to the supraaortic trunks and to the dome of the aorta. It is often necessary to divide several afferent vein branches to mobilize the brachiocephalic venous trunks. If these maneuvers are insufficient, as may be the case in aneurysms that grow towards the aortic dome, the brachiocephalic venous trunk is divided.

Ascending Aorta

The ascending aorta is exposed as soon as the pericardium is opened, from its origin to the origin of the innominate trunk which can be seen by retracting the brachiocephalic vein upwards. If necessary, the ascending aorta can be circled with a loop in the middle of its concavity 4 cm or 5 cm above the presumed site of origin of the coronary arteries. To accomplish this, an incision should be made using scissors on the fold of the pericardium on the left posterolateral face of the aorta in front of the right pulmonary artery. A finger is then passed behind the aorta from left to right. The tunneling and passage of tape is done using large, curved, blunt-ended forceps (Fig. 4) which exit between the aorta and the superior vena cava. Towards the top, the superior reflection of the pericardium is split to both sides of the aorta. The brachiocephalic venous trunk is pulled upwards allowing exposure of two thirds of the ascending aorta. The origin of the innominate artery is easily dissected at the top of the field. It may be necessary to encircle the aorta, at the upper limit of its exposure, by sliding a finger into the areolar tissue opposite

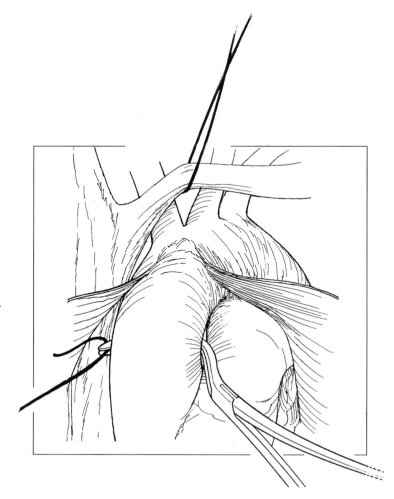

Figure 4. Encircling the ascending aorta.

the innominate artery. At this level aortic clamping is relatively easy.

Transverse Aorta

Following exposure of the ascending aorta and of the innominate artery, the dissection continues over the dome of the aorta. The left common carotid artery is freed easily with a finger, and the dissection is continued with scissors on the posterior surface of this vessel, once it is identified and retracted. Digital dissection continues towards the left subclavian artery. Exposure of the latter is more difficult due to its depth (Fig. 5). The phrenic nerve is rarely exposed because it is attached to the pleura and remains at some distance from the aorta. On the other hand, the vagus nerve crosses the left anterolateral surface of the aorta at this level; it is easily identified and is rarely freed as it is generally attached to the aortic wall particularly when the latter is aneurysmal. In practice, the dissection continues beyond the vagus nerve to reach and eventually surround the left subclavian artery. Once the supraaortic trunks are identified and isolated the dissection proceeds along the concavity of the arch. This is begun with scissors at the level of the reflection line of the pericardium of the pulmonary artery. This allows the inferior wall of the aortic arch to be mobilized away from the left pulmonary artery. The ligamentum arteriosum is next identified by its consistency. It is carefully divided using cautery staying close to the aorta, right at the adventitial level in order to protect the pulmonary artery which is a thin-walled, fragile vessel (Fig. 6). The conclusion of this dissection towards the posterior segment of the arch and around the isthmus of the aorta can only be done with fingers. The right index should hook around from front to back via the left side of the aorta to free the posterior surface; the left index completes the action by passing under the concavity along the right

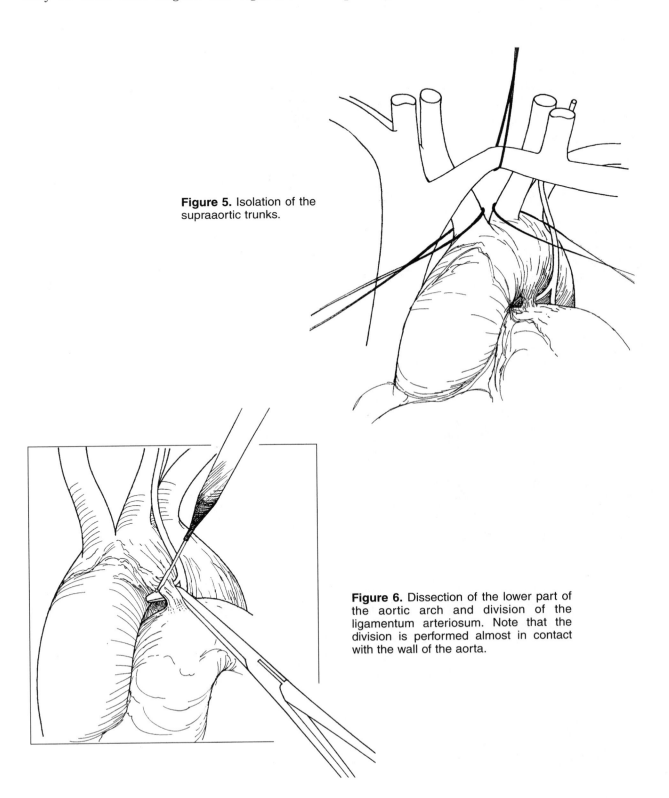

Figure 5. Isolation of the supraaortic trunks.

Figure 6. Dissection of the lower part of the aortic arch and division of the ligamentum arteriosum. Note that the division is performed almost in contact with the wall of the aorta.

edge to meet the right index. Once the freeing of the posterior surface is accomplished, the left index remains in place while a blunt-nosed curved clamp is introduced from the left (Fig. 7). This maneuver is difficult to accomplish when the tissues are infiltrated by hematoma. The freeing of the posterior part of the arch should not be attempted in aortic dissections. These maneuvers are facilitated by mild hypotension. In extreme cases, and particularly in aortic dissection, the exposure of the posterior segment of the aortic arch may not be possible, and is one of the indications for hypothermic circulatory arrest.

Extension

The median sternotomy can be complemented by a left anterolateral thoracotomy usually through the fourth intercostal space as far as the midaxillary line (Fig. 2D). This approach gives ample surgical exposure and permits control of the isthmus of the aorta and the first few centimeters of the descending thoracic aorta. Its repair is tricky, with the sternum cut into three fragments, and therefore it is rarely used. The sternotomy can be enlarged towards the neck by a right cervical incision, which gives excellent exposure of the innominate trunk and its branches (Fig. 2B), or by a transverse cervical incision cutting the subhyoid muscles that provides excellent exposure of the thoracic outlet (Fig. 2E).

Bilateral Submammary Thoracotomy[5,6]

This is an anterior, symmetric thoracotomy performed in the supine position from one axilla to the other. The thoracic wall is open in both sides through an intercostal space cutting

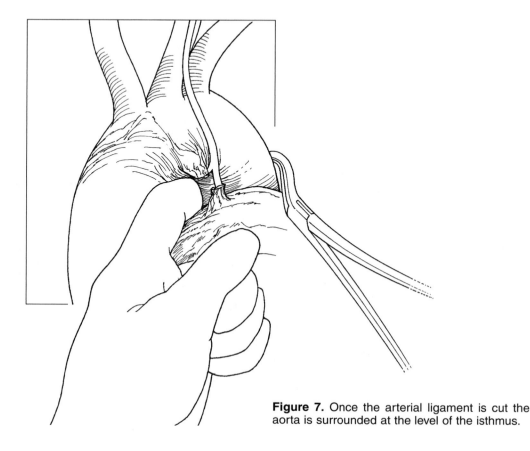

Figure 7. Once the arterial ligament is cut the aorta is surrounded at the level of the isthmus.

the sternum between the two intercostal incisions (Fig. 2C). The aortic arch is best exposed when the third or fourth intercostal space are used.

Patient Position

The patient is in the supine position and a roll is slipped under the scapulae. The arms are restrained along the body by means of a sheet. The lower lateral part of the thorax, both sides of the neck, and the left groin are included in the field. The surgical team is in the same position as described for the sternotomy.

Superficial Plane

The incision goes from one axilla to the other. In males it follows the fourth intercostal space, located by palpation, and corresponds roughly to the edge of the pectoral muscles. In females, it passes under the breasts in the submammary fold to reach the fourth intercostal space at the level of the axilla. The muscular layer is divided with cautery. The lower insertions of the pectoral muscles and, laterally, those of the anterior serratus muscle are cut. The anesthesiologist stops ventilation for a few seconds while the intercostal space is entered in order to open the pleura without injury to the lung. Once ventilation is restarted, the lung is protected using a right angle clamp while cutting the pleura. The sternum is horizontally cut using an oscillating saw.

Hemostasis is achieved with cautery and wax. Once the drapes are in place, two retractors are usually placed at the level of the two intercostal spaces. It is mainly the upper part of the incision which separates during opening.

Deep Planes

Opening the pericardium follows the same steps as described for the median sternotomy. The different segments of the aorta are also exposed in the same way, but the exposure may be extended through the left thoracic cavity for the entire length of the descending thoracic aorta from the aortic isthmus to the diaphragm. An alternative incision is a bilateral thoracotomy with an oblique sternotomy leading from the second right intercostal space to the fourth or fifth left intercostal spaces with the patient in right lateral decubitus (Fig. 2F).

Posterolateral Thoracotomy[7]

Patient Position

The patient is in lateral decubitus lying on the side opposite the thoracotomy. The transverse axis of the pelvis is perpendicular to the table and the patient is secured to the table at this level in order to leave the thorax free. An axillary roll is placed (Fig. 8). The ipsilateral arm is left hanging off the table above the

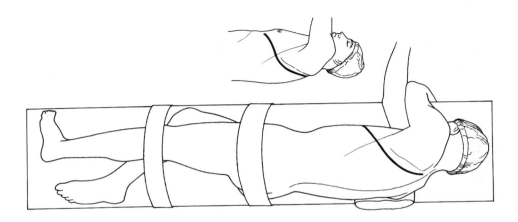

Figure 8. Patient position and skin incision for a posterolateral thoracotomy.

contralateral shoulder so as to pull the scapula as far forward as possible. The surgeon is behind the patient, the nurse at his side, and the assistants are opposite. The leg that rests on the table is flexed and the other is extended to improve stability.

Superficial Planes

The skin incision begins at the anterior axillary line and follows the ribs close to the nipple. It passes 2 cm below the lower end of the scapula and reaches a higher point located equidistant from the posterior angle of the scapula and the midline. After dividing the subcutaneous tissue with the electric cautery the two muscular layers, superficial and deep, are cut. The superficial layer is made up of the lattisimus dorsi anteriorly and by the trapezius posteriorly. The latter is involved little, or not at all, by the incision. The deeper plane consists of the rhomboid muscle posteriorly and the serratus anteriorly. Beyond this is the space between the serratus and the thoracic cage which is easily freed and which allows direct access to the ribs. One hand slipped into this space can count the ribs. The fourth intercostal space where the thoracotomy will be placed is easily identified. After dividing the intercostal muscles at the level of the upper edge of the fifth rib, the pleura is opened after stopping ventilation for a few seconds. Drapes and a retractor are placed on the posterior axillary line. The retractor is opened slowly.

Vascular Plane

The left lung is retracted. The transparency of the parietal pleura permits identification of the isthmus of the aorta, the first few centimeters of the descending aorta, the left subclavian artery, the vagus nerve, and the sympathetic chain (Fig. 9). The mediastinal pleura is opened vertically over the aorta going slightly anterior over the left subclavian artery. The first intercostal vein which crosses the aorta transversely at the level of the origin of the subclavian artery is divided. The descending aorta can easily be encircled with a finger followed by a curved clamp. During this maneuver care must be taken to avoid damag-

ing the intercostal arteries. The encircling of the aorta is done above or below those intercostals encountered (Fig. 10).

The anterior and posterior surface of the subclavian artery is freed with scissors which allows the artery to be encircled with a loop. Traction on the latter towards the surface and towards the back permits freeing the right lateral wall of the aortic arch towards the left common carotid artery. The arterial ligament is cut close to the aortic wall in order to avoid damaging the pulmonary artery. The dissection then proceeds upwards using scissors and a finger, staying in contact with the aortic arch. This procedure is facilitated by opening the pericardium between the aorta and the pulmonary artery. The aorta is surrounded using a finger followed by a forceps either between the subclavian arteries and the left common carotid artery or between the common carotid artery and the innominate trunk (Fig. 11). This procedure is always carried out in a relatively blind fashion using fingers and instrument; thus it should be performed with prudence.

Cardiopulmonary bypass reduces aortic pressure and facilitates the manipulation of the arch. Hemostasis should be meticulous because of the heparinization needed for cardiopulmonary bypass. In difficult cases hypothermic circulatory arrest avoids the need to encircle the aorta to clamp it at this level. This upward dissection of the aortic arch is always hindered by the presence of the vagus nerve which at this level gives origin to the left recurrent nerve. Cutting the vagus below the origin of the inferior laryngeal nerve has no adverse consequences and helps mobilization of the aorta. If the vagus nerve is grossly stretched and there is already a documented recurrent nerve palsy preoperatively, it can be cut if necessary.

Discussion

The approach used to expose the aortic arch is of utmost importance because it determines the ease with which the aorta can be accessed and, consequently, the quality of

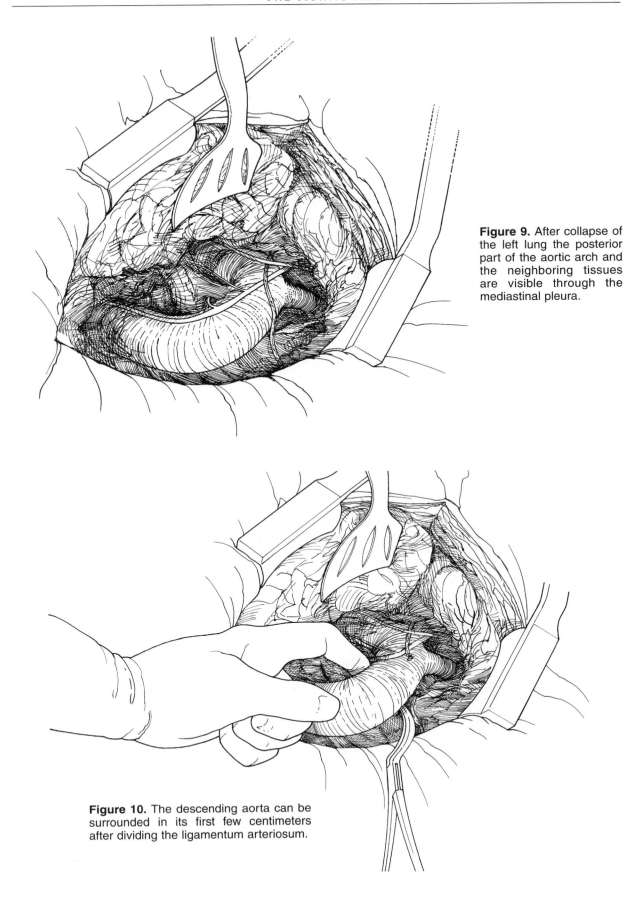

Figure 9. After collapse of the left lung the posterior part of the aortic arch and the neighboring tissues are visible through the mediastinal pleura.

Figure 10. The descending aorta can be surrounded in its first few centimeters after dividing the ligamentum arteriosum.

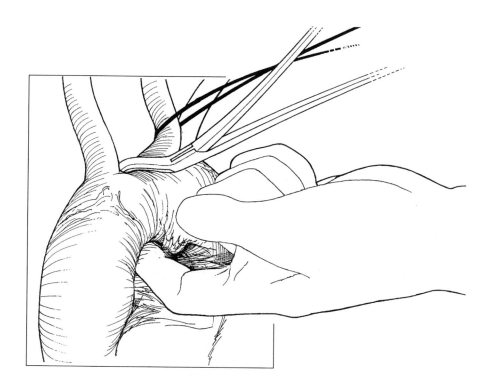

Figure 11. Encircling the transverse segment of the arch between the left common carotid artery and the innominate artery.

the vascular repair done. We prefer a median sternotomy because it provides excellent exposure of the aortic arch and has low morbidity. The anteroposterior location of the aortic arch and the possible proximal or distal extensions of its lesions bring into discussion the choice of an anterior or posterior approach.

The anterior approaches are the median sternotomy and the anterior bilateral thoracotomy. Both of these techniques allow excellent access to the ascending and transverse aorta as far as the isthmus. They also permit control of the origin of the supraaortic trunks,[8] access to the vena cava, cannulation of the supraaortic trunks, and performance of cardioplegia. Finally, they permit replacement of an aortic valve or simultaneous coronary revascularization. The drawback of these two anterior approaches is their limited accessibility to the distalmost portion of the arch and descending thoracic aorta. So, if clamping the descending aorta, as required in the case of femoral perfusion, is difficult, then one must consider using hypothermic circulatory arrest. The latter does not require a distal clamp since the distal anastomosis is

performed from inside the lumen. When unforeseen difficulties arise in the distal portion of the arch in a patient who has had a sternotomy, the only solution is to expand the sternotomy with an anterolateral incision opening the fourth intercostal space. This allows, after collapsing the left lung, access and control of the descending aorta.

An anterior bithoracotomy provides the same quality of access at the level of the ascending and transverse segments of the aortic arch. It also allows, after collapsing the lung during cardiopulmonary bypass, access to the whole descending aorta as far as the diaphragm. It thus provides access to the whole thoracic aorta and permits its entire replacement. The accessibility of the supraaortic trunks is more limited than in the median sternotomy to the extent that if there is a need for cannulation of the carotid arteries, the latter are exposed by two short cervical incisions at the base of the neck. Finally, this approach is both traumatic and painful; it compromises lung function and has a higher morbidity than the other thoracotomies that have been described.

A posterolateral thoracotomy gives excellent access to the aortic isthmus and to the first centimeters of the descending aorta. It allows clamping as far proximally as the space between the left common carotid artery and the innominate artery. This approach is best when one intends to reconstruct the left subclavian artery but it is not adequate for the other supraaortic trunks. In addition, the posterolateral approach limits the options for cardiopulmonary bypass. The inferior vena cava is only accessible from the femoral vein which limits the drainage output and implies a partial cardiopulmonary bypass. The other possibilities include cannulation of the pulmonary artery, or an atriofemoral shunt after cannulation of a pulmonary vein or of the left atrium. Hypothermic circulatory arrest is possible and is often the only solution for the most difficult lesions. Finally, it is not possible to perform cardioplegia using this approach.

Selective bronchial intubation with a double tracheal tube is often used during left posterolateral thoracotomy. It allows the left lung to be completely collapsed which improves exposure. Its drawbacks are the difficulties inherent to this technique which require an experienced anesthesiologist, and the problem of low oxygen saturation which may be caused by ventilating only the right lung, particularly in the right lateral decubitus position. The problem of low oxygen saturation is eliminated when the operation takes place under cardiopulmonary bypass with an oxygenator included in the circuit. Our team and certain others do not exclude the lung from ventilation; the latter is simply retracted.

Control of the circumference of the aortic isthmus during sternotomy and the horizontal aorta during posterolateral thoracotomy are the most difficult maneuvers. Circulatory assistance, by reducing the intraaortic pressure, facilitates these maneuvers. On the other hand, hypotension makes the vessels softer and more vulnerable to instrumentation. This can be dangerous in the case of the pulmonary artery. If control of the aorta is difficult because of its adhesions, hematoma, or fragility, as in the case of aortic dissection, it is best to avoid surrounding the aorta and to resort to either clamping with minimal exposure or to hypothermic circulatory arrest.

The choice of approach mainly depends on the topography and the extent of the lesions. For lesions of the ascending and transverse portions of the aorta, the anterior sternotomy approach is the choice. For lesions of the isthmus involving the left subclavian artery, the posterolateral thoracotomy technique is preferable. For lesions of the transverse portion of the aorta, the posterolateral thoracotomy can be used only if there is a healthy segment of the aorta allowing cross-clamping between the innominate and the left common carotid artery. If the aorta at the level of the left common carotid artery is diseased, an anterior approach such as a sternotomy or bithoracotomy should be chosen. This last approach, with the drawback described above, allows total access to the aortic arch and, if necessary, to the descending aorta.

References

1. Kamina P. *Dictionnaire Atlas d'anatomie.* Paris, Maloine, 1984, p 49.
2. Berguer R, Kieffer E. *Surgery of the Arteries to the Head.* New York, Springer-Verlag, 1992, pp 5-31.
3. Blondeau Ph, Henry E. *Nouveau traité de technique chirurgicale.* Vol 4. Coeur. Gros vaisseaux. Péricarde. Paris, Masson, 1972, pp 30-54.
4. Cooley DA. *Techniques in Cardiac Surgery.* Philadelphia, WB Saunders, 1984, pp 13-18.
5. Tran Viet T, Grunenwald D, Neveux JY. Sternotomies verticales et horizontales. *Encycl Méd Chir.* Paris, Techniques chirurgicales, Thorax 42210, 4.11.03.
6. Monod R, Germain A. La thoracotomie antérieure transversale bilatérale avec sternotomie: Indications et technique. *J Chir* 1956; 72, 593-611.
7. Noirclerc M, Chauvin G, Fuentes P, et al. Les thoracotomies. *Encycl Méd Chir,* Paris. Techniques Chirurgicales, Thorax, 42205, 4.5.11.
8. Laborde MN. Double canulation carotidienne et chirurgie de la crosse aortique. *Arch Mal Coeur* 1995.

16

Descending Thoracic and Thoracoabdominal Aorta

Edouard Kieffer, Fabien Koskas,
Amine Bahnini, Didier Plissonnier, Patrick Brami

Surgery of the descending thoracic and thoracoabdominal aorta requires the careful selection of the approach. This choice, although often simple, can become difficult when the lesions seem limited and/or when the poor general condition of the patient leads to a compromise between obtaining the ideal surgical exposure and limiting the trauma needed to achieve it. The aim of this chapter is to describe the thoracic, abdominal, and thoracoabdominal approaches to the descending thoracic and thoracoabdominal aorta.

Thoracic Approaches

Posterolateral Thoracotomy

The posterolateral thoracotomy is the preferred approach for the descending thoracic aorta. The patient is in the right decubitus, the pelvis slightly turned to the left in order to have access, if necessary, to the left femoral vessels. A roll is placed at the level of the tip of the scapula. A double-lumen tracheal tube is used for individual lung ventilation. The exclusion of the left lung greatly facilitates the operation while avoiding the potential complications of retracting a ventilated lung: lung contusion with the risk of serious hemorrhage if the operation is performed with cardiopulmonary bypass and heparinization, or displacement of the mediastinum with the risk of cardiac failure. In cases of an intrapulmonary or left bronchial hemorrhage, either spontaneous or iatrogenic, it avoids flooding the right lung. Rather than completely excluding the left lung, it should be ventilated with continuous positive airway pressure (CPAP) to avoid atelectasis and to reduce the shunt effect of lung exclusion without ventilation. The surgeon is to the left of the patient.

From Vascular Surgical Approaches, edited by Alain Branchereau and Ramon Berguer. ©1999, Futura Publishing Co., Inc., Armonk, NY.

Depending on the level of the thoracotomy, the skin incision (Fig. 1A) reaches from the interscapular-vertebral space following the angle of the scapula to the chondral margin (at the anterior limit of the sixth or seventh intercostal space) or to the sternum (at the anterior limit of the fourth or fifth intercostal space). Extensive muscular division (latissimus dorsi and anterior seratus muscles in front and rhomboid and serratus behind) is necessary to obtain sufficiently wide access.

The level of the thoracotomy (Fig. 1B) depends on the topography of the aortic lesions. The fourth intercostal space is used to reach lesions of the aortic isthmus. The sixth intercostal space is used for lesions of the midsection of the descending thoracic aorta and the seventh is used for lesions of the lower part of the descending thoracic aorta. In this latter case, a simple division of the cartilage at the anterior end of the thoracotomy allows better opening of the lower chest wall which, combined with pulling back the diaphragm with the help of a large retractor (avoiding injury to the spleen) gives excellent access to the lower thoracic aorta.

Access to the entire descending thoracic aorta is traditionally described through a combination of two thoracotomies, one in the fourth and the other in the seventh intercostal space.[1] Except in certain young, rangy patients with a straight thorax, this technique should be avoided wherever possible because of its length, its lack of direct access, and its risk of local complication (necrosis of the chest wall), particularly in the case of fractures of the intermediary ribs in elderly patients. In general, good access to the descending thoracic aorta is obtained by a posterolateral thoracotomy in the sixth intercostal space with division of chondral margin and the neck of the sixth rib (Fig. 1C).

The thoracotomy is usually intercostal. Resection of the inferior rib is only advised in case of a redo thoracotomy, when there is a history of pleural involvement requiring extrapleural detachment and in elderly patients with a rigid thorax. The detachment of pleural adhesions is performed intrapleurally or, occasionally, extrapleurally. Frequently the external surface, the apex, and the base of the

lung need to be freed. However, adhesions of the internal surface of the lung to the aorta should not be freed or should be freed only to a minimum, and only after the aorta has been controlled above and below.

With the lung retracted forward, the thoracic aorta is seen under the mediastinal pleura which is vertically incised. To access the aortic isthmus necessitates division of the left superior intercostal vein, which crosses transversally the left wall of the aortic isthmus. After this procedure, the left vagus nerve is identified and retracted, along with the overlying pleura. It gives off the left inferior laryngeal nerve around the arterial ligament while the vagus nerve drops behind the left pulmonary pedicle. The phrenic nerve crosses the lateral side of the vagus nerve, in relation to the supraaortic trunks, and lies forward against the pericardium before descending in front of the pulmonary hilum (Fig. 1D). The middle part of the descending thoracic aorta is approached by opening the mediastinal pleura. The approach to the lower part of the descending thoracic aorta is facilitated by dividing the left pulmonary ligament which leads from the bottom up to the lower edge of the left inferior pulmonary vein. Control of the distal descending thoracic aorta may require an isolated vertical incision of the left crux of the diaphragm, while leaving intact the crown of the diaphragm which is simply pulled back by a large retractor.

The left posterolateral thoracotomy is the only approach which allows direct and immediate exposure of the complete descending thoracic aorta (Fig. 1E); thus, it is by far the most frequently used approach. After vertical opening of the pericardium in front of the phrenic nerve, this approach also gives satisfactory access to the heart and the large vessels, allowing their cannulation (left atrium, left pulmonary veins, apex of the left ventricle, proximal aorta) or cardiac resuscitation (massage, defibrillation). Myocardial revascularization using a venous bypass is possible through a left thoracotomy, except at the level of the trunk of the right coronary artery. Finally, this incision exposes the subclavian artery before the left scalenus anticus muscle and a few centimeters of the left common carotid artery. A more distal approach to the

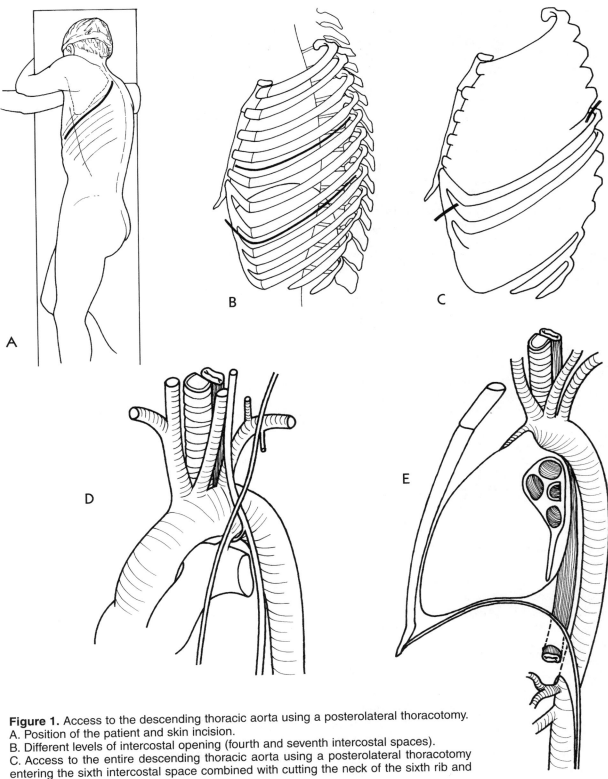

Figure 1. Access to the descending thoracic aorta using a posterolateral thoracotomy.
A. Position of the patient and skin incision.
B. Different levels of intercostal opening (fourth and seventh intercostal spaces).
C. Access to the entire descending thoracic aorta using a posterolateral thoracotomy entering the sixth intercostal space combined with cutting the neck of the sixth rib and chondral edge.
D. Anatomic relationships of the aortic isthmus: vagus nerve, inferior laryngeal nerve, pulmonary artery, and ligamentum arteriosum.
E. Left lateral view of the mediastinum showing the anatomic relationship of the descending thoracic aorta to the esophagus and the left pulmonary hilum.

subclavian artery may require resecting the first rib from inside the thorax,[2] unless an approach using the axillary artery through a separate incision is chosen, (the left upper extremity having been included in the operative field). The left posterolateral thoracotomy may be contraindicated in the case of a hostile thorax due to a previous thoracotomy and/or preexisting pleural pathology, in particular tuberculosis. In fact, these antecedents require extensive extrapleural detachments and result in multiple pulmonary injuries which may give rise to serious hemorrhage, particularly when using cardiopulmonary bypass with complete heparinization. The possibility of extension is relatively limited to the two extremities of the descending thoracic aorta. Vertical opening of the pericardium in front of the phrenic nerve allows access to the transverse and ascending sequence of the aortic arch for cannulation and/or clamping, but proximal aortic reconstruction remains difficult without hypothermic circulatory arrest.[3] It must be stressed that this procedure concerns only the arch and the distal part of the ascending aorta, and that once the aortic reconstruction is declamped, control of hemorrhage at the suture lines can be particularly difficult.

Anterior Approaches

Anterolateral Thoracotomy and Median Sternotomy

The anterior approaches to the descending thoracic aorta, whether an anterolateral thoracotomy or a median sternotomy, are rarely used and only in specific cases. These approaches provide restricted access to the descending thoracic aorta and above or below the pulmonary pedicle (Fig. 1E). The use of a double-lumen tracheal tube is not essential as the possibilities for retracting the lung are limited. The patient is in supine position with the left side slightly raised. The left arm is flexed and fixed either upwards on an arm rest or behind the back. The choice of position depends on the surgeon's preference, and on the need for a cervical incision to access the supraaortic trunks. The surgeon is to the left of the patient in the case of an anterolateral

thoracotomy and to the right for a median sternotomy.

The upper anterolateral thoracotomy is begun by a skin incision situated, in males, directly in the fourth intercostal space and in females, in the inframammary fold. The greater pectoral muscle is divided as well as the anterior part of the serratus muscle, avoiding its nerve which runs from top to bottom at the level of the midaxillary line. The thorax is opened through the fourth intercostal space. Access to the aortic isthmus is, however, limited. A satisfactory opening can be obtained by cutting the underlying adjacent chondral cartilage. Access to the aortic arch requires the combination of either a median sternotomy or an oblique transversal sternotomy with a right anterolateral thoracotomy in the third intercostal space.[4]

Dividing the triangular ligament of the lung after an anterolateral thoracotomy in the seventh intercostal space allows access to the descending thoracic aorta below the level of the pulmonary hilum. Exposure is improved by cutting the corresponding chondral edge with further retraction of the thoracic cage.

A median sternotomy gives access to the aortic isthmus because of a few technical maneuvers: asymmetrical opening of the sternotomy (for example, using an internal mammary retractor), vertical opening of the pleura just behind the costomediastinal recess, and surrounding the aortic arch with a loop between the common carotid and left subclavian arteries; this allows pulling the aorta forward and to the right. With the lung already excluded and retracted inferiorly, the vagus and phrenic nerves are identified, and the ligamentum arteriosum can be cut, taking care to preserve the left recurrent laryngeal nerve. Access to the descending thoracic aorta is limited at the lower end by the left pulmonary pedicle. Distal control of the aorta is often difficult and may be complicated by injury to an intercostal artery, the treatment of which may be difficult.

The combination of a median sternotomy with an anterolateral thoracotomy opening the third intercostal space can greatly improve access (Fig. 2). This should be foreseen and the

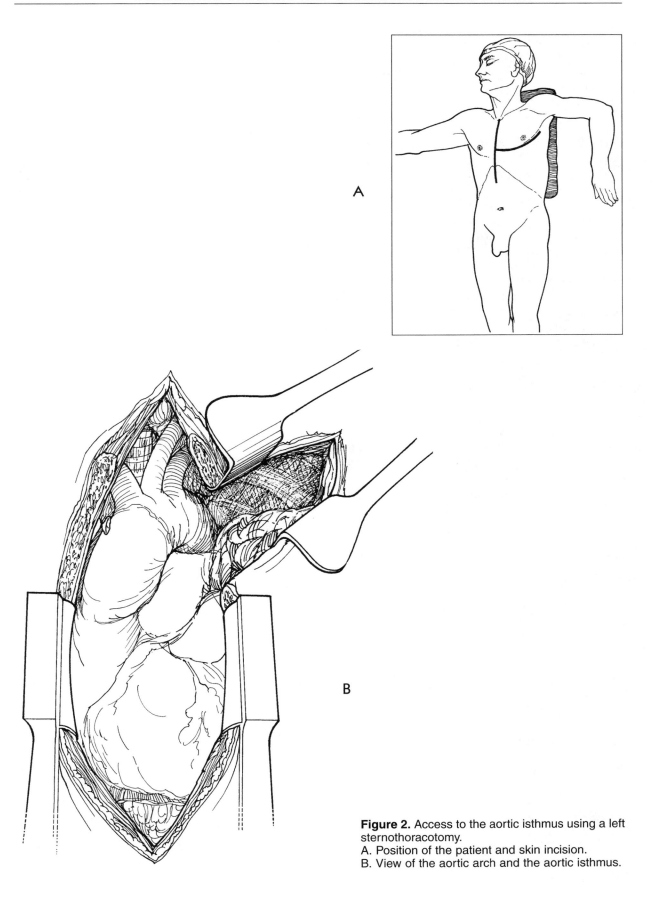

A

B

Figure 2. Access to the aortic isthmus using a left sternothoracotomy.
A. Position of the patient and skin incision.
B. View of the aortic arch and the aortic isthmus.

patient should be positioned in such a way that this combined approach may be used. This combined approach is recommended by certain authors who consider it the best access to the aortic isthmus.

Access can be gained to the lower thoracic aorta using a median sternotomy combined with a vertical incision of the posterior surface of the pericardium (Fig. 3A). After isolating the esophagus to one side or the other, the aorta is directly accessible. This procedure requires that the heart be pulled forward which can only be performed if one uses cardiopulmonary bypass or, in the case of an emergency, after a brief cardiac arrest, by clamping the superior and inferior vena cava.[5] The combination of a median laparotomy allows more direct access while leaving the heart in place (Fig. 3B). After vertical division of the diaphragm, of the pericardium, and of the left triangular ligament of the liver, the aorta can be exposed directly from the middle part of the descending thoracic aorta to the origin of the celiac trunk.

The anterior approaches to the descending thoracic aorta provide only deep, narrow, and incomplete access and are only recommended for limited procedures and in very specific cases. However, they do have the advantage of being quickly performed on patients in the supine position, and may also be useful in emergencies or during procedures associated with the upper supraaortic trunks, cervical arteries, or lower limbs. These approaches remain, however, a compromise solution. If the multiple lesions allow it, it is preferable to perform the reconstruction in two steps with an interval between them, or during the same operation by changing the position of the patient.

Abdominal Approaches

The abdominal approaches permit access only to the distal part of the descending thoracic aorta and to the upper abdominal aorta.

Laparotomy

The distal part of the descending thoracic aorta, or the supraceliac aorta may be accessed by a supraumbilical midline incision.[6,7] A roll is placed at the junction of the thoracic and lumbar spine. The surgeon is to the left of the patient. The procedure begins with the division of the left triangular ligament of the liver as far as the left suprahepatic vein, which can be seen, and displacing the left lobe of the liver to the right. The small omentum is dissected and a small left hepatic artery, originating from the left gastric artery, is cut to allow the esophagus to be pushed to the left. The right crux of the diaphragm is divided longitudinally, giving direct access to the aorta for approximately 10 cm, and avoiding the pleural cavities and the thoracic duct.

Visceral rotation is necessary to access the upper abdominal aorta. The aorta is approached from either in front of or behind the left kidney[8,9] depending on the lesions being treated, previous operation or anatomic abnormalities (left retroaortic renal vein) (Fig. 4). The aorta is approached above the celiac trunk after dividing the left crux of the diaphragm and dissected from top to bottom.

The laparotomy is well-tolerated. Since it is performed in the supine position, it permits all other associated surgical maneuvers in the neck, abdomen, or legs. Nonetheless, access to the distal part of the descending thoracic aorta remains limited. A possible proximal extension can be achieved by combining the median laparotomy with an anterolateral thoracotomy in the sixth intercostal space. However, this procedure is traumatic and the additional exposure is poor because of the canopy created by the ribs. It is largely preferable to perform a partial vertical sternotomy as far as the fourth intercostal space (Fig. 5A). This incision, which preserves the pericardium and the pleura at the thoracic level, is well-tolerated and allows the descending thoracic aorta to be accessed without displacing the heart.

Lumbar Approach

This technique, extraperitoneal and extrapleural, has become widely used in recent years for surgery of the supra- and interrenal abdominal aorta and has become the standard approach for many surgical teams.[10,11]

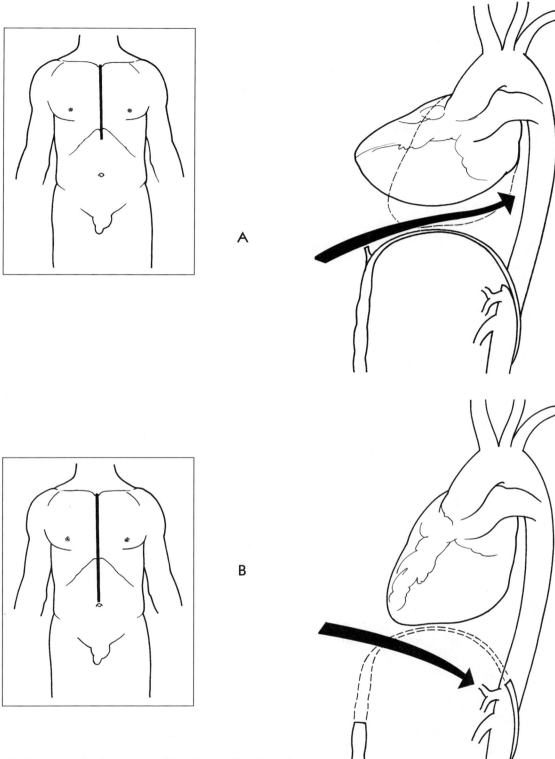

Figure 3. Access to the lower part of the descending thoracic aorta using an anterior approach.
A. Sternotomy alone requires an incision of the posterior surface of the pericardium and luxation of the heart.
B. Combined with a midline laparotomy; this allows direct access and avoids heart luxation.

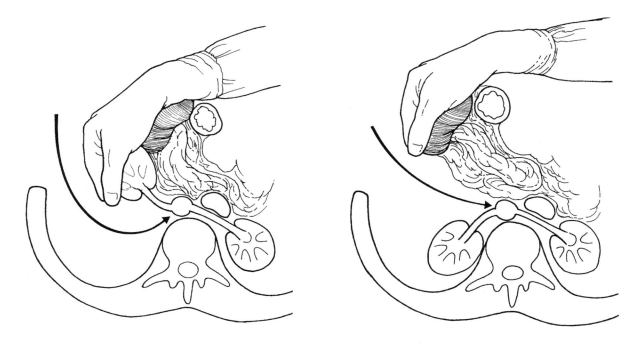

Figure 4. Cross-section of the abdomen showing the retrorenal approach to the upper abdominal aorta and the prerenal approach with detachment of the posterior mesogastrium.

The patient is in right lateral decubitus with a roll under the lumbar region (Fig. 6). The surgeon is to the left of the patient. The incision overlies the eleventh rib which is removed or left in place. The oblique muscles of the abdomen are divided as far as the external edge of the rectus muscle. The incision is followed by a transverse section of the anterior and posterior sheath of the aponeurosis of the rectus muscle which allows the muscle to be pulled to the right. Alternatively, the incision may be extended inferiorly by cutting the aponeuroses of the large muscles of the abdomen following the lateral edge of the rectus muscle. The visceral mass is detached from the lateral muscles of the abdomen, the psoas muscle, and the left posterior part of the diaphragm by dissecting the left retrocolic and retrorenal spaces. This leads directly to the abdominal aorta (Fig. 6B). The left renal artery is fully accessible after dividing the renoazygolumbar venous trunk. After dividing the inferior diaphragmatic artery, the left crux of the diaphragm is divided, which allows the lower descending thoracic aorta to be controlled by pushing back

the pleural fold and avoiding injury to the thoracic duct. The first few centimeters of the splanchnic arteries are exposed. The right renal artery is inaccessible.

Access is extended downwards towards the bifurcation of the aorta. The origin of the right common iliac artery and the entire left iliac axis are easily attained by enlarging the incision as far as the pubis along the lateral edge of the rectus muscle, by dividing the left epigastric artery and leaving the left ureter in contact with the visceral package. Access to the right iliac artery, including its bifurcation, is gained after dividing the inferior mesenteric artery at its origin. Extension towards the lower descending thoracic aorta requires a peripheral section of the diaphragm which transforms the lumbar incision into a thoracophreno-lumbar approach. If access to the thoracic aorta is inadequate, it may be improved by cutting the neck of the tenth rib. Access to the visceral arteries may also be improved by enlarging the incision anteriorly, and cutting the left, or even both, rectus muscles. Extending access to the superior mesenteric artery is possible by

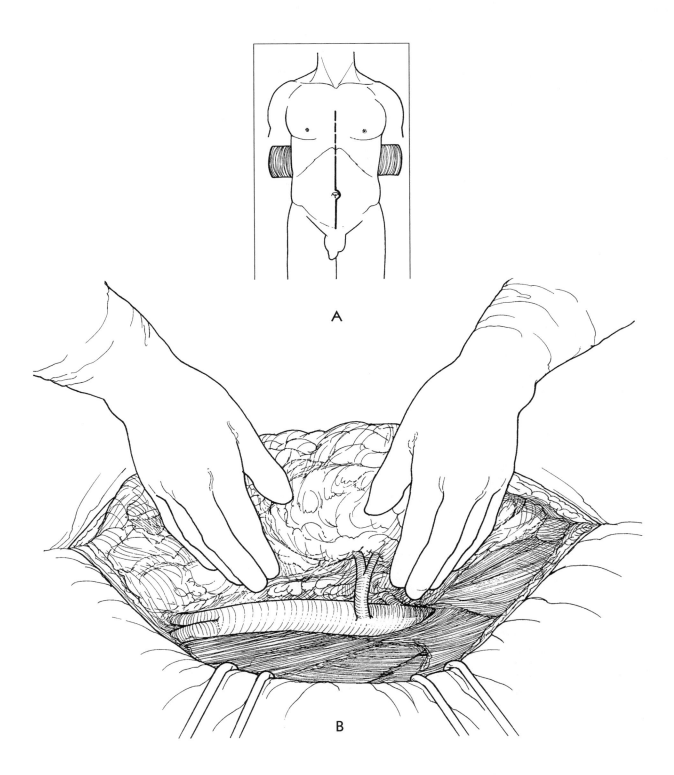

Figure 5. Access to the distal descending thoracic aorta and to the abdominal aorta using a midline laparotomy approach.
A. Position of the patient and skin incision including the extension by partial sternotomy.
B. Exposure after retrocolic and left retrorenal mobilization.

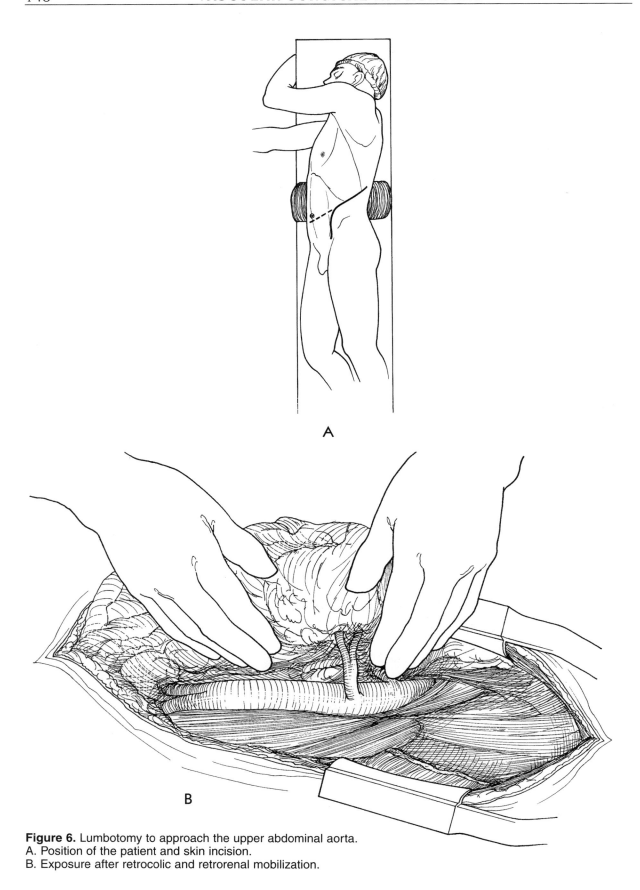

Figure 6. Lumbotomy to approach the upper abdominal aorta.
A. Position of the patient and skin incision.
B. Exposure after retrocolic and retrorenal mobilization.

detaching the posterior mesogastrium in front of the left kidney. Duodenopancreatic block rotation is required to access the right renal artery.

Thoracoabdominal Approaches

Thoracophreno-Lumbar Approach

After having employed the classic thoracophreno-laparotomy for many years,[12-15] we now prefer to use a thoracophreno-lumbar incision for surgery of the thoracoabdominal aorta (except for those lesions that involve only the distal part of the descending thoracic aorta). The thoracophreno-lumbar incision combines a complete lateral posterior thoracotomy entering the sixth intercostal space with a vertical extraperitoneal pararectal approach and a complete section of the diaphragm (Fig. 7A).[16,17]

The patient is in a right lateral decubitus position with the pelvis turned slightly towards the left, to permit access to the left femoral vessels, if necessary. A double-lumen tracheal tube is used. The surgeon is to the left of the patient. The procedure is begun by making the thoracic and abdominal incisions. The chondral edge is cut and hemostasis of the external branches of the internal mammary artery is achieved (Fig. 7B). The periphery of the diaphragm is incised using electric cautery for approximately 10 cm, while about 5 cm away from the costal margin (Fig. 7C). The inferior segment of the chondral margin and the seventh rib are retracted towards the lower left while the peritoneal sac is retracted towards the midline. Using a finger, retrocolic detachment is performed as far as the infrarenal aorta and the left common iliac artery. While an assistant continues to widen the thoracic opening by retracting the cut costal margin towards the lower left, the central segment of the diaphragm is grasped, using strong forceps, and pulled upwards. Using the left fist, the surgeon pushes into the retroperitoneal space behind the left kidney as far as the diaphragm, to detach and raise all the

abdominal viscera and to put some tension on the visceral peritoneal reflection for the length of the diaphragm (Fig. 7D). The diaphragm is divided from the lower edge to the top using the electric cautery and avoiding the spleen and the stomach. The viscera may then be completely rotated without difficulty as far as the midline. This procedure avoids any manipulation of the spleen during the detachment of the visceral rotation, and avoids an accidental splenectomy.

The left part of the abdomen is completely emptied. The division of the diaphragm is completed using the cautery approximately 5 cm from the costal insertions and reaches as far as the left crux of the diaphragm (Fig. 7E). The left crux of the diaphragm is divided using scissors. A ratchet thoracic retractor is placed with the transverse bar at the posterior part of the thoracotomy. The diaphragm is then suspended from the upper arm of the retractor using a U-shaped stitch on a pledget to avoid tearing the muscle fibers. The abdominal viscera are covered with damp drapes and pushed back as far as the midline either by using a deep retractor or by the assistant's hands.

Access to the descending thoracic aorta is easy in the absence of pleural adhesions. The use of a double-lumen tracheal tube allows complete exclusion of the lung. In the case of pleural adhesions because of an associated pathology or previous thoracic surgery, freeing the lung may be difficult. Adhesions are worse at the level of the diaphragm and the lateral part of the thorax while generally the anterior costomediastinal sinus and the paraspinal space remain free. Freeing of the lung should therefore begin at this level. Adhesions at the apex and pulmonary base should be freed only as required to access the aorta, since cutting the diaphragm allows retraction of the lung without difficulty. In order to achieve hemostasis, particularly when using cardiopulmonary bypass with heparinization, the extrapleural approach should only be used when it is impossible to use an intrapleural approach. Lung lacerations must be absolutely avoided.

Once the lung is pushed forward, the descending thoracic aorta appears immediately

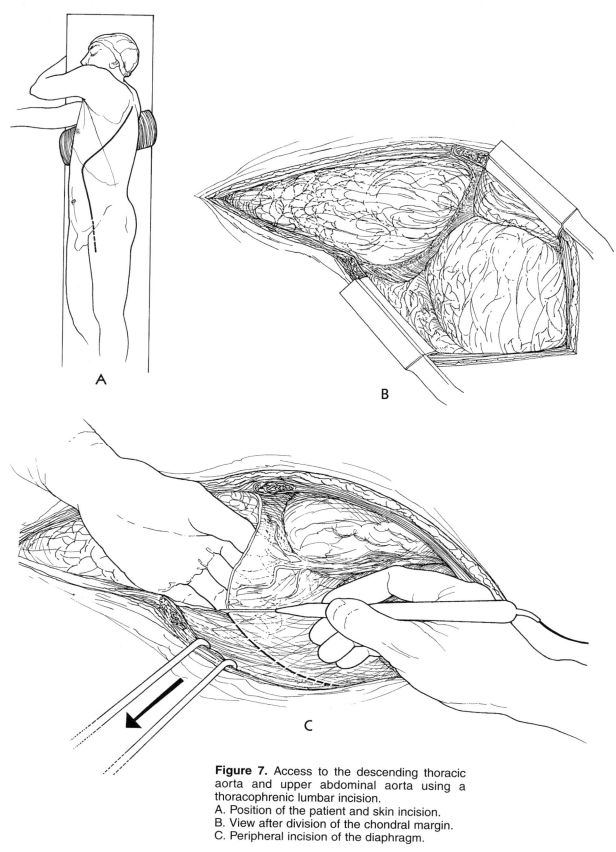

Figure 7. Access to the descending thoracic aorta and upper abdominal aorta using a thoracophrenic lumbar incision.
A. Position of the patient and skin incision.
B. View after division of the chondral margin.
C. Peripheral incision of the diaphragm.

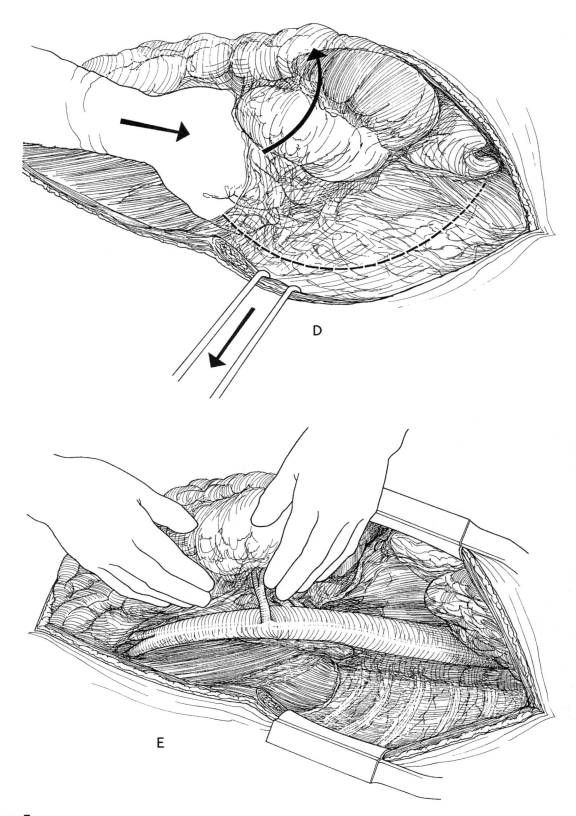

Figure 7.
D. Retrocolic and retrorenal detachment
E. Exposure of the aorta distal to the left subclavian artery.

under the mediastinal pleura. The posterior aspect of the left pulmonary hilum, with its bronchus easily located by palpation, and the lower third of the esophagus, (with a gastric tube or a transesophageal echo catheter) can be identified. A vertical incision of the pleura, with or without division of the left pulmonary ligament, gives access to the descending thoracic aorta. The upper part of the aorta is often crossed transversally by the left superior intercostal vein which must be divided.

Access to the lower part of the aorta, directly under the diaphragm, presents no difficulty once the section of the diaphragm has been performed and the left crux of the diaphragm is divided. Once the viscera have been detached as far as the midline, access to the abdominal aorta is often straightforward. The only tissues that are divided are, from top to bottom: the external roots of the solar plexus (splanchnic nerves), which cross the crux of the diaphragm, and an anteroposterior vein (the trunk of the renoazygos lumbar vein) which makes up part of the inferior hemiazygos vein. These structures may be cut without problems, after ensuring that the anteroposterior vein is not a left retroaortic renal vein. If the preoperative computed tomographic (CT) scan does not resolve the question, it may be useful to do a prerenal dissection to identify the left renal vein. In the absence of a normal left preaortic renal vein, the left kidney should be left posteriorly. In this situation the aortotomy is performed in front of the left renal artery. In the case of a double renal vein leading to a periaortic collar, the smallest vein is cut (generally the posterior one) and the aorta is approached either from in front or more frequently from behind the left renal artery.

The infrarenal aorta is surrounded by thick fatty tissue which bleeds. Hemostasis must be achieved before opening the aneurysm. When this covering is very dense, the left ureter may be pulled towards the midline where it may be at risk when the aneurysm is opened. In this case, the ureter must first be exposed for the complete length of its lumbar segment, from the point where it crosses the left iliac artery.

This extended approach which avoids opening the peritoneum allows direct and immediate access to the entire descending thoracic and abdominal aorta. The iliac axis and the left renal artery are directly accessible. Only the first centimeters of the splanchnic arteries can be exposed along with the aorta but their distal segments may be approached separately by detaching the posterior mesogastrium. It is difficult, if not impossible, to access the right renal artery using a pre- and then lateroaortic approach. In the case of an aneurysm it is possible, however, to control the first centimeters of the trunk of the right renal artery thanks to the following maneuver: after opening the aneurysm, the ostium of the renal artery is closed using an X-shaped stitch which allows sufficient traction to externalize the artery after incising the wall of the aneurysm surrounding its origin.[14] Clamping the renal artery using a large instrument keeps the renal artery well exposed.

The right common iliac artery and its bifurcation may be exposed retroperitoneally after dividing the inferior mesenteric artery at its origin. The hypogastric artery and the right external iliac artery can only be accessed using an additional right retroperitoneal approach. The left femoral artery may be accessed using a separate incision or by continuing the vertical incision towards the groin, either sectioning or retracting the inguinal ligament (Fig. 7A). Access to the right femoral artery is difficult if not impossible. Access to the left subclavian artery may require cutting the neck of the fifth rib.

The diaphragm should be carefully closed to avoid postoperative dehiscence. U-shaped polypropylene 0 stitches are recommended as well as Teflon pledgets leading to an inversion suture of the diaphragm towards the abdomen in order to avoid any postoperative thoracic bleeding. The pleural cavity is drained by two large tubes, one low, the other apical, while the retroperitoneal space is drained by two or three suction catheters.

Thoracophreno-Laparotomy

The classic thoracophreno-laparotomy is used only in very specific cases. This approach combines a posterolateral thoracotomy, entering the sixth intercostal space with a midline laparotomy, and complete section of the diaphragm. This consists of an evisceration of the small bowel towards the right which may be the source of significant liquid depletion and of traction on the mesentery. It allows more satisfactory access to the visceral arteries, the right renal artery, and the branches of the right iliac artery than a thoracophrenolumbar incision. The lower thoracophrenolaparotomy, which combines an anterolateral thoracotomy through the seventh intercostal space, a laparotomy, and a short peripheral section of the diaphragm (Fig. 8A) gives excellent access to the lower third of the descending thoracic aorta and the whole abdominal aorta including its branches.[13] The patient is supine with the left side raised by a longitudinal roll. The left arm is placed above and behind and is fixed by an arm rest. The anterolateral thoracotomy in the seventh intercostal space is extended by dividing the left rectus muscle as far as the midline. This incision may be continued by a median laparotomy or by an extension following the same line with division of the contralateral right rectus muscle.

If access is required only to the upper abdominal or supraceliac aorta, the diaphragm is radially incised for approximately 10 cm and fixed at the edges of the thoracic incision. The lower part of the thoracic aorta is easily controlled by a separate longitudinal incision of the left crux of the diaphragm (Fig. 8B). The interest of this technique is that it is less damaging to the diaphragm and especially to the branches of the phrenic nerve. If the abdominal aorta and the lower half of the descending thoracic aorta need to be accessed directly, a complete peripheral division of the diaphragm is used as in the previous procedure. In both cases, the thoracic abdominal aorta is reached using a retroperitoneal approach, either by detaching the posterior mesogastrium or by a retrocolic and retrorenal approach (Fig. 8B).

The posterior mesogastrium is entered and the spleen, the tail of the pancreas, and the stomach are rotated to the front and right leaving the left kidney behind. This gives sufficient access to the left side of the supra- and juxtarenal aorta and to the origin of the splanchnic arteries. The left renal vein crosses the anterior face of the aorta below the origin of the superior mesenteric artery and the two renal arteries. Downward displacement of the renal vein requires cutting the suprarenal vein, and allows control of the infrarenal aorta, the retrocava segment of the right renal artery, and the entire left renal artery. Better access to the infrarenal aorta requires either a classic lateroduodenal approach (with the transverse mesocolon separating both fields) or a left colic mobilization which provides direct access. In both cases, access to the distal part of the right renal artery remains limited. This should be approached separately by a duodenopancreatic rotation which is easily achieved with the patient in the supine position and the operating table rotated to the left. Access to the superior mesenteric artery is sufficient as far down as the duodenojejunal junction. Access to the most distal part may be achieved by an intramesenteric approach.

Complete retrocolic and left retrorenal visceral rotation allows easy and rapid access to the entire abdominal aorta. Access to the entire length of the left renal artery is easier than in the previous technique, but access to the right renal artery is not possible and the approach of the superior mesenteric artery is limited to its first few centimeters. In addition, this technique requires retraction of the viscera towards the midline even more so than in the previous procedure, with a small, but real, associated risk of severe pancreatic trauma. Downward extension of the exposure to the aorta, the splanchnic, and right renal arteries is performed as required, using the same technique as in the previous procedure. With the patient in the supine position, access to the femoral arteries, particularly the right femoral artery, presents no difficulty.

Conclusion

While the purely thoracic and abdominal approaches to the aorta are fundamentally different, the thoracoabdominal techniques are very similar. The differences, which relate to the choice of intercostal space, the type of visceral rotation, and the opening of the diaphragm are, nonetheless, very important. The ease and quality of access and, in part, the

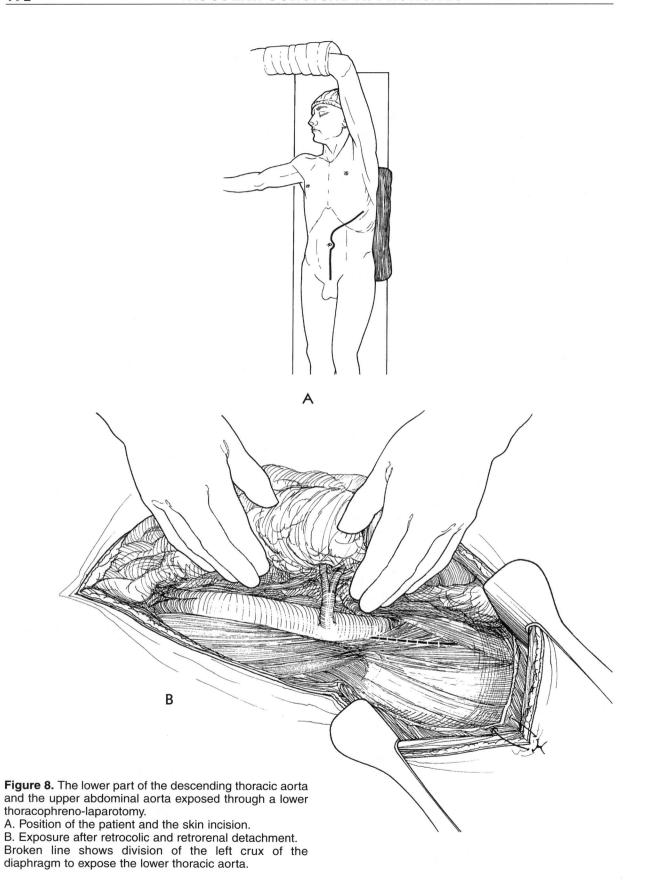

A

B

Figure 8. The lower part of the descending thoracic aorta
and the upper abdominal aorta exposed through a lower
thoracophreno-laparotomy.
A. Position of the patient and the skin incision.
B. Exposure after retrocolic and retrorenal detachment.
Broken line shows division of the left crux of the
diaphragm to expose the lower thoracic aorta.

general consequences of the operation depend on these details. Taking into account the severity of the superficial trauma in operations on the thoracoabdominal aorta, the choice of access is of great importance and should be considered along with the anatomy of the lesions and the general status of the patient.

References

1. Cooley DA. *Surgical Treatment of Aortic Aneurysms.* Philadelphia, WB Saunders, 1986, pp 81-97.
2. Mathey J, Binet JP, Menage C. Résection endothoracique de la première côte dans la chirurgie des lésions cervico-thoraciques. *J Chir* 1963; 85: 541-554.
3. Kieffer E, Koskas F, Walden R, et al. Hypothermic circulatory arrest for thoracic aneurysmectomy through left-sided thoracotomy. *J Vasc Surg* 1994; 19: 457-464.
4. Villard J, Vial P, Dureau G, et al. La thoraco-bi-sternotomie en chirurgie cardio-vasculaire. *Nouv Presse Med* 1982; 11: 3647-3649.
5. Ergin MA, O'connor JV, Blanche C, Griepp RB. Use of stapling instruments in surgery for aneurysms of the aorta. *Ann Thorac Surg* 1983; 36: 161-166.
6. Barral X, Youvarlakis P, Boissier C. Revascularisation des membres inférieurs à partir de l'aorte supra-coeliaque. *Ann Chir Vasc* 1986; 1: 30-35.
7. May J, Patrick W, Harris J. Transabdominal exposure of the thoracic aorta. *Surg Gynecol Obstet* 1980; 151: 803-805.
8. Mattox KL, McCullum WB, Jordan GL, et al. Management of upper abdominal vascular trauma. *Am J Surg* 1974; 128: 823-828.
9. Reilly LM, Ramos TK, Murray SP, et al. Optimal exposure of the proximal abdominal aorta: a critical appraisal of transabdominal medial visceral rotation. *J Vasc Surg* 1994; 19: 375-390.
10. Butler PE, Grace PA, Burke PE, et al. Risberg retroperitoneal approach to the abdominal aorta. *Br J Surg* 1993; 80: 971-973.
11. Williams GM, Ricotta J, Zinner M, Burdick J. The extended retroperitoneal approach for treatment of extensive atherosclerosis of the aorta and renal vessels. *Surgery* 1980; 88: 846-855.
12. Crawford ES, Crawford JL. *Diseases of the Aorta.* Baltimore, Williams & Wilkins, 1984, pp 78-133.
13. Elkins RC, Demeester TR, Brawley RK. Surgical exposure of the upper abdominal aorta and its branches. *Surgery* 1971; 70: 622-627.
14. Kieffer E. Chirurgie des anévrysmes de l'aorte thoracoabdominale. Editions techniques. *Encycl Med Chir* (Paris, France) Techniques chirurgicale, Chirurgie Vasculaire 43-150 et 43-151. 1993, 18 et 32 p.
15. Rutherford RB. *Atlas of Vascular Surgery: Basic Techniques and Exposures.* Philadelphia, WB Saunders, 1993, pp 186-233.
16. Stoney RJ, Wylie EJ. Surgical management of arterial lesions of the thoracoabdominal aorta. *Am J Surg* 1973; 126: 157-164.
17. Pokrovsky AV, Karimov SI, Yermolyuk RS, et al. Thoracophrenolumbotomy as an approach of choice in reconstruction of the proximal abdominal aorta and visceral branches. *J Vasc Surg* 1991; 13: 892-896.

17

The Abdomen: The Celiac Aorta

Jean-Baptiste Ricco, Frederic Dubreuil

The difficulties in approaching the celiac aorta arise from its intermediary position between the descending thoracic aorta and the infrarenal abdominal aorta. This anatomic region is deep and accessing it is difficult. Access to the celiac aorta may be achieved by a direct midline intraperitoneal approach with visceral rotation or by a retroperitoneal approach.

Surgical Anatomy

The aorta enters the abdomen via a fibrous inextensible orifice between the crus of the diaphragm. The upper limit of this orifice is at the level of the twelfth thoracic vertebra. Behind the aorta, rising towards the thorax there are two lumbar lymphatic trunks which continue to the satellite lymph nodes of the abdominal aorta. The intestinal lymphatics drain into the left para-aortic trunk. Sometimes the two lumbar trunks join together below the aortic orifice to form a dilated reservoir: the cisterna chyli, which marks the origin of the great thoracic duct. The contributors to the azygos veins or the left inferior hemiazygos vein may pass through the same orifice of the diaphragm. The sympathetic nerves descend behind the arcuate ligament and in front of the psoas. The inferior phrenic arteries originate from the celiac aorta and supply the diaphragm.[1]

Direct Intraperitoneal Approach

The patient is in the supine position with a roll placed at the level of T12 to raise the spine (Fig. 1). The midline xiphopubic approach begins above the xiphoid process dividing the insertions of the sheath of the rectus muscles. The round and the falciform ligaments are divided and a subcostal retractor is placed under the costal margin. The left lobe of the liver is mobilized by cutting the triangular and then the coronary ligament as far as the left suprahepatic vein. The left lobe of the liver is then pushed to the right and retained by a retractor with an articulated autostatic arm. After checking the absence of a left hepatic artery, the small omentum is opened through the pars flacida (Fig. 2). Opening the epiploic cavity at this level gives access to the celiac region. The esophagus, identifiable by a

From Vascular Surgical Approaches, edited by Alain Branchereau and Ramon Berguer. ©1999, Futura Publishing Co., Inc., Armonk, NY.

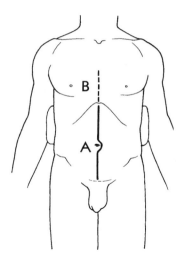

Figure 1. Direct approach to the celiac aorta.
A. Midline xiphopubic laparotomy. The patient is in the supine position with a roll below the base of the thorax.
B. Upwards extension by a partial median sternotomy.

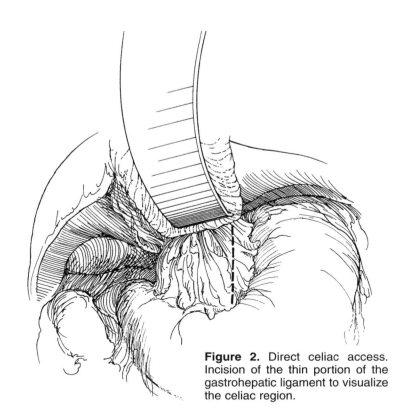

Figure 2. Direct celiac access. Incision of the thin portion of the gastrohepatic ligament to visualize the celiac region.

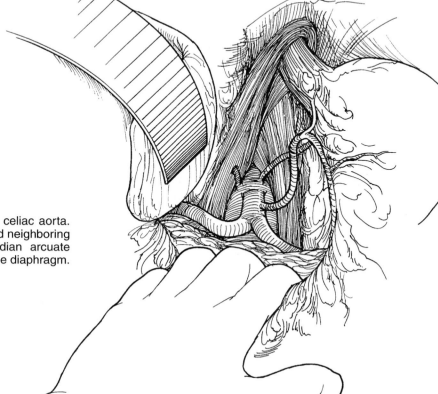

Figure 3. Direct access to the celiac aorta. Exposure of the celiac trunk and neighboring aorta before dividing the median arcuate ligament and the right crus of the diaphragm.

nasogastric tube, and the two vagus nerves are pushed to the left. Pulling the stomach downwards allows identification of the arcuate ligament. This ligament is divided while a blunt right angle clamp pushes the celiac trunk and the aorta backwards, protecting the arteries during the division of the ligament. The aorta is exposed by cutting the right crus of the diaphragm (Fig. 3).

Most frequently[1] the right crus of the diaphragm is made up of two layers; the superficial consists of the main bundle of the right crus and a second deeper one is formed by a crossed bundle which covers the aorta. The superficial bundle is freed by dividing the median arcuate ligament, which attaches it to the left crus, and is then pushed back. The deep bundle is then cut using the electric cautery. The anterior wall of the aorta is freed for 8-10 cm. The right and left inferior phrenic arteries are exposed, ligated distally, suture ligated close to the aorta, and then cut. When exposed in this manner, the aorta can be cross-clamped. The right pleural cul-de-sac is pushed upwards to allow access to the supraceliac aorta. In the case of a bypass from the celiac aorta, the tunnel for the bypass and for an eventual omentoplasty should be prepared before clamping the aorta. The anterior leaf of the transverse mesocolon is lifted and a tunnel is made across the base of the transverse mesocolon to the left of the midcolic artery.

There are three possible complications linked to this approach. The first is the risk of opening the pleura in the posterior infra-mediastinal region, which is a minor problem that requires negative pressure drainage. The second is the risk of postoperative pancreatitis, which has been described by Cormier et al.[2] The third complication, the possibility of gastroesophageal reflux, is more theoretical than real although it can happen after dividing the right crus of the diaphragm in a patient with a preexisting cardioesophageal anomaly.

Comments

This direct intraperitoneal approach is narrow and deep. In obese patients with a narrow thorax it should be strictly avoided. It can, nonetheless be extended through a partial median sternotomy (Fig. 1B).[2] This approach allows clamping of the celiac aorta during resection of difficult juxtarenal aortic aneurysms which is preferable to immediate suprarenal clamping adjacent to the aneurysm. Cross-clamping may not be possible when there is occlusive and heavily calcified athero-sclerotic disease of the juxtarenal aorta. This approach allows the implantation of a pros-thesis in the celiac aorta in order to revas-cularize the hepatic artery, the superior mesenteric artery, the renal arteries, or the femoral arteries.

Intraperitoneal Approach by Abdominal Visceral Rotation

This approach, popularized by Stoney[3] was first described by Shirkey et al. in 1967[4] and then revived by Blaisdell et al.[5] in the treatment of traumatic injuries of the upper abdominal aorta and visceral arteries. This approach uses a median xiphopubic incision eventually prolonged by a partial inferior median sternotomy. The patient is in the supine postion with a roll placed under the base of the thorax (Fig. 1). The small bowel is lifted from the abdomen towards the right and protected by damp drapes. Mobilization of the left colon is begun by cutting the peritoneal reflexion line from the sigmoid mesocolon upwards (Fig. 4). The phrenocolic ligament is cut rotating the spleen and the caudal pancreas from left to right (Fig. 5). The dissection plane is between the pancreas, in front, and the prerenal fascia behind (Fig. 6A). To have wider access to the celiac aorta one can approach it from behind the left kidney (Fig. 6B). This posterior retrorenal approach allows complete access to the interrenal aorta, the suprarenal and the celiac aorta (Fig. 7).

If the preferred access is in front of the kidney and, if there are difficulties in finding the plane of dissection in an obese patient, the left ureter may be used as a guide, following it from bottom to top. The ureter is easily identified in the lower part of the incision after mobilizing the sigmoid colon. The dissection continues, staying in front of the left ureter and

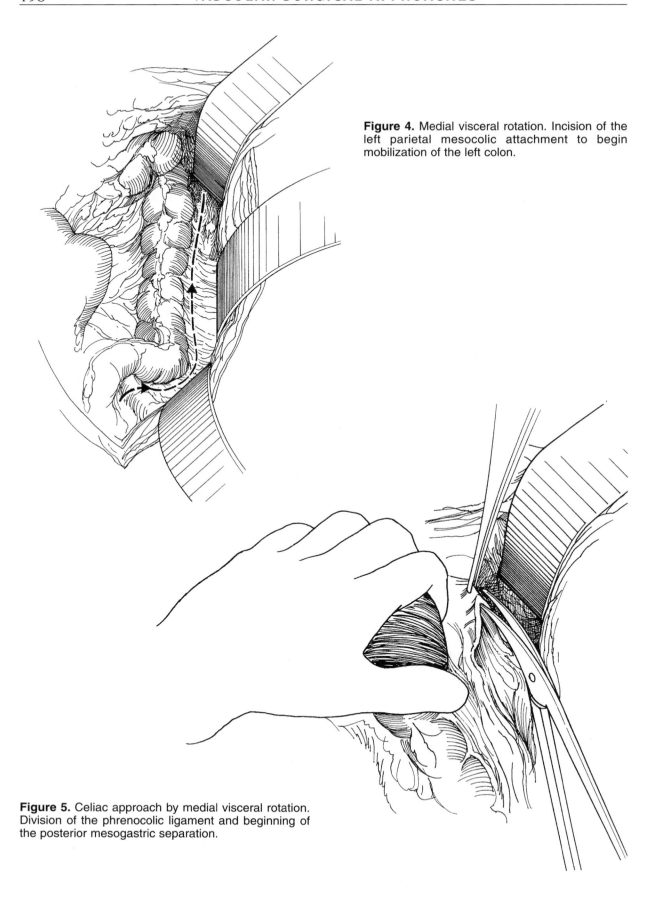

Figure 4. Medial visceral rotation. Incision of the left parietal mesocolic attachment to begin mobilization of the left colon.

Figure 5. Celiac approach by medial visceral rotation. Division of the phrenocolic ligament and beginning of the posterior mesogastric separation.

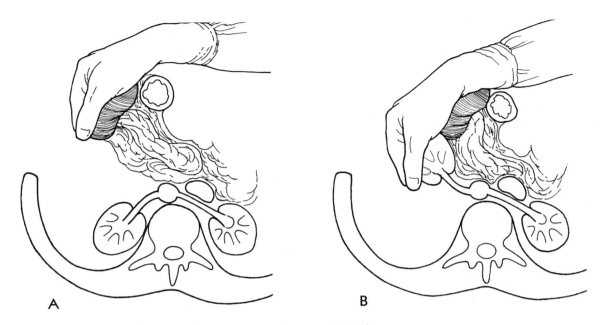

Figure 6. Celiac approach by visceral rotation.
A. Prerenal approach detaching the posterior mesogastrium.
B. Retrorenal approach.

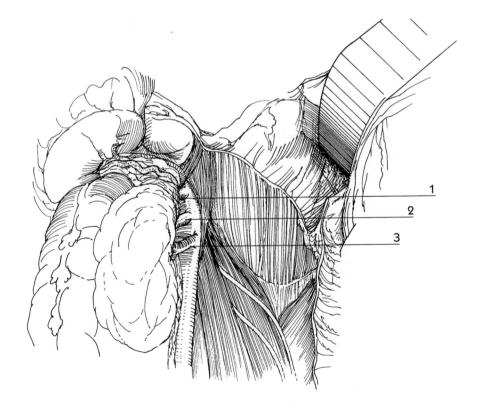

Figure 7. Celiac approach by visceral rotation. Retrorenal detachment allows access to the entire abdominal aorta and the left anterolateral wall of the celiac aorta. The left kidney and ureter have been rotated forward.
1. Celiac trunk.
2. Superior mesenteric artery.
3. Left renal artery.

over the anterior wall of the aorta as far as the left renal vein. The plane is easily extended in front of the left kidney joining the plane developed after mobilization of the spleen and the tail of the pancreas. The dissection continues to the right by rotating the stomach, and then dividing the left triangular ligament to rotate the left lobe of the liver to the right. This maneuver allows complete exposition of the abdominal aorta (Fig. 8).

The arcuate ligament and then the crus of the diaphragm may be divided in order to access the supraceliac aorta and open the posterior inframediastinal space (Fig. 9). In the case of a partial inferior median sternotomy, the lower part of the descending thoracic aorta may be accessed using an extrapericardiac approach by sectioning the phrenic center and retracting the pericardium upwards.

Comments

One of the advantages of this approach is the possibility of gaining extensive access, without additional dissection on a patient in the supine position, from the celiac aorta to the iliac arteries and the common femoral arteries. The dissection is, however, extensive and heparinized patients are at risk for serious intraoperative blood loss. The risk of splenic trauma is substantial, reaching 21% in a study by Reilly[6] on 108 procedures of this type. The possibility of acute pancreatitis must also be taken into account as there were five cases of this in Reilly's study, two of which resulted in death.

This procedure is recommended in emergency cases of suprarenal abdominal aortic traumatism.[5] It may also be used in suprarenal transaortic endarterectomies to treat stenosis at the origin of the celiac/mesenteric arteries.[6]

Celiac Access Using a Retroperitoneal Approach

Retroperitoneal access to the celiac and supraceliac aorta may be achieved by a lumbotomy or a thoracophreno-lumbotomy.

Lumbotomy (Retroperitoneal Lumbar Approach)

The patient is in right lateral decubitus. A roll is placed transversally under the lumbar region. The incision is made over the eleventh rib, which is removed (Fig. 10), and the large muscles of the abdomen are divided as far as the lateral edge of the left rectus muscle. From here the incision may be extended in two ways. The first involves following the same direction towards the midline, and dividing the anterior and posterior sheath of the left rectus muscle, and sometimes the left rectus itself, after detachment of the peritoneal sac. This method of enlarging the incision gives improved access to the suprarenal aorta and to the visceral arteries. The second alternative is to extend the incision following the edge of the left rectus muscle downwards disinserting the large muscles of the abdomen; this method improves access to the bifurcation of the aorta and to the origin of the common iliac arteries. The retrocolic and retrorenal dissection allows the visceral mass to be rotated forward leaving to the rear the lateral muscles of the abdomen, the psoas, and the left posterior part of the dome of the diaphragm. The division of the left crus of the diaphragm, raised by a dissector, is the key to this procedure; it allows direct access to the celiac aorta by pushing back the left pleural sinus. The right renal artery is difficult to access using this approach.

Comments

This approach is particularly well-adapted to suprarenal abdominal aortic surgery and to treat type IV thoracoabdominal aneurysms.[7] The approach is simple, the celiac aorta is relatively superficial and surgical maneuvers are easy, in particular anterograde revascularization of the left renal artery. In addition, this retroperitoneal and extrapleural approach is usually well-tolerated by frail patients and results, arguably, in a faster return of bowel activity.[8,9]

Extension of this approach towards the lower thoracic aorta is possible by performing a peripheral division of the diaphragm which transforms the lumbotomy into a thoraco-phreno-lumbotomy.

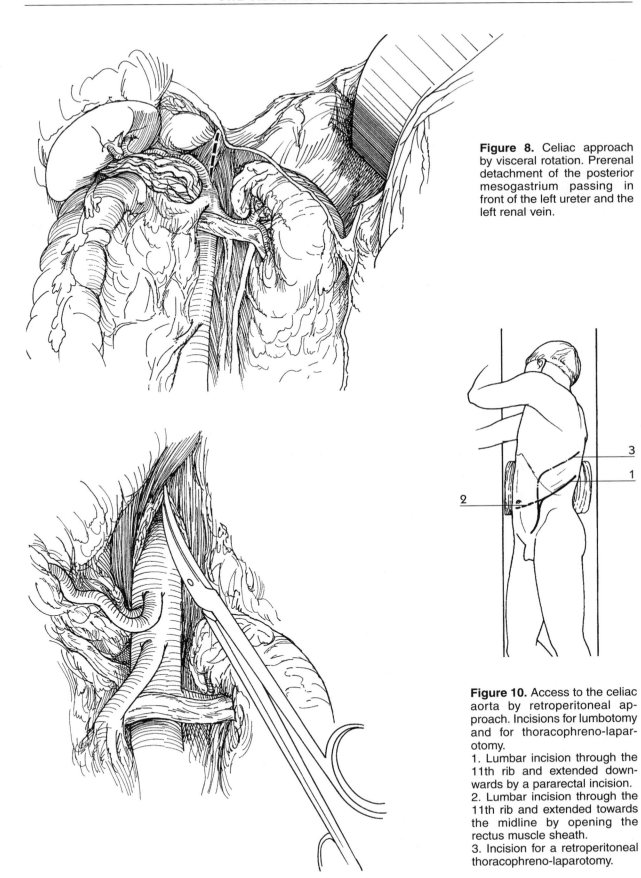

Figure 8. Celiac approach by visceral rotation. Prerenal detachment of the posterior mesogastrium passing in front of the left ureter and the left renal vein.

Figure 10. Access to the celiac aorta by retroperitoneal approach. Incisions for lumbotomy and for thoracophreno-laparotomy.
1. Lumbar incision through the 11th rib and extended downwards by a pararectal incision.
2. Lumbar incision through the 11th rib and extended towards the midline by opening the rectus muscle sheath.
3. Incision for a retroperitoneal thoracophreno-laparotomy.

Access by Thoracophreno-Lumbotomy

This extraperitoneal approach gives direct access to the lower thoracic aorta, the celiac aorta, and the complete abdominal aorta. It is performed with the patient in a 70 degree right lateral decubitus. It combines an eighth intercostal thoracotomy with an extraperitoneal pararectal abdominal incision (Fig. 10). The chondral edge is cut and the lateral branches of the internal mammary artery are ligated. The diaphragm is divided peripherally a few centimeters from its chest wall insertion leaving marker sutures to allow easier closure later (Fig. 11). At this stage in the dissection the chondral edge is retracted to the left and the left colon towards the midline. The parietal mesocolic attachment of the peritoneum is cut. Dissection is continued behind the left colon as far as the suprarenal aorta passing in front of or behind the left kidney. Detachment of the posterior mesogastrium, passing in front of the left kidney, gives access to the left margin of the suprarenal aorta (Fig. 12). The left renal vein crosses the anterior face of the aorta; its mobilization requires cutting an adrenal vein and the gonadal vein. The lower thoracic aorta is exposed by dividing the left inferior phrenic artery and the arcuate ligament of the diaphragm and by making a vertical incision of the left crus. Access to the first 3 cm of the right renal artery is achieved by this prerenal detachment.

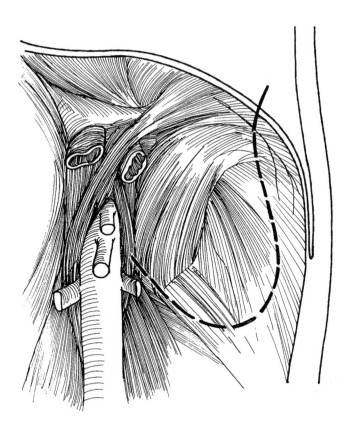

Figure 11. Thoracophreno-laparotomy. The diaphragm is cut a few centimeters from its chest wall attachment. The diaphragmatic incision ends behind the left crus of the diaphragm.

Left retrorenal detachment allows unhindered access to the abdominal aorta. However, access to the first part of the right renal artery is difficult, and the superior mesenteric artery can only be exposed near its origin (Fig. 13).

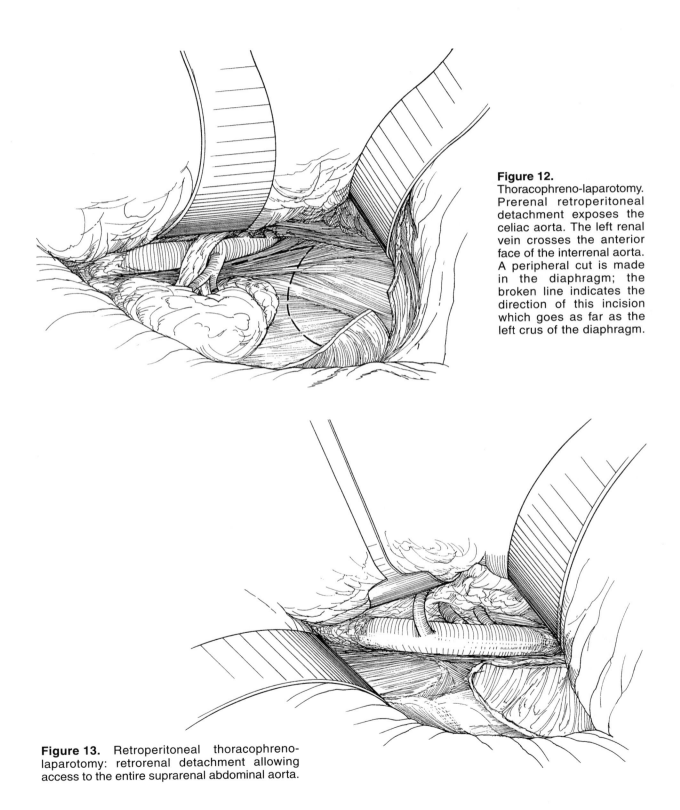

Figure 12. Thoracophreno-laparotomy. Prerenal retroperitoneal detachment exposes the celiac aorta. The left renal vein crosses the anterior face of the interrenal aorta. A peripheral cut is made in the diaphragm; the broken line indicates the direction of this incision which goes as far as the left crus of the diaphragm.

Figure 13. Retroperitoneal thoracophreno-laparotomy: retrorenal detachment allowing access to the entire suprarenal abdominal aorta.

Comments

Whether the thoracophreno-lumbotomy is pre- or retrorenal, it allows complete access to the lower thoracic aorta and the celiac aorta. The left renal artery is clearly visible. The advantage of the extraperitoneal approach is that it is better tolerated than a thoracophreno-laparotomy and allows extended access to the lower thoracic and celiac aorta in type IV aneurysms and in calcified and occlusive lesions of the thoracoabdominal aorta.

References

1. Couinaud C. *Anatomie de l'Abdomen.* Paris, Doin & Cie, 1963, 398 p.
2. Cormier JM. Revascularisation aortique supra-cœliaque par voie transpéritonéale. *Encycl Méd Chir* Paris, Techniques chirurgicales, Chirurgie Vasculaire, 43060, 4.11.11, 7 p.
3. Stoney RJ, Wylie EJ. Surgical management of arterial lesions of the thoracoabdominal aorta. *Am J Surg* 1973; 126: 157-164.
4. Shirkey AL, Quast DC, Jordan JL. Superior mesenteric artery division and intestinal function. *J Trauma* 1967; 7: 7-24.
5. Buscaglia LC, Blaisdell FW, Lim RC Jr. Penetrating abdominal vascular injuries. *Arch Surg* 1969; 99: 764-769.
6. Reilly LM, Ramos TK, Murray SP, et al. Optimal exposure of the proximal abdominal aorta: A critical appraisal of transabdominal medial visceral rotation. *J Vasc Surg* 1994; 19: 375-390.
7. Kieffer E. Chirurgie des anévrysmes de l'aorte thoracoabdominale (I). *Encycl Méd Chir* Paris. Techniques chirurgicales, Chirurgie Vasculaire 43-150. 1993, 18 p.
8. Sicard GA, Freeman MB, Vanderwoude JC, Anderson CB. Comparison between the transabdominal and retroperitoneal approach for reconstruction ot the infrarenal aorta. *J Vasc Surg* 1987; 5: 19-27.
9. Cambria RP, Brewster DC, Abbott WM, et al. Transperitoneal versus retroperitoneal approach for aortic reconstruction: A randomized prospective study. *J Vasc Surg* 1990; 11: 314-325.

18

Retroperitoneal Approach to the Intraabdominal Aorta

Gregorio A. Sicard, Boulos Toursarkissian

Exposure of the abdominal aorta is frequently performed by vascular and general surgeons via the intraabdominal approach. Although the retroperitoneal approach to the aorta is not a new technique, it has recently gained increased popularity based on studies demonstrating certain advantages of this approach when compared to the customary transabdominal approach.[1,2] The retroperitoneal approach should be part of the surgical armamentarium of all vascular surgeons and general surgeons who perform aortic surgery.[3,4]

Anatomic Review

After crossing the diaphragmatic hiatus, the abdominal aorta can be found in front and slightly to the left of the lumbar vertebrae (Fig. 1). The aortic bifurcation is usually located around the 4th lumbar vertebra. The autonomic nervous plexus is intimately associated with the aorta along its length. The suprarenal aorta gives rise from its anterior surface to the celiac axis at the level of L_1, and to the superior mesenteric artery approximately 1 cm more distally. The suprarenal aorta also supplies a number of visceral arteries, including, from top to bottom, the inferior phrenic arteries, the suprarenal vessels (whose number and origin are variable), and the gonadal vessels.

The renal arteries mark the point of transition to the infrarenal aorta. This point is also marked by the passage of the left renal vein anterior to the aorta in 90% of patients; in the remaining 10%, the left renal vein may be retroaortic or a venous circumaortic collar may be present. The infrarenal aortic segment, which is located between the top of L_2 and the bottom of L_4, gives rise in its anterior surface to the inferior mesenteric artery, and from both posterolateral walls to a number of lumbar vessels, and to a middle sacral artery at the level of the aortic bifurcation. The lumbar

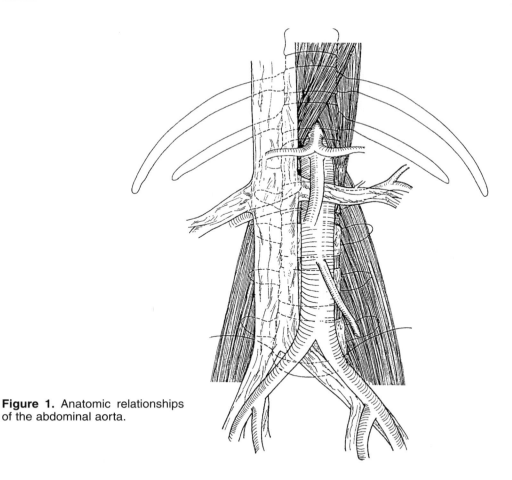

Figure 1. Anatomic relationships of the abdominal aorta.

vessels (arteries and veins) are found posterior to the aorta and vena cava, between the lumbar vertebrae and the psoas muscles.

The inferior vena cava is normally located to the right of the aorta. A translocated left-sided cava can be found in 0.2% to 0.5% of patients which crosses from left to right, anterior to the aorta, at the level of the renal arteries. A duplicated vena cava is noted in 0.2% to 3% of patients, with formation of a common trunk at the level of the renal arteries.

The aortic bifurcation is separated from the 4th lumbar vertebra by the left iliac vein, which courses from left to right behind the right common iliac artery. The ureters and gonadal vessels stand parallel to the aorta and vena cava, with the ureters occupying a more lateral position.

General Considerations

The retroperitoneal approach to the abdominal aorta offers a number of advantages over the standard midline transabdominal approach.[5] In fact, it has been associated with less intraoperative hypothermia, less fluid loss, a lower incidence of ventilatory difficulties, and a shorter postoperative ileus duration.[6,7] Because the peritoneum is not violated, the risk of postoperative adhesive intestinal obstruction is reduced or eliminated, and the long-term risk of an aortoenteric fistula seems also to be greatly diminished.

The retroperitoneal exposure is the approach of choice to the aorta for patients with a so-called *hostile* abdomen, such as patients with multiple previous intraabdominal procedures, prior abdominal and/or pelvic irradiation and gastrointestinal or urologic stomas. It can also be very useful in massively obese patients, patients with ascites and patients undergoing peritoneal dialysis. It also provides an excellent approach for uncommon, but difficult aortic problems such as aortic pathology associated with horseshoe kidney, inflammatory aneurysms, and juxtarenal or pararenal aortic occlusive or aneurysmal disease.[8]

The underlying discussion relates mainly to the left retroperitoneal approach to the infrarenal aorta. Besides providing excellent access to the infradiaphragmatic aorta, this approach also provides excellent exposure of the left renal artery for left renal revascularization alone or in combination with aortic reconstruction. Although aortic and right renal reconstruction can be carried out from a left retroperitoneal approach, the need for right renal revascularization in infrarenal aneurysmal disease with a short proximal neck has been considered a relative contraindication to this approach and is best carried out through a midline transabdominal approach or through a right retroperitoneal approach.[4] In aortic replacement for aortoiliac occlusive disease, mobilization of the proximal 1.5-2 cm of the right renal artery can be frequently performed using a left retroperitoneal approach. On the other hand, in a large infrarenal abdominal aortic aneurysm with a short infrarenal neck, this mobilization can be cumbersome unless the neck of the aorta is completely transected allowing for left lateral and downward retraction of the neck. This facilitates the exposure of the proximal right renal artery for its anastomosis of the latter to a prosthetic graft or to a bypass from the aortic prosthesis. A second contraindication to the left retroperitoneal approach has been the infrarenal aortic rupture, except in situations of a chronic contained rupture. Recent reports have shown that using a high incision and mobilizing the left kidney anteriorly can allow for safe proximal infra- or juxtarenal cross-clamping in this situation. Despite these reports, we feel that the entry into the retroperitoneal hematoma can occur, and we still consider the presence of a ruptured aneurysm to be a contraindication to using the retroperitoneal approach, except for very selected situations in

which the transabdominal approach would be considered too risky, such as in patients with a *hostile* abdomen. Another relative contraindication is the need for aortic replacement in a patient with a duplicated inferior vena cava (IVC) or a left-sided IVC; however, careful mobilization of the cava in the juxtarenal location should allow for safe clamping and aortic revascularization.[9] Finally, the distal portion of the right common iliac artery is difficult to access, especially in large infrarenal aortic aneurysms from a left retroperitoneal approach, requiring a counter incision in the right lower quadrant. On the other hand, the retroperitoneal approach can be easily modified (by using a higher incision) to allow access to the suprarenal aorta, or extended into a thoracoretroperitoneal incision to allow access to the thoracic aorta.

Positioning and Incisions for Retroperitoneal Aortic Exposure

For infrarenal aortic reconstruction in which an adequate infrarenal aortic neck is expected, the patient is positioned over a self-molding, vacuum-operated, plastic bean bag (Olympic Medical, Seattle, WA) with the shoulders elevated 45 to 60 degrees off the table and the hips allowed to fall back as parallel to the table as possible. The left arm is extended superiorly and anteriorly and supported on a Mayo stand or secured to an operating table-mounted screen. In order to provide maximal separation of the iliac crest from the postero-lateral costal margin, the kidney rest is elevated with the patient in the lateral position and then the bean bag is suction aspirated, providing a stable patient position (Fig. 2). At this point, the patient is flexed to a jackknife position which further opens the costal margin superior iliac crest angle. It is important to secure an appropriate anterior rotation of the torso in order not to limit the posterior exposure. For juxtarenal or suprarenal aortic pathology, the patient is rotated 45 to 60 degrees , the left arm is elevated more cephalad, and the same steps as described above are followed. This more

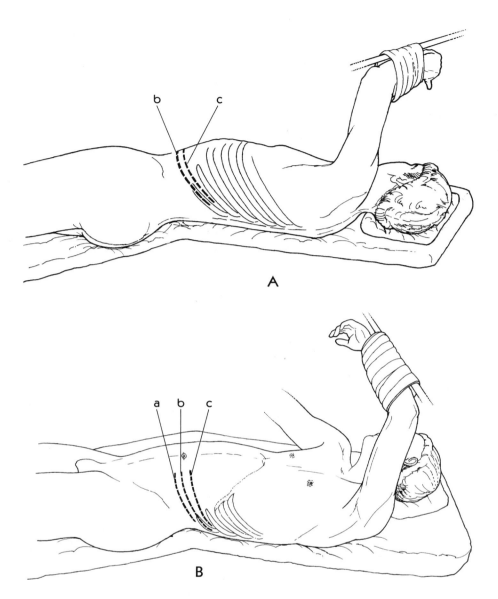

Figure 2. Patient's position for retroperitoneal exposure of the iliac arteries and the infrarenal aorta. Incision A is used for iliac artery exposure, incision B for aortic exposure, and incision C for infrarenal aortoiliac exposure.

posterior positioning expands the left retroperitoneal exposure, providing easier access to the juxta- or suprarenal aorta (Fig. 3).

The incision to be chosen depends on the proximal extent of the aortoiliac pathology. For left iliac surgery, our preferred incision is a curvilinear incision starting approximately 4 cm above the symphysis pubis at the left

rectus border and extended laterally to the level of the midaxillary line (Fig. 2A). For infrarenal aortic cross-clamping, the most common incision we utilize is a curvilinear incision starting medial to the left border of the rectus abdominis muscle about the level of the umbilicus and extended laterally to the tip of the 12th rib (Fig. 2B). At this point, depending on the extent of the infrarenal aortic neck, as

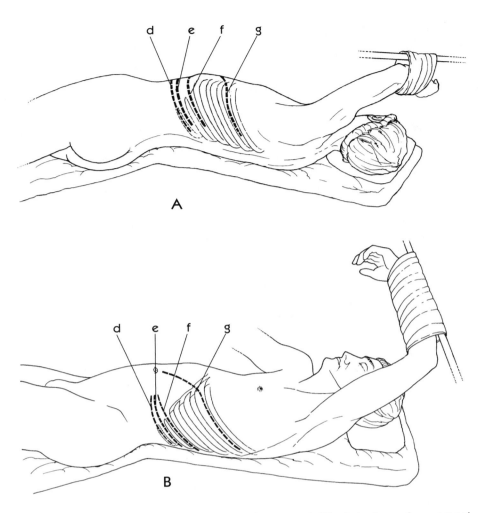

Figure 3. Patient's position for retroperitoneal exposure of the in juxta- and suprarenal aorta and the different incisions based on the extent of disease. Incision D is used primarily for juxtarenal aneurysm repair, incision E for suprarenal aneurysm repair with cross-clamp above the superior mesenteric artery, incision F for supraceliac aortic cross-clamping, and incision G for mid- and lower-thoracic aortic cross-clamping.

well as the patient's body habitus, the incision can be extended into the 11th intercostal space or the 12th rib can be resected (Figs. 2C and 3D). In thin patients with an infrarenal aortic aneurysm in which a tube graft can be placed, the incision can be started in the lateral border of the rectus sheath and carried posteriorly with resection of the 12th rib (Fig. 2B). For left iliac endarterectomy, a lower and shorter incision suffices (Fig. 2A). In thin patients with a wide costal iliac angle, a J-type of incision can be a useful option. This incision is started 2-4 cm below the umbilicus and extended laterally and superiorly along the left lateral rectus abdominis border to the 9th costochondral border. In patients with an inflammatory or juxtarenal aortic aneurysm, the preferred incision is the standard curvilinear incision extended into the 11th or 10th intercostal space depending on the level of infradiaphragmatic aortic cross-clamping required (Fig. 3E or 3F). If supraceliac aortic cross-clamping is required, the 10th intercostal incision with intrapleural extension provides the best exposure to the suprarenal infradiaphragmatic aorta. For type III thoracoabdominal aortic aneurysms a thoracoretroperitoneal incision in the 7th or 8th intercostal space is made (Fig. 3G).

Surgical Exposure of the Retroperitoneal Aorta

Except for markedly obese patients, excellent exposure of the retroperitoneal aorta can be achieved by division of the lateral abdominal wall muscles without the need to divide the left rectus abdominis muscle except in its most lateral aspect (lateral to the inferior epigastric vessels). The retroperitoneal space is best entered at the lateral junction of the left rectus abdominis muscle by dividing the transversalis fascia and mobilizing the peritoneal sac medially and cephalad. This approach permits excellent exposure of the infrarenal aorta and the left iliac arteries and permits access to the proximal right iliac artery in most instances. After entering the retroperitoneal space the peritoneal sac is mobilized medially until the left ureter and gonadal vein (attached to the peritoneal envelope) are visualized. The left ureter is then mobilized with its normal periureteral fat and encircled with a vessel loop. The ureter is dissected with its associated periureteral fat superiorly to the renal pelvis and inferiorly to just below the bifurcation of the left common iliac artery. The ureteral mobilization facilitates exposure of the infrarenal aorta at the level of the renal vein and avoids traction injury to the left ureter during aortic reconstruction. It is important to avoid skeletoning the ureter during its mobilization in order to prevent ischemic stricturing. If the patient has excess perirenal fat, Gerota's fascia is entered inferiorly allowing for easier mobilization of the kidney posteriorly. The left kidney itself is not routinely mobilized anteriorly, unless suprarenal clamping is anticipated. At this point, the left gonadal vein is ligated at the level of its junction to the left renal vein. This maneuver allows for a better exposure of the juxtarenal aorta (Fig. 4). In a significant number of cases, ligation of any lumbar(s) vein(s) draining into the posterior aspect of the left renal vein further improves the exposure of the juxtarenal aorta, and of the left renal artery. A chest

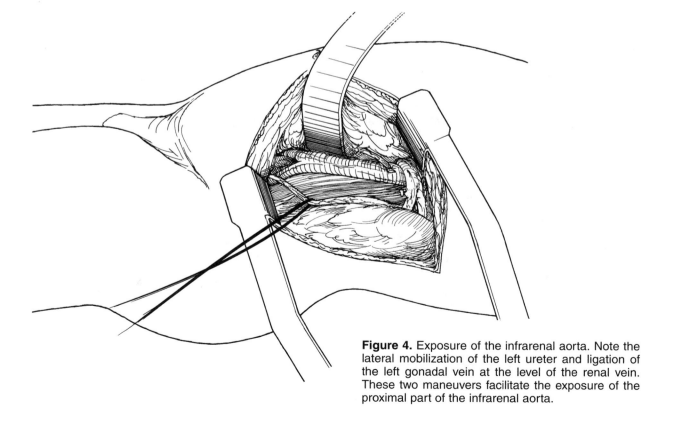

Figure 4. Exposure of the infrarenal aorta. Note the lateral mobilization of the left ureter and ligation of the left gonadal vein at the level of the renal vein. These two maneuvers facilitate the exposure of the proximal part of the infrarenal aorta.

retractor is sutured to the abdominal wall with #2 silk suture and the retractor opened, providing excellent separation of the costal margin-iliac crest angle. The use of a self-retaining multiadapter retractor, such as the Stoney-Omni retractor, provides excellent static retraction and virtually eliminates the accidental injury to intraabdominal organs such as the spleen and pancreas.

The proximal position of the left common iliac artery can be easily mobilized for clamping. On the other hand, in patients with large abdominal aortic aneurysms which extend to the aortic bifurcation, circumferential dissection of the proximal right common iliac can be difficult and hazardous since it can lead to injury to the left iliac vein-vena cava confluence. In these situations, control of the right iliac system is best achieved endoluminally with an occluding balloon catheter after the left common iliac and infrarenal aorta have been cross-clamped and the aortic aneurysmal sac opened. The aorta is opened on its posterolateral aspect to avoid the vascular and neural plexus. The inferior mesenteric artery (IMA) is usually suture ligated from within the aneurysmal sac, thereby avoiding injury to the left colic arterial branches that may join the IMA close to the IMA aneurysm junction. After suture ligation of back-bleeding lumbar vessels, an aortic tube or bifurcation graft is anastomosed end-to-end proximally with 2-0 or 3-0 nonabsorbable monofilament suture. The distal aortic anastomosis is similarly carried out in aortic tube grafts.

In aortobiiliac grafts, the anastomosis to the proximal common iliacs can be easily performed to the proximal right common iliac through the same exposure. If a bifemoral anastomosis is needed, the left limb is tunneled retroureterally into a previously made femoral incision. To tunnel the graft to the right femoral area, blunt finger dissection from the femoral triangle, as well as *directly over* the right common iliac artery, assures a retroureteral graft position (Fig. 5). This index finger blunt dissec-

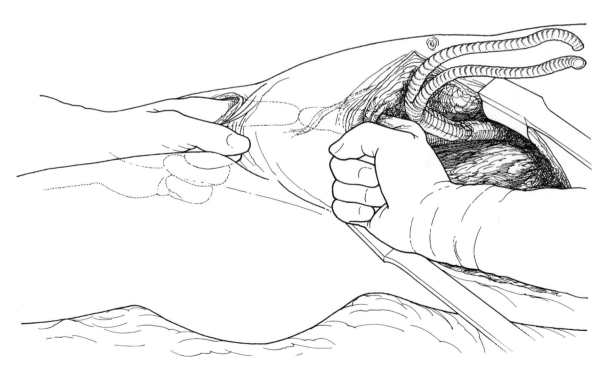

Figure 5. End-to-side aortobifemoral graft for aortoiliac occlusive disease. Note the blunt retroureteral dissection to create the iliofemoral tunnel where the right limb of the graft will be passed. Prior to passing a blunt clamp, two index fingers must touch each other.

tion from the femoral approach (right index finger) and the anterior face of the right iliac system (left index finger) must create a tissue free tunnel. Prior to passing a blunt tip clamp through this tunnel, the tip of both index fingers must touch *without* interposed tissue. This assures that a right ureteral injury does not occur. A blunt instrument (i.e. large Crafoord clamp) is passed from the femoral area gently until it touches the right index finger which should be under the right ureter and superior to the anterior wall of the external iliac artery (Fig. 6). The blunt instrument should not be passed unless it directly touches the right index finger and there is no tissue between them. The left limb of the aorto-bifemoral is similarly passed retroureteral and into the left femoral area. This technique allows for an aortobifemoral bypass without the need for a counter incision in the right lower quadrant.

In patients with juxtarenal aneurysms or inflammatory aneurysms, the incision is carried more posteriorly into the 11th interspace with or without removal of the 12th rib depending on the patient's body habitus. In most circumstances, the left kidney is mobilized from Gerota's fascia, specifically its superior and posterior attachments to the inferior surface of the left hemidiaphragm. This allows for the juxtarenal aortic dissection to be carried out with the kidney mobilized anteriorly or posteriorly as indicated. Once the peritoneal envelope has been mobilized to the level of the aortic hiatus, the left crux of the diaphragm is divided with the electrocautery easily exposing the suprarenal aorta to a level of 5-8 cm above the celiac axis (Fig. 7). In most cases, suprarenal cross-clamping of the aorta is performed between the SMA and the renals (if sufficient space is available) (Fig. 8) or in the supraceliac aortic position; the latter requires division with electrocautery of the left crux of the diaphragm. This maneuver is best performed with the left kidney mobilized anteriorly, although it can be performed with the left kidney in its posterior position but fully mobilized from Gerota's fascia (Fig. 7 A and B, and Fig. 8 A and B). When the suprarenal aorta is opened, the back-bleeding from the celiac and superior mesenteric arteries is best controlled with balloon catheters. The renal arteries are routinely cannulated with an

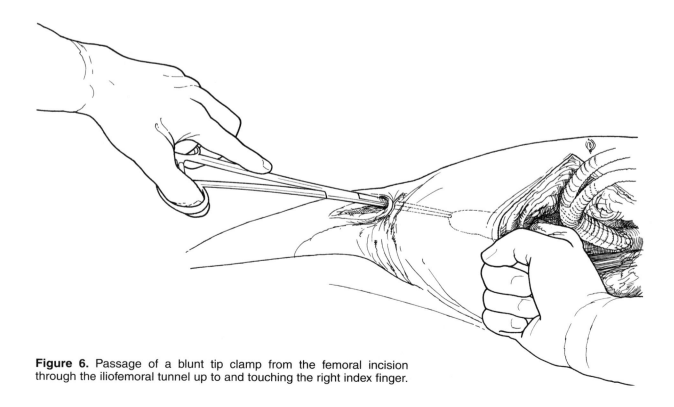

Figure 6. Passage of a blunt tip clamp from the femoral incision through the iliofemoral tunnel up to and touching the right index finger.

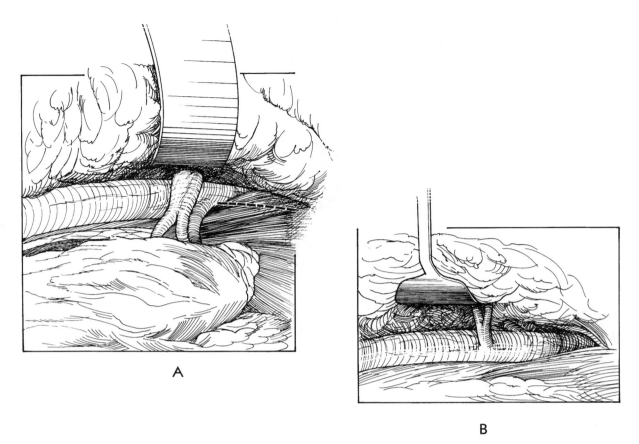

Figure 7. A. Thoracoretroperitoneal incision for exposure of the suprarenal aorta. Note that Gerota's fascia has been mobilized from the under surface of the left hemidiaphragm which causes the descent of the left kidney. The hatch marks show the line of division of the left diaphragmatic crux. Although the kidney can lie posteriorly, in most suprarenal procedures, the left kidney is rotated anteriorly (B).

irrigating balloon catheter and the kidneys perfused with cold (4° C) heparinized saline during the revascularization of the mesenterorenal arteries.

In aortoiliac occlusive disease in which an aortobifemoral bypass is going to be performed, the iliac vessels usually do not need mobilization if an end-to-side or an end-to-end aortic anastomosis is to be performed. In selected cases of localized aortic bifurcation disease, an *aorto-common iliac endarterectomy* can be performed through a left retroperitoneal approach since, in most cases of occlusive disease, the right common iliac artery can be mobilized to its bifurcation allowing for distal

intimal tacking sutures with excellent visualization. If the disease extends into the right external iliac artery, the procedure should be converted to an aortobifemoral bypass (Figs. 5 and 6), or the endarterectomy can be extended to the right femoral artery by using retrograde ring endarterectomy strippers from the femoral artery.

The Right Retroperitoneal Approach

This approach is excellent for right iliac and iliofemoral endarterectomy, right renal

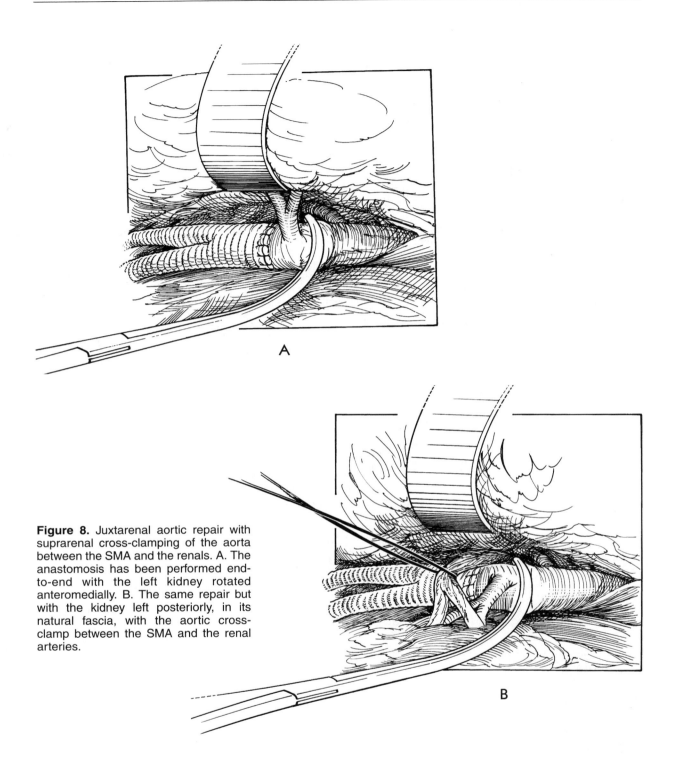

Figure 8. Juxtarenal aortic repair with suprarenal cross-clamping of the aorta between the SMA and the renals. A. The anastomosis has been performed end-to-end with the left kidney rotated anteromedially. B. The same repair but with the kidney left posteriorly, in its natural fascia, with the aortic cross-clamp between the SMA and the renal arteries.

revascularization and, in selected cases, for aortic reconstruction. It is applicable in patients having undergone prior left retroperitoneal surgical procedures (such as nephrec-

tomy) or in whom a left approach is contraindicated because of abdominal wall infection or the presence of a stoma. The major contraindication to using the right retroperitoneal approach is the presence of a large infrarenal aneurysm, or one with a very short neck or juxtarenal/suprarenal aortic pathology. In such cases, the cross-clamping from a right retroperitoneal approach is virtually impossible and, therefore, not recommended. Patient positioning is analogous (mirror image) to that used for the left retroperitoneal approach. For infrarenal aortic exposure, the incision starts below the umbilicus and is extended toward the 11th interspace. Entry into the retroperitoneum is carried out similar to the left retroperitoneal approach: at the junction of the rectus sheath and lateral abdominal wall muscles. The right kidney is left in its bed. It is also helpful to divide the right gonadal vein at its junction into the vena cava. This approach is very useful for aortobifemoral bypass in

selected cases with aortoiliac occlusive disease (Fig. 9), and is an excellent approach for unilateral right renal revascularization to the native aorto-right iliac system or to an aortic prosthetic graft.

Conclusion

The left retroperitoneal approach to the aorta is useful for aortic, mesenteric, renal (left), and iliac revascularizations. The right retroperitoneal approach is an excellent surgical strategy for isolated right renal revascularization and, in selected cases, a good alternative for aortic reconstruction. One can always enter

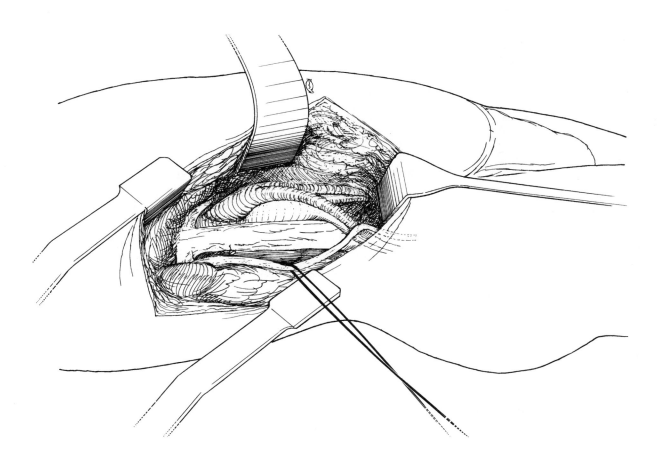

Figure 9. Right retroperitoneal approach for aortoiliac occlusive disease. Note the aortobifemoral bypass graft tunneled retroureterally on both sides. The proximal anastomosis can be performed end-to-side or end-to-end.

the peritoneal cavity if needed by simply incising the peritoneum. A need to examine the peritoneal contents should not, therefore, constitute a contraindication to utilizing this approach in aortic or renal reconstruction or aortomesenteric endarterectomy.

References

1. Darling RC III, Shah DM, Chang BB, Paty PSK, Leather RP. Current status of the use of retroperitoneal approach for reconstruction of the aorta and its branches. *Ann Surg* 1996; 224(4): 501-508.
2. Sicard GA, Reilly JM, Rubin BG, et al. Transabdominal versus retroperitoneal incision for abdominal aortic surgery: Report of a prospective randomized trial. *J Vasc Surg* 1995; 21; 174-183.
3. Sicard GA, Reilly JM. Left retroperitoneal approch to the aorta and its branches. Part I. *Ann Vasc Surg* 1994; 8(2): 12-19.
4. Reilly JM, Sicard GA. Right retroperitoneal approach to the aorta and its branches. Part II. *Ann Vasc Surg* 1994; 8(3): 318-323.
5. Shepard AD, Tollefson DFJ, Reddy DJ, et al. Left flank retroperitoneal exposure: A technical aid to complex aortic reconstruction. *J Vasc Surg* 1991; 14: 283-291.
6. Leather RP, Shah DM, Kaufman JL, et al. Comparative analysis for retroperitoneal and transperitoneal aortic replacement for aneurysms. *Surg Gynecol Obstet* 1989; 168: 387-393.
7. Hudson JC, Wurm WH, O'Donnell TF, et al. Hemodynamics and prostacyclin release in the early phases of aortic surgery: Comparison of transabdominal and retroperitoneal approaches. *J Vasc Surg* 1988; 7: 190-198.
8. Sicard GA, Freeman MB, VanderWoude JC, et al. Comparison between transabdominal and retroperitoneal approach for reconstruction of infrarenal abdominal aorta. *J Vasc Surg* 1987; 5: 19-27.
9. Giordano JM, Trout HH III. Anomalies of the inferior vena cava. *J Vasc Surg* 1986; 3: 294-298.

19

Transperitoneal Approach to the Infrarenal Aorta

Alain Branchereau, Jean-Pierre Mathieu

Infrarenal aortic reconstructive surgery has undergone rapid development since Oudot, and then Dubost, performed the first techniques. Aneurysms situated at this level are the most frequent of the arterial aneurysms; their surgical treatment has been well-established for many years and continues to demonstrate its efficacy in improving life expectancy. Aortobifemoral bypasses have some of the longest follow-ups and demonstrate the best long-term patency rates: 74% to 79% at 10 years.[1,2] For these reasons, infrarenal aortic surgery has become one of the most frequently performed and most stereotyped approaches in the range of vascular surgery. Although the thoracophreno-laparotomy was used initially in this type of surgery, the median laparotomy quickly became the preferred technique and by far the most frequently used. Currently there is an upsurge in interest in other approaches and their potential benefits, either for performing particular techniques or adapting to the varied types of patients. Although the median laparotomy remains the basic technique in dealing with the majority of situations, it is important that vascular surgeons be familiar with the alternative approaches in order to implement them in situations where they are more suitable and of greater benefit to the patient.

Median Transperitoneal Access

Patient Position

The patient is placed in decubitus with the upper limbs in 90 degree abduction on arm-rests and accessible to the anesthesiology team. To raise the aortic area a transverse roll is placed under the inferior angles of the scapulae or the operating table is angulated. The entire abdomen and both groins are in the surgical field. The surgeon is to the right of the patient with two assistants opposite.

From Vascular Surgical Approaches, edited by Alain Branchereau and Ramon Berguer. ©1999, Futura Publishing Co., Inc., Armonk, NY.

Laparotomy

The skin incision begins at the xyphoid process and descends, following the midline, then circles the umbilicus to the left and ends at or near the pubic symphysis. The subcutaneous tissue and the linea alba are entered above the umbilicus and the incision is then continued vertically to open the peritoneum. Once opened, the wall is raised and the laparotomy completed by a single cut upwards and downwards. An autostatic retractor is helpful in this type of incision. The simplest method is to use a retractor in which the valves resting on the edges of the laparotomy are combined with a subcostal retractor which improves upward opening and exposure. Autostatic frame-mounted retractors are becoming more and more popular with surgeons: they allow simultaneous opening of the abdominal wall and retraction of the viscera.

If it is decided to eviscerate the patient, which is frequently the case, the transverse colon is lifted upwards and covered with moist laps. Alternately, it can be retracted under the rib cage.

The intestinal loops are exteriorized to the right and protected by damp compresses or by a bowel bag. To avoid the exteriorized intestines obstructing the view of the surgical site, a retractor is placed to hold the intestinal loops. Care should be taken during evisceration to avoid disrupting hemodynamics. When the intestines are not exteriorized the loops are carefully laid in bundles under the rib cage and against the right side of the abdomen; they are protected by several layers of moist laps on which the retractor blades can rest.

Exposure

The posterior peritoneal fascia must be opened in order to expose the aorta. The primary marker is the duodenojejunal angle which should be clearly identified once the loops of the small intestine have been displaced. Any duodenal folds which may be present are detached in order to give clear exposure of the fourth portion of the duodenum and the beginning of the first jejunal

loop. With the surgeon or an assistant pulling the latter slightly upwards and to the right, the wall of the peritoneum is incised along the left side of the fourth duodenum and above the angle which it makes with the jejunum (Fig. 1). This incision is extended downwards as required, perpendicular to the abdominal aorta, which is identified by its pulse and consistency when calcified. Freeing of the duodenojejunal angle is followed by division of the ligament of Treitz which allows the fourth portion of the duodenum to be mobilized to the right and the duodenopancreatic block to be displaced upwards.

A large deep retractor or preferably two retractors are placed at the top of the peritoneal incision to widen the retroperitoneal cavity in a V-shape. One retractor rests on the duodenopancreatic block which is displaced upwards to the right, the other holds onto the peritoneal fold which underpins the inferior mesenteric vein (Fig. 2). Depending on the case and/or the need to improve exposure upwards and to the left, the inferior mesenteric vein may be sectioned between two ligatures without adverse consequence. The next step consists of identifying the left renal vein which marks the upper limit of the aortic dissection.

In thin patients the left renal vein can be seen once the deep retractors are placed at the edges of the peritoneum (Fig. 2). In more obese patients the left renal vein can only be seen after the anterior surface of the aorta has been dissected. It is identified with a finger before the fat tissue that covers it is incised with scissors. After the aortic wall is identified, the tissue covering it is dissected from the bottom upwards to the lower edge of the renal vein, which marks the upper limit of this dissection. The dissection between the aorta and the surrounding fat tissue is easily done. There is occasional bleeding that can be controlled by electrocoagulation or by a few minutes of pressure with warm saline-soaked laps. When the lower edge of the left renal vein is reached, it is freed, exposing the anterior hemicircumference of the aorta.

In most cases, it is at this level below the left renal vein that the aorta is clamped. This dissection generally involves only the anterior and lateral walls of the aorta. Any possible polar

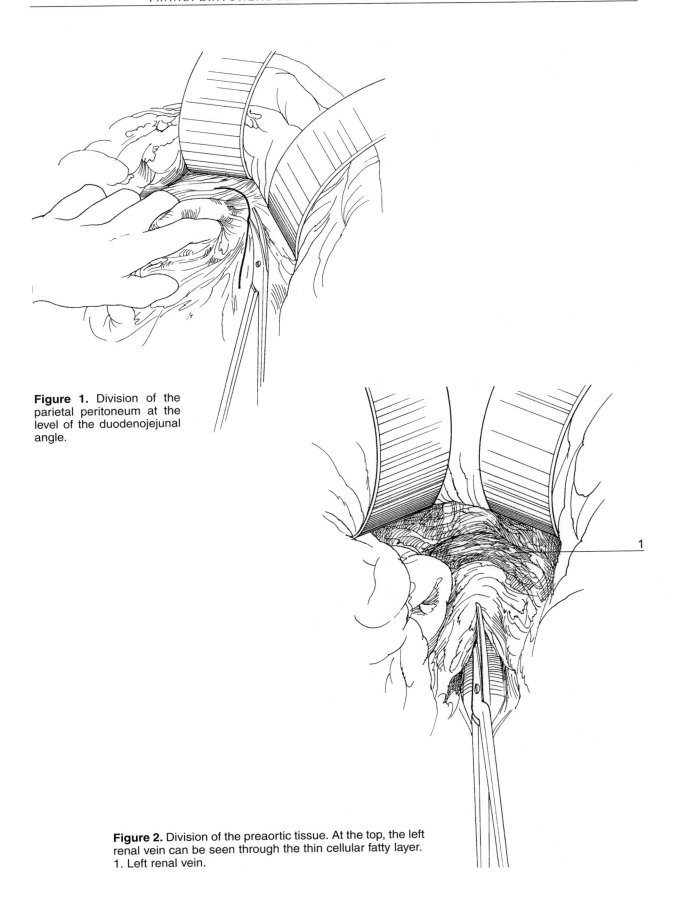

Figure 1. Division of the parietal peritoneum at the level of the duodenojejunal angle.

Figure 2. Division of the preaortic tissue. At the top, the left renal vein can be seen through the thin cellular fatty layer.
1. Left renal vein.

arteries, previously identified by arteriography, should be isolated and preserved. The small lymphatic collaterals are coagulated or ligated and then cut. The posterior wall and the origin of the lumbar arteries are not dissected other than in special cases. The lower part of the dissection generally continues as far as the inferior mesenteric artery. The origin and first centimeters of this are always exposed. Depending on the case, this artery is isolated and clamped, or it is held within the clamp which occludes the distal segment of the infrarenal aorta.

Extension

When doing a bypass, exposure of the aortic segment between the left renal vein and the inferior mesenteric artery is generally sufficient because the aorta immediately below the renals is relatively uninvolved by atherosclerosis. In addition, this limited approach best preserves the periaortic plexus in males. In certain cases, the extent of the lesions or tactical considerations requires either upward or downward extension of the approach.

Upward Extension

The aim of upward extension is to gain access to the inter- or suprarenal aorta and it requires a subcostal retractor. The main hindrance is the left renal vein which must be either mobilized or temporarily sectioned and restored after aortic reconstruction. In practice, a choice between these two maneuvers must be made from the start, because the ligation and division of the branches of the main renal vein is relatively incompatible with dividing, even temporarily, the main renal vein. Mobilization of the renal vein necessitates dividing some of these venous affluents, especially the suprarenal and gonadal veins, to permit dissection of the origin of the two renal arteries and placement of a clamp above them. Sectioning the left renal vein gives an excellent view of the entire inter- and suprarenal aorta (Fig. 3). To do this,

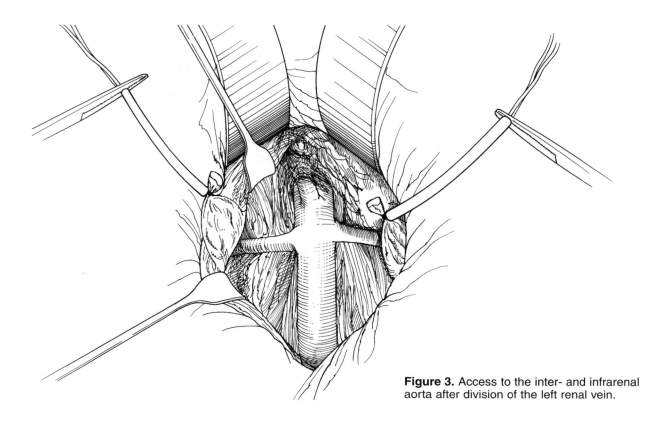

Figure 3. Access to the inter- and infrarenal aorta after division of the left renal vein.

preservation of the branches emptying into the left main renal vein is desirable since they provide venous drainage and lessen venous renal hypertension. Rather than dividing the main renal vein between clamps, we usually perform two circular purse-string sutures on the vein, near its caval junction. After division, these purses are secured with rubber tourniquets (Rummels) which assure hemostasis and separate the two venous ends to expose the aorta. The vein continuity is restored by anastomosis once the aortic reconstruction is completed.

Downward Extension

There are two potential problems in accessing the aortic segment situated below the inferior mesenteric artery (IMA): the presence of the superior hypogastric plexus and the iliocava venous confluence which closely adheres to the posterior ward of the artery. Access to the anterior wall of the aorta is performed by direct incision of the covering tissue along the midline. The nerve fibers are best preserved by performing a strictly median, clean section and by laterally rolling back all the fatty tissue containing the sympathetic nervous fibers.

However, as soon as the aortic dissection reaches beyond the level of the IMA, it is inevitable that certain nerve fibers will be divided with some adverse consequences particularly if the arterial dissection extends through the first centimeters of the common iliac arteries. Dissection between the venous and arterial planes at this level is difficult and may result in venous injuries difficult to control. Freeing the posterior wall of the aorta at this level should be avoided. In cases where it is necessary, we prefer to divide the aorta across and then dissect from top to bottom dividing the lumbar arteries. In practice and in most cases, freeing the posterior face of the aortic bifurcation is unnecessary. The iliac arteries are either clamped at a lower level or occluded endoaortically.

Variations of Aortic Exposure

During a median laparotomy, the aorta is generally exposed by opening of the posterior peritoneum. However, it is possible and even useful in certain cases to approach the aorta by detaching the right or left colon.

The right laterocolic approach begins with an incision of the posterior parietal peritoneum from the right colic angle and continues along the right colic gutter (Fig. 4). The right colon is freed as far as the cecum and displaced to the left along with the mass of the intestinal loops. This maneuver is followed by retroduodeno-pancreatic detachment. The inferior vena cava (IVC) is approached at the level where it joins the renal veins behind the second portion of the duodenum (Fig. 5). The next step consists of freeing and exposing the entire anterior wall and the left lateral border of the IVC ligating and dividing several branches, including the left gonadal vein. The aorta is exposed below the left renal vein dissecting its anterior wall, from top to bottom. The infrarenal aorta is exposed as far as its termination using this approach which gives excellent exposure of the IVC, renocaval confluent, right renal pedicle, right kidney, and the right iliac artery.

The left laterocolic approach consists of freeing the posterior mesogastrium with medial rotation of the viscera. A peritoneal incision, which should allow freeing of the left parietal mesocolic attachment, begins at the level of the left colic angle and continues upwards following the posterior edge of the spleen and then on the diaphragm towards the triangular ligament of the liver (Fig. 6). Freeing of the splenic adhesions followed by mobilization of the spleen is the most delicate part of this procedure. The colon, the spleen, and the tail of the pancreas are displaced upwards and to the right in one block. This leaves the kidney, adrenal gland, and the veins draining into the cava to the back of the dissection (Fig. 7). The ureter separated from the peritoneum remains to the rear with the kidney. The stomach is mobilized and is displaced to the right along with the visceral mass. In this way access is gained to the anterior wall of the aorta, which is crossed by the left renal vein, as far as the left crux of the diaphragm (Fig. 8). Access to the posterolateral wall of the aorta and to the left renal artery is helped by using the retrorenal plane of detachment (Fig. 7). This technique (see Chapter 17) is used mainly to access the suprarenal aorta but also gives adequate access to the entire infrarenal aorta.

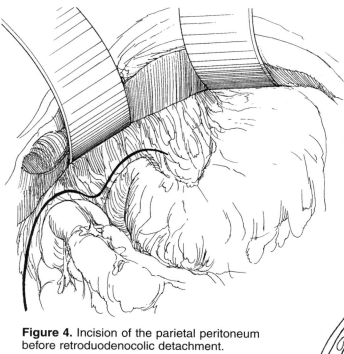

Figure 4. Incision of the parietal peritoneum before retroduodenocolic detachment.

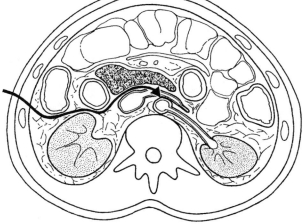

Figure 5. Pathway to the aorta using a right-sided approach with retroduodenocolic detachment.

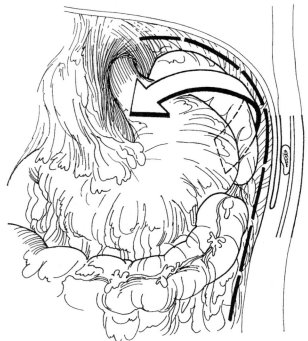

Figure 6. Incision of the parietal peritoneum for aortic exposure through a left retroperitoneal approach. The arrow indicates the direction of the medial visceral rotation.

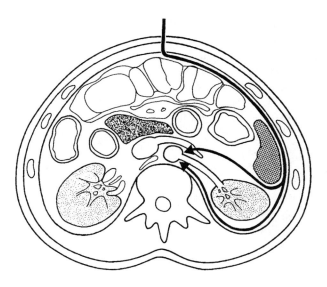

Figure 7. Pre- or retrorenal pathway to the aorta in a left retroperitoneal approach.

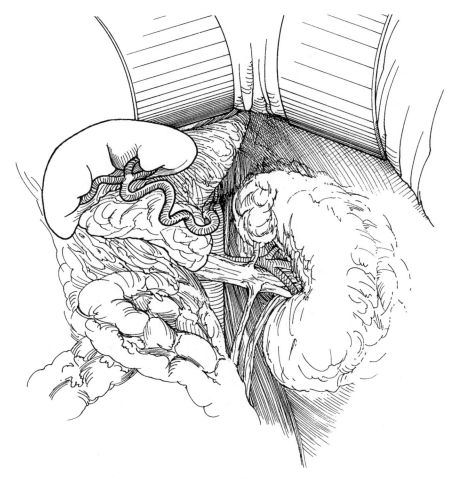

Figure 8. Access to the supra-or infrarenal aorta using a left retroperitoneal approach with prerenal detachment and medial visceral rotation.

Horizontal Transperitoneal Approach

The patient is placed on the table as in the previous descriptions. It is important to place a transverse roll under the inferior angles of the scapulae or, better yet, to tilt the operating table 20 to 30 degrees. The peak of the angle should lie midway between the umbilicus and the xiphoid process. This maneuver raises the aortic region and helps retraction of the edges of the incision.

Laparotomy

A transversal rectilinear skin incision is most frequently used and is situated 2 cm or 3 cm above the umbilicus (Fig. 9). Laterally, it terminates 2 cm beyond the lateral edge of the rectus muscle. The subcutaneous cellular tissue and the anterior muscular aponeurosis are incised simultaneously. The anterior sheath of the rectus muscle is transversally incised. This incision extends laterally onto the anterior face of the aponeurosis of the great oblique muscle in the same direction as its fibers. Sectioning of the aponeurosis reveals the recti which are cut across transversally using cautery after liberating their posterior

attachments (Fig. 10). This dissection requires meticulous electrocoagulation of the vascular pedicles, the largest of which may necessitate division between ligatures. Once this maneuver is completed, the deep plane, consisting of the posterior sheath of the rectus muscles attached to the peritoneum, is incised. The two edges of the incision are raised by hooking the fingers on either side of the sheath of the rectus muscle in order to detach the wall of the underlying viscera (Fig. 11). The peritoneum is opened at the midline and the division is completed across using cautery and extending it 1-2 cm beyond the lateral edge of the sheath of the rectus muscle.

Patient Position

Generally this procedure is performed without intestinal exteriorization. The greater omentum, the transverse colon, and its mesocolon are displaced upwards under the rib cage. The intestinal loops are separated into three bundles and are positioned respectively: upwards to the right, in the right parietocolic groove, and downwards to the right. The sigmoid colon is displaced downwards and to the left. Damp intestinal compresses protect and retain the viscera in this position (Fig. 12).

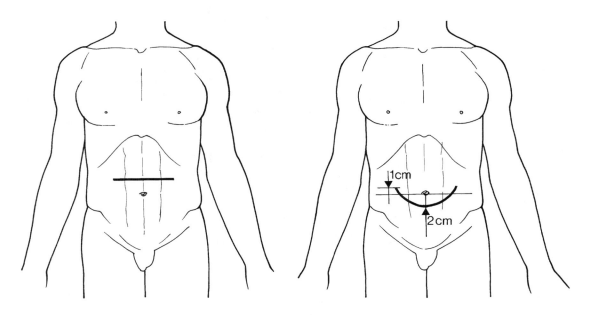

Figure 9. Two incisions for transverse laparotomy.

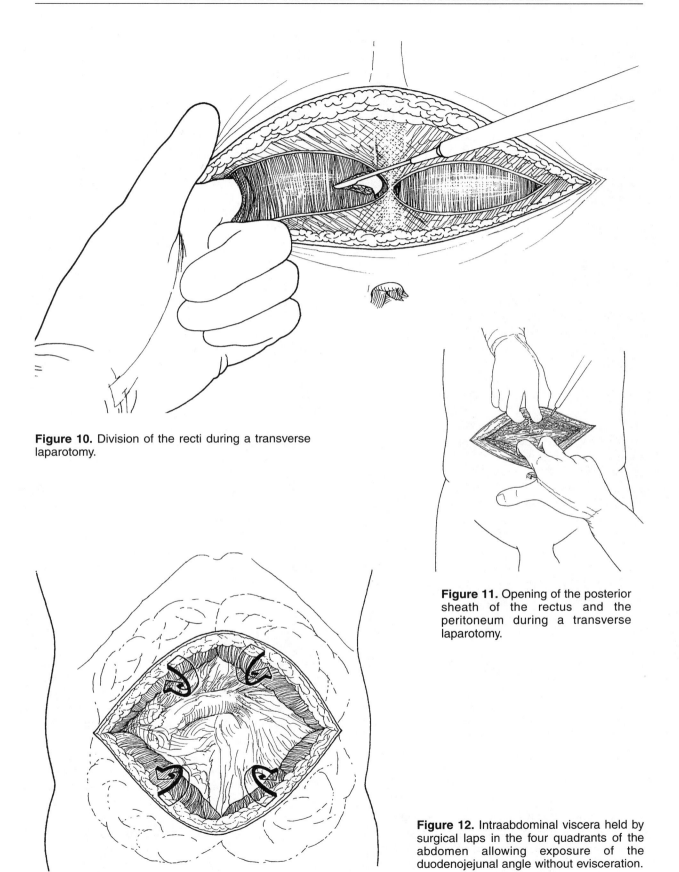

Figure 10. Division of the recti during a transverse laparotomy.

Figure 11. Opening of the posterior sheath of the rectus and the peritoneum during a transverse laparotomy.

Figure 12. Intraabdominal viscera held by surgical laps in the four quadrants of the abdomen allowing exposure of the duodenojejunal angle without evisceration.

Two retractors placed near the top allow the displaced viscera to be pulled upwards along with the duodenopancreatic block. A retractor placed laterally, with a flexible curved blade, on the right edge of the incision, retains the intestinal loops. Towards the bottom, a large retractor separates the bladder and the sigmoid colon which are protected by moist laps. Autostatic frames with multiple valves are helpful for this exposure. Exposure of the aorta is performed as described for the median laparotomy.

Technique Variations

The skin incision may extend well beyond the lateral edge of the rectus muscle. This helps in exposing the aorta in obese patients or if a simultaneous renal revascularization is planned.

The cutaneous incision may be arc-shaped with an upward curve in order to improve exposure of the iliac arteries down to their bifurcation. The incision passes 2 cm or 3 cm below the umbilicus and rises laterally as far as a point situated beyond the lateral edge of the rectus muscle at a level situated 1-2 cm above the umbilicus (Fig. 9). The upper abdominal wall canopy is held by a transfixion stitch to the epigastric wall. If after all exposure is completed, intestinal evisceration is required, this is performed as in the median laparotomy. In this case this approach loses one of its major advantages.

Discussion

The most serious complication associated with infrarenal aortic exposure is a large venous injury. This may be the consequence of a congenital anomaly, of which the most common example is the retroaortic renal vein, or of dissection injury, due to the close venous relationship which normally exists. A CT scan allows identification of venous anomalies preoperatively. When CT scan is not available, the first step should be to identify the left renal vein before any aortic clamping is performed.

The sexual functional problems associated with dissection of the nerve plexus, in males, are difficult to avoid. The anatomic grouping of the nerve fibers is highly variable and their role in ejaculation and erection is still uncertain. The variations and the density of this nerve plexus make an anatomic solution to this problem almost impossible.

When exposing the aorta or aortoiliac function the only preventive measure is to remain as far as possible from these elements. Of the techniques used for aortic exposure, two appear to better preserve sexual function: the median or transverse transperitoneal approach when exposure is limited to the segment of the aorta between the renal arteries and the IMA, and the retroperitoneal approach when limited to exposure of the aorta without dissection of the origin of the iliac arteries.

Advantages and Inconveniences of Different Techniques

The median laparotomy is the basic technique. It allows upward extension and if necessary, separate clamping of the supraceliac aorta via the lesser omentum. It allows downward access to the two iliac arteries, and finally, with some difficulty, it permits control of the visceral arteries with more or less difficulty. In emergency cases where lesion assessment and surgical approach may not be totally established preoperatively, this technique is the obvious one to select.

Conversely, its important respiratory complications include a reduction in vital capacity in the order of 50%.[3] Evisceration, which is generally required, disturbs intraoperative hemodynamics and increases postoperative ileus.[4] Finally, this approach results in a substantial number of long-term eventrations.[5]

The transverse laparotomy without evisceration is reported to be less traumatic. This has never been scientifically proven but has seemed obvious to surgical teams that employ this technique. Respiratory complications and abdominal wall pain are decreased and there is less intestinal ileus in the postoperative period. The biomechanic characteristics of the abdominal wall explain the advantages of this approach. The oblique muscles of the abdomen exert strong traction towards the sides. This traction is greatest at the midline.

The rectus muscles may be considered as rigid supports on which the previously mentioned muscles exert traction but they themselves exert minimal or no traction from top to bottom (Fig. 13). This explains why closure of a transverse laparotomy is performed without traction and results in less postoperative pain and a reduced risk of secondary eventration. Contrarily, this approach satisfactorily exposes only the infrarenal aorta. Exposure of the renal arteries is limited and may only be sufficient to treat ostial lesions. Extension to the iliac arteries is also limited; the use of an arched approach allows access to the iliac bifurcations but extension of this approach remains problematic. Finally, upward extension is very limited and is extremely difficult, if not impossible.

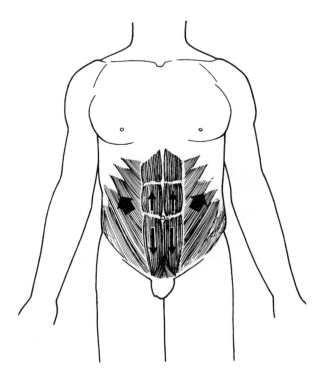

Figure 13. Lines of force of the muscles of the abdominal wall.

Extraperitoneal approaches have fewer respiratory and intestinal complications than a median transperitoneal approach and result in abdominal closures which are less painful and more reliable, as long as the intercostal nerves are preserved. These approaches give excellent access to the infrarenal aorta and even to the left renal artery. They also allow convenient access to the suprarenal aorta and its mesenteric branches.

Criteria for Choice

Lesions to Be Treated

If the operation is limited to the infrarenal aorta (aortobifemoral bypass or simple aortic aneurysm), the choice is generally either a median transperitoneal or a transverse approach. Although the first is simpler and faster, we prefer the second for its smoother postoperative recovery and the reduced risk of eventration. In the case of upward extension, if the celiac aorta needs to be clamped, a laparotomy is sufficient. If one needs to control the suprarenal aorta and the origin of the visceral arteries, a thoracoretroperitoneal approach should be chosen. For the latter the entry should be between the 11th and 9th intercostal space depending on the lesions. In general, access to the suprarenal aorta is improved the higher the incision. Another possibility is to use a median laparotomy with medial visceral rotation. This technique is more traumatic than those previously described and has the additional risk of splenic rupture and pancreatitis. Compared to a retroperitoneal approach it gives better access to the visceral arteries and especially to the right renal artery. In the case of downward extension, i.e., if a complex procedure is planned at the level of the iliac bifurcations or beyond, a median laparotomy is more suitable.

Associated Lesions

In the case of planned simultaneous restoration of bilateral renal lesions, a transperitoneal approach should be chosen. In our experience a transverse approach is appropriate where the procedure is relatively simple whereas a median approach is more suitable if difficulties in exposure are anticipated. Temporary sectioning of the left renal vein improves simultaneous access to the aorta and the two renal arteries and is generally indicated in this situation. In the case of simultaneous reconstruction of the aorta and the left renal artery, the retroperitoneal approach gives excellent access to the left renal artery and infrarenal aorta; it also allows easy suprarenal clamping but its distal exposure is limited.

In simultaneous restoration of the right renal artery, the standard midline transperitoneal approach is generally sufficient.

If a complex and/or distal procedure on the right renal artery is planned, autotransplantation, or if associated nephrectomy is involved, two alternative approaches can be considered. One is a vertical transperitoneal approach with mobilization of the right colon and duodenum, which gives good access to the renal pedicle and the right kidney as well as the infrarenal aorta. The other is performing a right retroperitoneal approach to expose the right renal pedicle and right kidney and the infrarenal aorta.

If mesenteric artery revascularization is planned, the transverse transperitoneal approach allows distal access to the superior mesenteric and hepatic arteries. If control of the first few centimeters of these arteries is necessary, the best solution is to access the suprarenal aorta and its branches by a left retrocolic detachment and medial visceral rotation. The exposure is superior to that obtained by a retroperitoneal approach which gives access only to the origin of these arteries.

Local Conditions

Transperitoneal approaches should be avoided in obese patients with a hostile abdomen, colostomies, or urinary derivations. Low retroperitoneal approaches provide limited exposure, and the incisions are close to the areas where most of the ostomies are placed. A high posterior retroperitoneal approach with resection of the 11th or 12th rib is generally the best solution. In practice there is no single solution; it is important, however, to know the range of options in this situation in order to choose the most suitable.[6]

Conclusion

Access to the infrarenal aorta is easy and description of the various techniques may seem unnecessary. However, the small benefit gained by the choice of an unusual approach but one that is well suited to an individual case contributes to the success of the procedure. Vascular surgeons should be aware of the multiplicity of alternatives.[6]

References

1. Nevelsteen A, Wouters I, Suy R. Aortofemoral Dacron reconstruction for aortoiliac occlusive disease: A 25 year survey. *Eur J Vasc Surg* 1991; 5: 179-186
2. Crawford ES, Bomberger RA, Glaeser DH, et al. Aortoiliac occlusive disease: Factors influencing survival and function following reconstructive operation over a twenty five year period. *Surgery* 1981; 90: 1055-1067.
3. Gouin F, Martin C, Auffray JP. Principes généraux d'anesthésie réanimation en chirurgie abdominale chez l'adulte. *Encycl Med Chir.* Paris. Anesthésie réanimation 36560 A10 3-1984.
4. Hudson JC, Wurm WH, O'Donneill TF, et al. Hemodynamics and prostacyclin release in the early phases of aortic surgery: Comparison of transabdominal and retroperitoneal approaches. *J Vasc Surg* 1988; 7: 190-198.
5. Lord RSA, Crozier JA, Snell J, Meek AC. Transverse abdominal incisions compared with midline incisions for elective infrarenal aortic reconstruction: Predisposition to incisional hernia in patients with increased intraoperative blood loss. *J Vasc Surg* 1994; 20: 27-33.
6. De Natale RW, Crawford ES, Safi HJ, Coselli JS. Graft reconstruction to treat disease of the abdominal aorta in patients with colostomies, ileostomies and abdominal wall urinary stomata. *J Vasc Surg* 1987; 6: 240-247.

20

The Iliac Arteries

Pierre Tournigand

Reconstructive surgery of the iliac arteries is less frequent since the advent of transluminal angioplasty. The iliac veins are rarely the site of reconstructive surgery. In fact, of all the vascular approaches those to the iliac vessels are now some of the least used. Exposure of the iliac arteries is not particularly traumatic and it can be done extraperitoneally. The disadvantage, however, is the limitation of their exposure, particularly the difficulty in extending it proximally. Iliac approaches may be either oblique or vertical; the latter may be lateral or medial.

Anatomic Background

The first parietal layer is the aponeurosis of the greater oblique muscle which at the lateral margin of the rectus muscle becomes the anterior sheath of this muscle. The next layer is the transverse and lesser oblique muscles whose aponeurosis is fused to form the posterior sheath of the rectus muscle as far inferiorly as the linea arcuata. Below this, the common aponeurosis of both the lesser oblique and transverse muscles join the anterior sheath of the rectus muscle. A detachable space is found posterior to the transverse muscle to which the peritoneum adheres. This adhesion is less the further it is from the midline. Conversely, it is densely adherent at the lateral margin of the rectus muscle and behind it. Therefore, the detachment of this layer begins at the outside. This detachable space leads to the laterovesical space which continues upwards with the perirenal fossa. The outline of the psoas muscle is the essential reference point: the iliac vessels follow its medial surface, the genitofemoral nerve runs over its superior surface, and the femorocutaneous nerve stays lateral to it. The twelfth intercostal nerve must be handled carefully as it runs between the lesser oblique and transverse muscles at the upper lateral abdominal wall.

Oblique Access

The incision follows a line that joins the tip of the twelfth rib to the midpoint between umbilicus and the pubis without crossing the

From Vascular Surgical Approaches, edited by Alain Branchereau and Ramon Berguer. ©1999, Futura Publishing Co., Inc., Armonk, NY.

midline (Fig. 1). The length of the incision varies according to the patient's morphology. The incision may be displaced upwards or downwards depending on the level of the iliac bifurcation, ascertained by arteriography. The aponeurosis is opened obliquely and the incision continues over the lateral half of the sheath of the rectus muscle. This exposes the fibers of this muscle and allows visualization of the lateral limit of the posterior surface of the rectus sheath. The lesser oblique muscle lies more laterally with its fibers running in the opposite diagonal. These muscle bundles are attached by a very short fibrous segment to the lateral edge of the sheath of the rectus muscle (Fig. 2). It is very easy to divide them by separating them with the fingers or retractors and to continue the same division of the

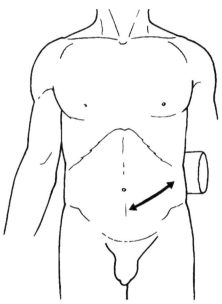

Figure 1. Skin incision for the oblique approach to the iliac arteries.

Figure 2. Oblique approach. The rectus muscle and the anterior sheath of the rectus muscle have been opened. A finger enlarges the opening by separating the fibers of the greater oblique muscle.
1. Greater oblique muscle.
2. Minor oblique muscle.
3. Rectus muscle.

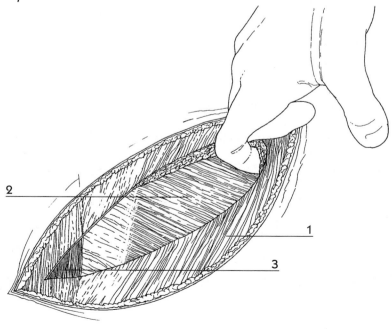

transverse muscle by simply changing the direction of the muscular retraction (Fig. 3). The transversalis fascia is raised with two forceps to be opened just enough to identify the peritoneum. For separation of the peritoneum it is easier to first use closed scissors and then a finger tip or a gauze moving in all directions, especially downwards about the posterior surface of the rectus sheath (Fig. 4). It is at this level in the process of detachment that the

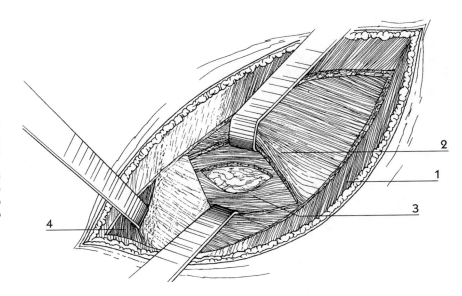

Figure 3. Oblique approach. At the bottom left of the diagram the rectus muscle is retracted. In the center, two retractors separate the fibers of the minor oblique muscle. This reveals the fibers of the deeper transverse muscle which have been separated to allow the retroperitoneal fat to appear.
1. Greater oblique muscle.
2. Minor oblique muscle.
3. Transverse muscle.
4. Rectus muscle.

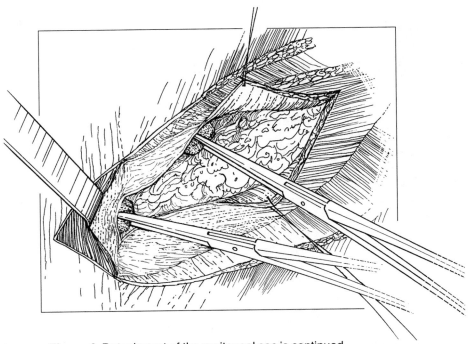

Figure 4. Detachment of the peritoneal sac is continued forwards and upwards with the aid of a gauze.

peritoneum is usually torn. Any tears must be immediately repaired; otherwise, they enlarge and the small bowel invades the operative field. Once detached, the peritoneal sac is progressively pushed back towards the midline. As this maneuver progresses, the fat of the laterovesical space appears towards the midline. Sometimes the space obtained with these maneuvers is insufficient and the medial internal part of the incision needs to be extended by cutting 2 cm or 3 cm into the posterior sheath of the rectus muscle after detaching the peritoneum from it (Fig. 5). Once the outline of the psoas muscle is identified, the dissection progresses towards the back with the surgeon's hand supinated, detaching the peritoneum from inside the psoas with the fingernails in contact with the freed anterior surface of the muscle. The ureter, attached to the peritoneal sac, is located. The vascular bundle is then identified. On the right side is the right edge of the common iliac vein, and the artery lies medially and anteriorly. On the left the iliac bifurcation is first palpated by the finger. One or two retractors maintain the exposure during dissection of the iliac bifurcation (Fig. 6). The role of the assistant is essential because it is not possible to use a self-retaining retractor here unless an Omnitract® retractor (Omnilaparo-Tract, Cardio-Choc, Nice, France) is used. The close relation between the arterial and the venous walls must be kept in mind, especially when the arteries are dilated. The artery may be lifted with forceps in order to see clearly the vein and its line of adhesion to the artery before placing a dissector around the artery.

Closing this access is very simple and follows the same anatomic planes. After placing a drain, the visceral sac is released and the aponeurotic muscles sutured. The transverse and the lesser oblique muscles are sutured together with the posterior sheath of the rectus muscle. The aponeurosis of the oblique muscle is then closed. The fascia superficialis is well-developed and permits good skin closure.

Incidents, Accidents, Limitations

The most frequent problem is opening the peritoneum. This is a minor inconvenience if it is a small rent but a major one if it tends to enlarge. Contusion of the ureter may follow strong retraction and can cause intraoperative hematuria. Rarely, it may lead to wall necrosis and leakage. Contusion of the genitofemoral nerve may be caused by the edge of a retractor applied to the anterior surface of the psoas. Eventrations occur but are rare if care is taken to suture each layer separately. This oblique access gives very good exposure of the iliac bifurcation and the external iliac artery but the exposure of the common iliac artery, particularly of its origin, is limited. Except in special circumstances (thin patient, very low bifurcation), control of the distal aorta and of the opposite iliac artery is impossible using this approach. This means that if such a need arises during this approach, there are only two solutions: to abandon the iliac approach and use a midline laparotomy, or to extend the incision upwards to the 12th rib and downwards beyond the midline. This extension transforms this limited approach into a low retroperitoneal Rob-type approach, with all the inconveniences linked to the required extensive muscular division and the possible trauma to the 11th and 12th intercostal nerves.

Suprainguinal External Iliac Approach

The incision resembles McBurney's incision but is placed lower and more medial, two or three finger widths above the line joining the anterior superior iliac spine to the pubic spine. It is centered in the middle of the inguinal ligament and is 3-4 cm long. After opening the aponeurosis of the oblique muscle, the muscle fibers which make up the conjoined tendon are pushed back, using a gauze, from the lower lip of the aponeurosis. This reveals the subperitoneal fat through which the artery is identified as it arises from the pelvic concavity (Fig. 7). Thanks to its flexibility, a loop passed around the artery allows it to be easily pulled to the surface giving sufficient length to perform an anastomosis. A few sutures on the aponeurosis reinforced by suture of the fascia superficialis are sufficient to close this incision. This approach has

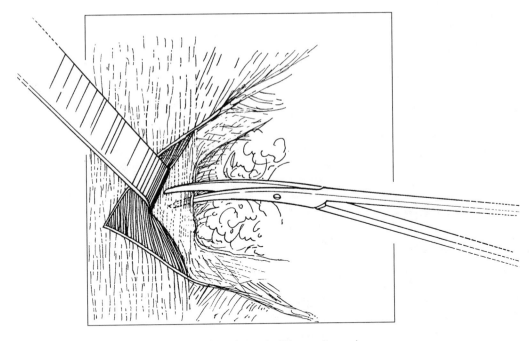

Figure 5. After detachment of the peritoneal sac the posterior sheath of the rectus muscle is cut.

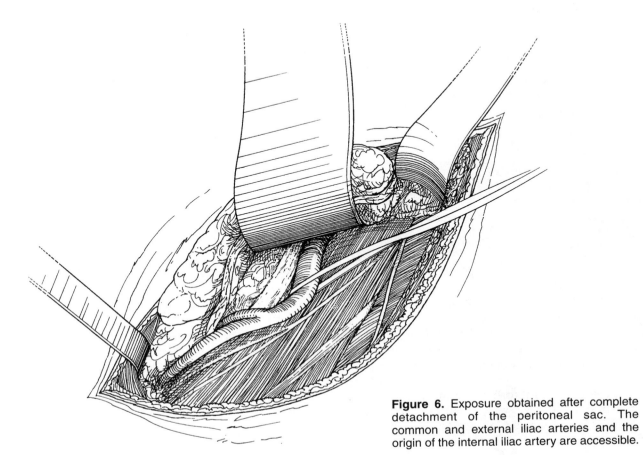

Figure 6. Exposure obtained after complete detachment of the peritoneal sac. The common and external iliac arteries and the origin of the internal iliac artery are accessible.

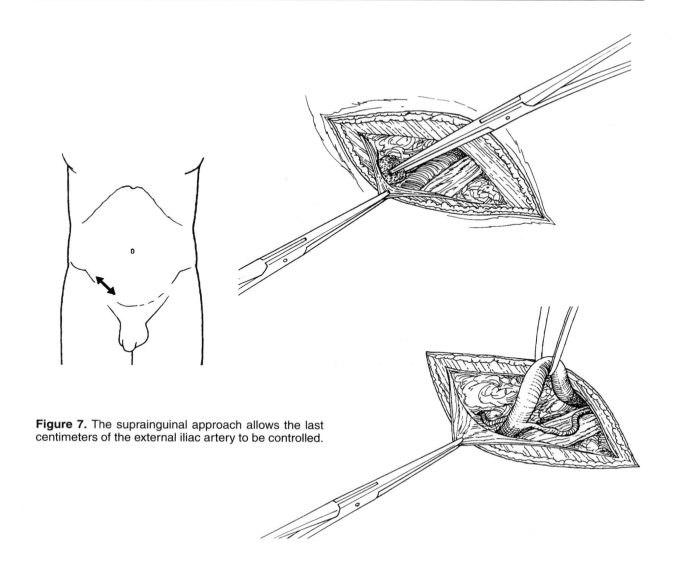

Figure 7. The suprainguinal approach allows the last centimeters of the external iliac artery to be controlled.

specific and restricted applications only. It allows proximal control of an aneurysm of the femoral artery or of traumatic or septic bleeding from the femoral artery. It allows construction of a cross-iliofemoral (subcutaneous or retromuscular) bypass. Such bypasses have a better anatomic lay than those of the femorofemoral type. Finally, it allows distal anastomosis of an aortic femoral bypass when patency of the common femoral artery is certain but one wishes to avoid a groin incision.

Vertical Approaches

The vertical subperitoneal approach is an upward extension of the incision used to expose the femoral artery in the groin[1] (Fig. 8). This procedure consists of cutting the inguinal ligament and extending the opening upwards from the external iliac artery over the iliac vessels. The vertical incision follows the external margin of the rectus muscle from the middle of the inguinal ligament. The latter is cut in front of the artery, first in its aponeurotic part and then in the muscular part of the conjoined tendon. This procedure opens the retroperitoneal space in front of the vessels; it is then easy to continue the detachment of the peritoneal sac by pushing it upwards away from the vessels. The muscular division is extended vertically as far as the site to be exposed. This easy access permits exposure from the common iliac artery to the femoral artery. This has a certain advantage when performing open endarterectomy of the iliofemoral segment. However, the extensive muscular division added to the division of the inguinal ligament often results in abdominal wall mechanical and neuritic problems. Due to its tension the inguinal ligament is difficult to repair satisfactorily. For these reasons, this approach has been more or less abandoned.

Extraperitoneal, Subumbilical Approach

This is a classic approach to the ureters. It can also be useful in iliac surgery as it allows simultaneous access to the two iliac arteries through the same incision.[2]

Anatomic Characteristics

The space used is the laterovesical space which extends from one side to the other crossing the midline. Its upper limit is marked by the two linea arcuata and by the umbilicus. At this level the posterior sheath of the rectus muscle has disappeared and the detachment of the peritoneal sac is extremely easy. In contrast, in the upper part of the field the exposure is hindered by the lateral fibrous attachment of the linea arcuata under which the peritoneum is found. The clivage plane is crossed by the spermatic cord which limits the detachment of the peritoneum towards the top. To have sufficient access, the spermatic cord must be isolated in order to detach the peritoneum and free the attachment of the linea arcuata to the transverse muscle.

Technique

The skin incision begins at the pubis and goes around the left of the umbilicus (Fig. 9). Care must be taken to remain well to the middle without straying into the muscular fibers. The anterior aponeurosis is opened from the upper edge of the pubis to the umbilicus. The two edges are then raised with Kocher clamps and the detachment begun at the posterior layer, from the midline to the side being exposed first, in contact with the fibers of the rectus muscle that has no posterior sheath at this level (Fig. 9). The psoas muscle appears but the clivage plane is hindered by the spermatic cord which closely anchors the peritoneal sac. Dissection continues above and outside it at the posterior surface and the lateral edge of the rectus muscle in order to continue the plane that ends at the level of the linea arcuata. At this point, the arcuate line must be carefully cut with scissors at the level of its parietal insertion. The peritoneum is identified and progressively detached (Fig. 10). A gauze helps finish freeing the anterior and medial surface of the psoas exposing the iliac vessels from the aortic bifurcation to the inguinal ligament (Fig. 11). The difference

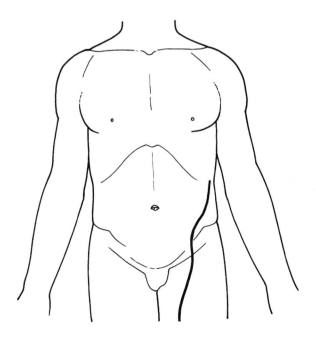

Figure 8. Vertical subperitoneal approach.

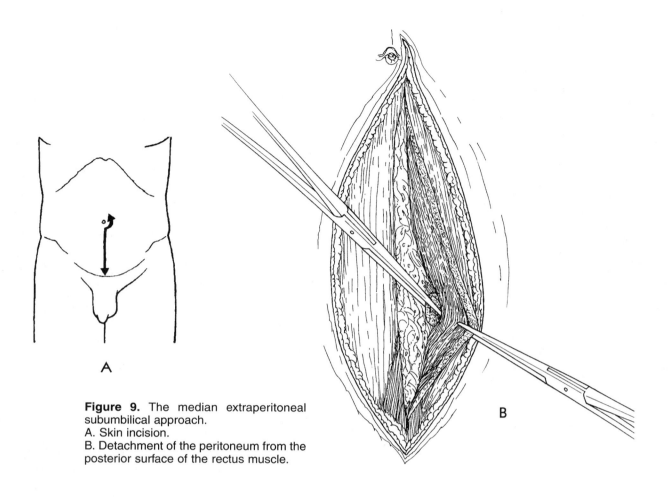

Figure 9. The median extraperitoneal subumbilical approach.
A. Skin incision.
B. Detachment of the peritoneum from the posterior surface of the rectus muscle.

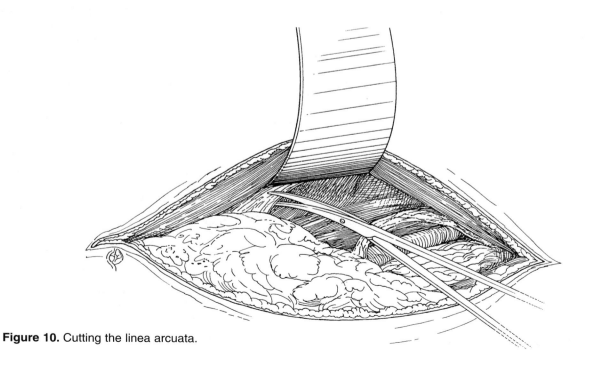

Figure 10. Cutting the linea arcuata.

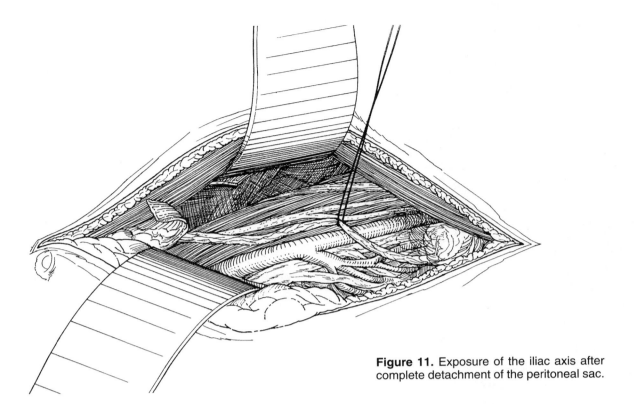

Figure 11. Exposure of the iliac axis after complete detachment of the peritoneal sac.

between this and the oblique approach is mainly that the iliac axis and especially the internal iliac artery are viewed differently: running away from the operator in the oblique approach or dropping away in the median approach. This angle allows all the branches of the hypogastric artery to be easily recognized and isolated into the minor pelvis without having to be concerned about the veins which are clearly exposed. The closure is the same as that of the subumbilical laparotomy.

Discussion

The oblique access is the traditional approach: it is simple, repairs are easy and it leads to few eventrations. The difficulty of its upward extension is its only drawback. This may be overcome by enlarging the incision and transforming the approach into a retroperitoneal aortic approach. The median subperitoneal approach is more complex but offers three distinct advantages. First, it allows synchronous access to bilateral iliac lesions especially

those of the external iliac arteries which are seen frequently. Second, it is time saving and has few abdominal wall sequelae. In case of unforeseen problems with the aorta, a rapid transperitoneal midline xiphopubic laparotomy can be performed. Third, it gives excellent exposure of the internal iliac artery and its branches which is of particular interest for the rare cases of aneurysm of the hypogastric artery. The vertical femoral iliac approach with division of the inguinal ligament, on the other hand, should no longer be used because of the abdominal wall neuromuscular deficits that may occur.

References

1. Cormier JM, Santot J, Frileux C, Arnulf G. *Nouveau traité de technique chirurgicale.* Artères, veines, lymphatiques. Tome V. Paris, Masson 1970 pp 208-212.
2. Shumacker HB Jr. Midline extraperitoneal exposure of the abdominal aorta and iliac arteries. *Surg Gynecol Obstet* 1972; 135: 791-792.

21

Mesenteric Arteries

*Jean-Michel Jausseran, Michel Ferdani,
Enrico Sbariglia, Jean Rezzi, Michel Reggi*

Surgery of the mesenteric arteries is done in 2-3% of procedures involving surgery of the abdominal aorta. The small number of studies published leads to a lack of consensus on the best approach or the best type of technique for reconstruction. The approach to the mesenteric vessels blends with those used for the upper abdominal aorta, but the specific techniques for their reconstruction, bypass, or endarterectomy, often require a different approach. A different approach is also used for acute embolectomy, for isolated mesenteric arterial revascularization and reconstruction and for mesenteric reconstruction combined with aortic surgery.

Anatomic Review

The celiac trunk and the superior mesenteric artery (SMA) originate from the subdiaphragmatic aorta below the diaphragm in the segment of abdominal aorta most difficult to access. The inferior mesenteric artery originates at the level of the infrarenal aorta. The approach to its origin is straightforward and commonplace for vascular surgeons but it is rarely the target of direct reconstruction.

The celiac trunk originates from the anterior wall of the aorta at the level of T12-L1 (Fig. 1). After 1-3 cm, it crosses the upper edge of the pancreas where it divides into three branches: the hepatic artery, the left gastric

artery, and the splenic artery which is the largest of the three branches. The origin of the celiac trunk is surrounded by lymph nodes and by the nerve fibers of the solar plexus. It is covered by the posterior parietal peritoneum and may be hidden by the upper edge of the pancreas.

The SMA, which is the largest of the mesenteric arteries, supplies a part of the pancreas, the small bowel, and the right half of the large intestine. It originates from the anterior wall of the aorta at about 1 cm below the celiac trunk. Proximally, it has a fixed supramesenteric segment which is difficult to access and is frequently the target in revascularization for atherosclerotic lesions. More distally, in its

From Vascular Surgical Approaches, edited by Alain Branchereau and Ramon Berguer. ©1999, Futura Publishing Co., Inc., Armonk, NY.

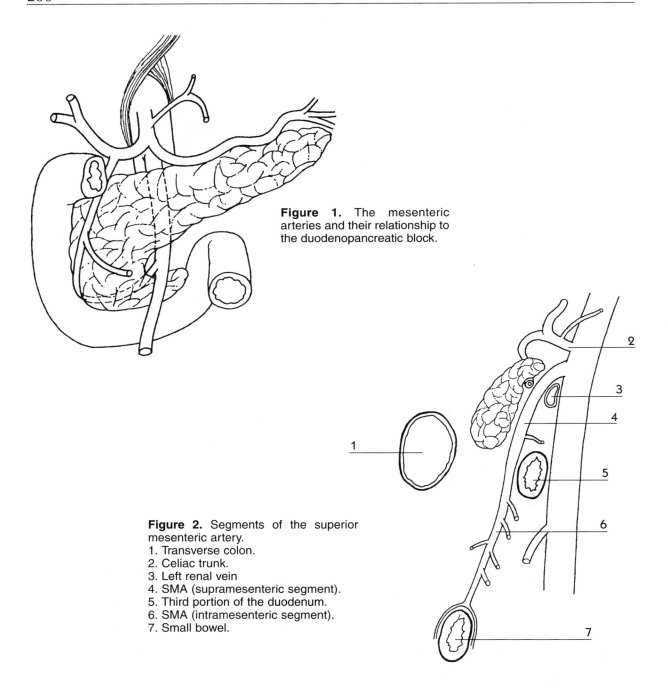

Figure 1. The mesenteric arteries and their relationship to the duodenopancreatic block.

Figure 2. Segments of the superior mesenteric artery.
1. Transverse colon.
2. Celiac trunk.
3. Left renal vein.
4. SMA (supramesenteric segment).
5. Third portion of the duodenum.
6. SMA (intramesenteric segment).
7. Small bowel.

intramesenteric segment, the artery is exposed to treat mesenteric embolization (Fig. 2). In its fixed segment the SMA is initially retropancreatic for the first 2 cm or 3 cm from its origin. The left renal vein separates posteriorly the SMA from the aorta. In this segment the SMA is surrounded, like the celiac trunk, by nerve fibers that form part of the aortomesenteric plexus. The artery then passes between the inferior edge of the pancreas and the third part of the duodenum. The superior mesenteric vein lies to its right. To its left, the ligament of Treitz suspends the duodenojejunal flexure from the left crus of the diaphragm. Before reaching the free intramesenteric segment, the artery runs in front of the duodenum covered by the submesocolic posterior parietal peritoneum. At this level an uncommon right hepatic branch may originate from the SMA in 8% to 15% of cases. This artery runs behind the pancreas and the portal vein. The right superior colic artery is one of the largest branches: it originates in the first segment of the SMA and runs transversely to the right. In the free intramesenteric segment, the SMA gives rise to the right colic arteries and the jejunal and ilial arteries.

The mesenteric arteries have important anastomoses between the celiac, superior mesenteric, and inferior mesenteric territories.[1] The connections between the celiac and SMA territories are via the anastomotic network of the duodenopancreatic block (Fig. 3). The connections between the superior and inferior mesenteric territories is via the paracolic anastomoses. The inferior mesenteric artery and the hypogastric territories are linked by the hemorrhoidal arteries. The prominent visualization of one of these anastomosis in an aortogram is a pathognomonic sign of an occlusive lesion of one of the origins of the mesenteric supply and calls for further arteriographic examination.

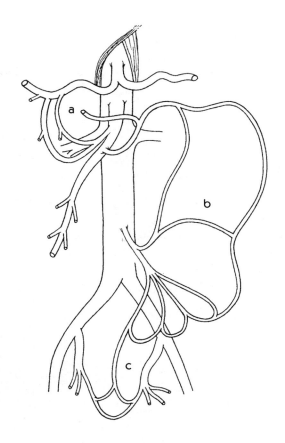

Figure 3. Anastomoses in the splanchnic arteries.
a. Between the celiac trunk and the SMA.
b. Between the superior and inferior mesenteric arteries.
c. Between the inferior mesenteric and hypogastric arteries.

Transperitoneal Approach

Patient Position and Incision

The classic approach to the aorta and the mesenteric arteries is the median laparotomy. The patient is supine for a transperitoneal approach. The arms are placed alongside the body. A roll is placed under the lower ribs. The drapes are laid out over a frame that separates the operative field from the anesthesiologist and which may be used to attach a subcostal retractor if needed. The fixation device of an Omnitract® retractor (Omnilaparo-Tract, Cardio-Choc, Nice, France) may also be attached to the lateral fixation bar of the operating table. Orthostatic retractors with interchangeable heads of varying size and depth greatly help with exposure of the suprarenal portion of the aorta and its visceral branches.

Celiac Trunk and Its Branches

The origin of the celiac trunk in the aorta is hidden by the muscular pillars of the aortic orifice of the diaphragm. For this reason access via a median xiphopubic approach is known sometimes as a transdiaphragmatic exposure. The exposure is facilitated by an orthostatic retractor which lifts the costal canopy.[2] The left lobe of the liver is retracted to the right after dividing the triangular ligament as far as the falciform ligament. After opening the lesser omentum, the esophagus, which is easily palpated with a nasogastric tube in place, is retracted to the left. The crura of the diaphragm are identified and the medial arcuate ligament is divided exposing the aorta. It is important to continue the dissection close to the aortic wall to avoid excursions into the periaortic nerve fibers which make up the celiac plexus (Fig. 4).

The origin of the celiac trunk is in the anterior wall of the aorta. Its wall is very thin, and consequently, it should be exposed with great care when dissecting it from the celiac plexus. If the aorta is to be used for an

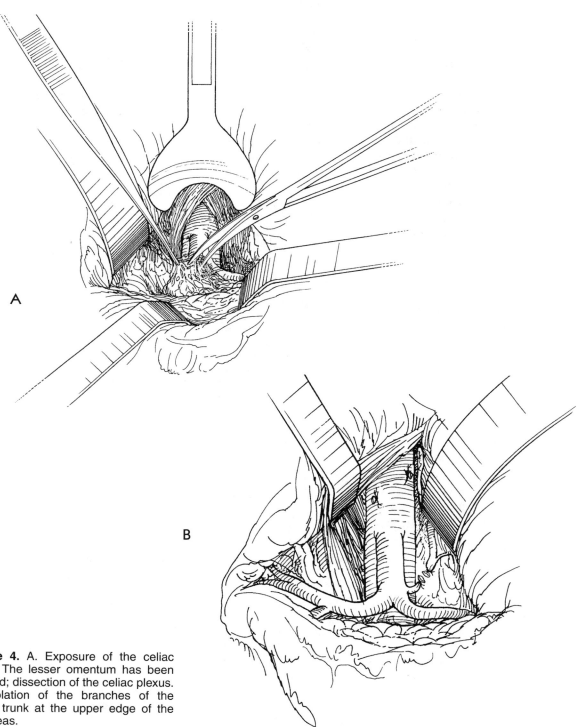

Figure 4. A. Exposure of the celiac trunk. The lesser omentum has been opened; dissection of the celiac plexus. B. Isolation of the branches of the celiac trunk at the upper edge of the pancreas.

anterograde bypass, the largest crus covering the anterior wall of the aorta must be almost completely divided and resected. This allows exposure of 5-8 cm of aorta, depending on the patient's morphology, and permits clamping of the aorta at its lowest intrathoracic portion. Occasionally, it is necessary to ligate and divide a diaphragmatic artery during this maneuver.

The hepatic artery is the branch of the celiac trunk most frequently used as a distal site for splanchnic revascularization. The left gastric artery is generally divided between ligatures to improve access to the celiac artery from the left. The hepatic artery is generally found at the upper edge of the pancreas before it penetrates the hepatic hilum. The upper edge of the pancreas is pulled downwards using two retractors and then the artery is dissected (Fig. 4A). The hepatic artery is tightly surrounded by nerve fibers. It is often useful to infiltrate the artery with Xylocaine in order to dilate it before its reconstruction. The gastro-duodenal artery must be identified in case of revascularization of the right renal artery. The dissection of the hepatic artery is continued towards the hepatic hilum as far as the division of the common hepatic artery (Fig. 4B). The gastroduodenal artery marks the right limit of the foramen of Winslow and then descends downwards and to the right behind the first segment of the duodenum to divide into two branches: the right inferior pancreatic duodenal artery and the right gastroepiploic artery. Ligature of the right superior pancreatic duodenal artery which originates behind the duodenum facilitates mobilization of the gastroduodenal artery. Detachment of the pancreatic duodenal block, from right to left, is also necessary for accessing the right renal artery. The gastroduodenal artery is then followed to the posterior wall of the duodenum as far as its division, where the possibility of using the artery at this level for anastomosis to the renal artery can be evaluated (Fig. 5).

Exposure of the splenic artery may be needed for treatment of an splenic aneurysm or to revascularize a renal artery (Fig. 5).[3] The splenic artery may be approached close to its origin by following the celiac trunk towards the left. It follows the upper edge of the pancreas. By dissecting it as far as the posterior wall of the pancreas and placing clips on its various pancreatic branches, it is possible to free the few centimeters of artery needed to perform a right splenorenal anastomosis. For the more traditional left splenorenal anastomosis, the splenic artery is approached by detaching the posterior mesogastrium and mobilizing the spleen upwards and to the right. The extent of this dissection depends on the caliber and quality of the artery needed for the renal revascularization.

Superior Mesenteric Artery

The origin of the SMA may be exposed by a median approach, dissecting below the celiac trunk and retracting the upper edge of the pancreas downwards. The origins of the celiac and SMA are very close: the dissection should stay close to the aortic wall separating the elements of the aortomesenteric plexus. At its origin the SMA adheres to the aorta; only 2 cm or 3 cm of the artery may be freed using this approach because traction on the pancreas should be limited to avoid tearing the hepatic and splenic arterial attachments of the latter. This approach is most useful when performing anterograde bypasses.

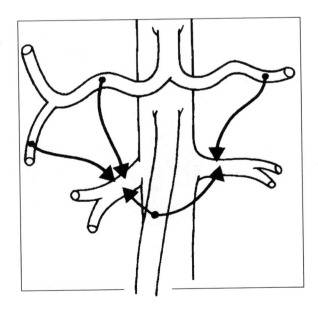

Figure 5. The splanchnic arteries as a source for revascularization of the renal arteries.

The preduodenal and infraduodenal segments of the SMA are exposed for embolectomy (Fig. 6). Exposure is achieved by pulling the transverse mesocolon upwards and using traction on the first jejunal loop which causes the mesenteric pedicle to stick out to the right of the mesentery, like a cord. The peritoneum is opened longitudinally along this cord and the dissection continues towards the artery after freeing the nerves that surround it. Upwards, the dissection may be carried out up to the right superior colic artery. Downwards, the dissection should be done with careful attention to the mesenteric branches, which

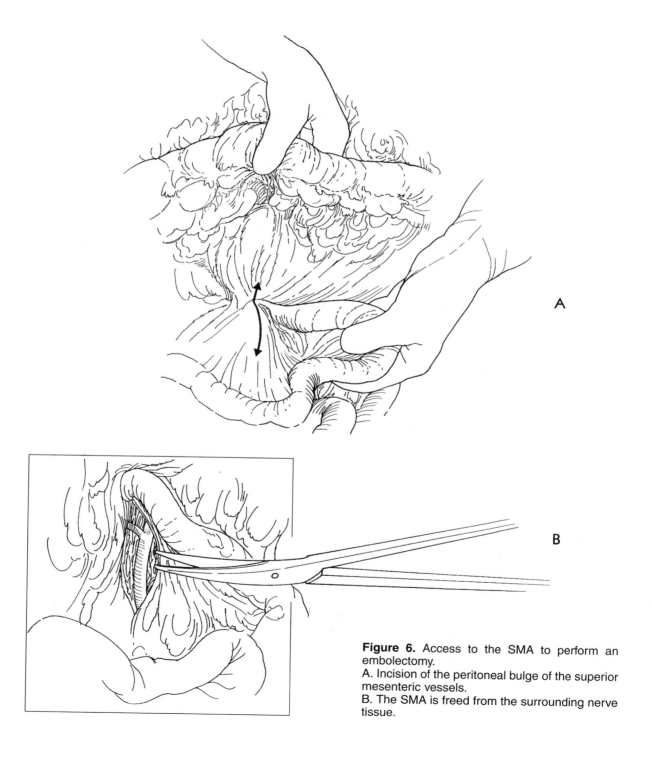

Figure 6. Access to the SMA to perform an embolectomy.
A. Incision of the peritoneal bulge of the superior mesenteric vessels.
B. The SMA is freed from the surrounding nerve tissue.

have very fragile walls, and the superior mesenteric vein, which runs very close and is often double.

The interduodenopancreatic approach to the SMA is more conventional (Fig. 7). After a midline laparotomy the transverse colon is pulled upwards and the small bowel is evis-

cerated. Manual traction on the first jejunal loop allows division of the peritoneum and the ligament of Treitz.[4] Freeing the third portion of the duodenum allows access to the SMA which is always surrounded by sympathetic nerves and lymph nodes. The superior mesenteric vein does not yet run alongside the artery at this level. Downward extension of the peritoneal

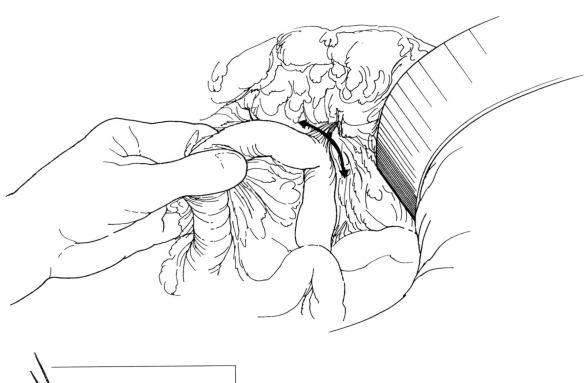

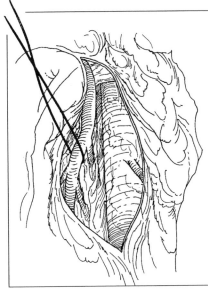

Figure 7. Interduodenopancreatic approach to the SMA. Detachment of the duodenojejunal angle and division of the ligament of Treitz. Inset: Inferior extension to expose the infrarenal aorta.

incision at the level of the posterior parietal peritoneum allows the infrarenal aorta to be exposed.

The duodenopancreatic detachment also allows the retropancreatic portion of the SMA to be accessed[5] (Fig. 8). Detachment begins at the right flexure of the colon and continues towards the duodenopancreatic block which allows the inferior vena cava and the left renal vein to be exposed. Dissection continues towards the aorta; the origin of the SMA is identified and dissected from the surrounding sympathetic nerves. This approach exposes the first 2-5 cm of the SMA and provides sufficient exposure of the aorta to perform a transposition of the SMA to the latter.

Inferior Mesenteric Artery

This artery is rarely approached on its own, but is regularly handled during surgery of the infrarenal aorta. After a midline laparotomy the transverse colon and the greater omentum are pulled upwards. The small bowel is pulled to the right which allows the posterior parietal peritoneum to be exposed. A vertical division at the level of the mesenteric insertion on the posterior parietal peritoneum and as far as the duodenojejunal angle allows access to the entire infrarenal aorta which is crossed at the top by the left renal vein. The origin of the inferior mesenteric artery is on the anterior or left lateral wall of the aorta. Running closely alongside the aorta at its origin and surrounded by nerve fibers and lymph nodes, the origin of the inferior mesenteric artery is usually situated halfway between the origin of the renal arteries and the bifurcation of the aorta.

Subcostal Approaches

Unilateral Subcostal Approach

This approach, extending from the midline to the tip of the 11th rib, is mainly used for

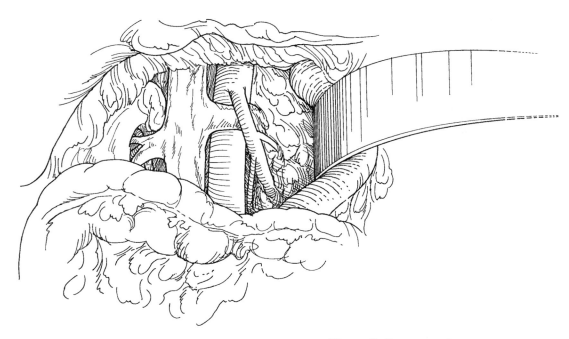

Figure 8. Exposure of the origin of the SMA by mobilization of the duodenopancreatic block.

surgery of the renal arteries (Fig. 9). It is a useful approach for the reconstruction of renal arteries using a splanchnic source; a splenic artery for the left or a hepatic artery for the right. The parietal incision is a fingerbreadth below the costal margin from the xiphoid process to the tip of the 11th rib. The hepatic artery or the gastroduodenal artery is approached from the right side as already described, and a duodenopancreatic detachment allows exposure of the right renal artery. On the left side, the splenic artery is exposed through the posterior mesogastrium.

When this exposure is extended behind the left colon it allows access to the left renal artery.

Bisubcostal Access

This approach combines two subcostal incisions at a certain distance from the xiphoid process. It gives good access to the supra-mesocolic compartment and is frequently used in hepatic surgery. Using a retractor to lift the costal canopy, access to the upper abdominal aorta and to the visceral vessels is excellent. This approach is particularly well suited to

celiac and mesenteric reconstructions. It is not used for surgery of the infrarenal aorta.

Midline Laparotomy with Mediovisceral Rotation

This approach described by Mattox[6] and popularized by Stoney,[7] marks a turning point in the surgical approach to that segment of the aorta, from diaphragm to the renal arteries which is difficult to expose (Fig. 10). After a midline xiphopubic laparotomy and placement of an orthostatic retractor with a subcostal blade, the procedure begins by dividing the triangular ligament which allows the left lobe of the liver to be freed and pushed to the right. The left colon is then detached and mobilized downwards freeing the spleen and the left flexure of their attachments to the diaphragm. The peritoneal incision is continued to the right at the level of the phrenicogastric ligament which allows mobilization of the pancreas. The spleen and the tail of the pancreas, the stomach, and the left colon are displaced to the right and held by retractors. There are two possible approaches to the left

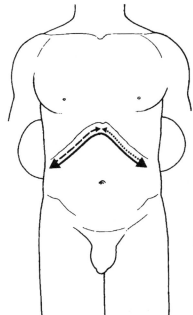

Figure 9. The subcostal approach.

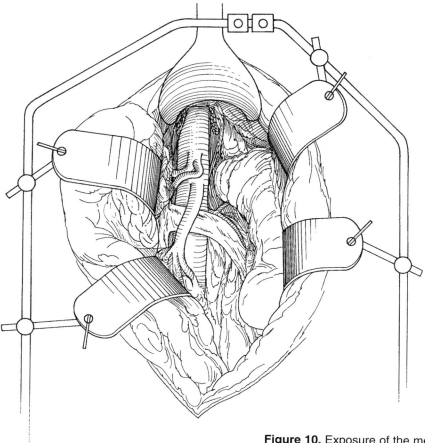

Figure 10. Exposure of the mesenteric arteries after prerenal medial visceral rotation.

kidney: it may be detached and retracted forward and to the right with the other viscera, or it can be left in place in the lumbar region. The latter allows exposure of a longer segment of the SMA. In this case, care must be taken when separating the kidney and the suprarenal gland from the pancreas to avoid any injury to any of these three organs. The left crus of the diaphragm bars access to the aorta as the latter exits the diaphragm; it may be cut or simply detached from the aorta after dividing the median arcuate ligament. Often a diaphragmatic artery needs to be divided. The left celiac ganglion, which covers the origin of the celiac trunk, is cut and the celiac arterial trunk is located by staying close to the aorta. The SMA is exposed and controlled 1 cm below; it may be freed for 4-6 cm beyond its origin. The left renal artery is easily located, with the kidney either being rotated forward or left in place.

The origin of the right renal artery and the perimeter of the infrarenal aorta may be encircled with loops. The dissection may be extended as far as the aortic bifurcation if required.

Retroperitoneal Approach

Patient Position

The patient lies on a bean bag (Olympic Medical Corporation, Seattle, Washington, USA). When a thoracolumbar approach is planned, the patient is in the supine position, a shoulder turned towards the right while the pelvis is maintained flat on the table. The left arm may be fixed to the anesthesia frame or left free in front and to the right. When a lumbar incision alone is planned, the patient is in right lateral decubitus with the bean bag acting as a roll under the lumbar region. The post of the Omnitract retractor is placed above and to the left of the patient.

Lumbar Incision (11th Rib)

This extrapleural retroperitoneal approach is becoming more popular in surgery of infrarenal aortic aneurysms and in approaches to the inter- and infrarenal aorta.[8-11] The lumbotomy begins at the 11th rib which is resected and then continues towards the umbilicus (Fig. 11). The greater and lesser oblique and the transverse muscles are divided as far as the edge of the rectus muscle. At this level the rectus muscle may be divided or the incision extended downwards between the greater and lesser oblique muscles and the

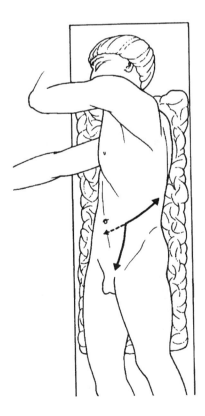

Figure 11. Extrapleural, extra-peritoneal lumbotomy.

lateral edge of the rectus muscle. The dissection starts in the retroperitoneum behind the left colon. It is easier to go behind the kidney while pushing the visceral mass forward but, when done in this manner, the length of SMA that can be exposed is more limited. To the rear of this cavity, which has been freed, lies the psoas muscle, and towards the top is the left crus and the dome of the diaphragm. Dividing the left crus of the diaphragm allows access to the suprarenal aorta; to perform this it is often necessary to tie the inferior left diaphragmatic artery. The mesenteric arteries may be dissected in their first few centimeters by staying in close contact with the aorta and resecting the nerve plexus that surrounds the latter. This approach may be extended forward by dividing the rectus muscle if a greater length of the mesenteric arteries needs to be freed. The infrarenal aorta may be exposed by extending the incision along the length of the rectus muscle and then freeing the peritoneal sac towards the pelvis.

Thoracophreno-Laparotomy Through the 8th Rib

A number of approaches begin by opening the thorax at the 8th intercostal space[11,12] (Fig. 12). The approaches may be extraperitoneal if the incision stops at the rectus edge or if they run downwards along its lateral edge. They become transperitoneal thoracophreno-laparotomies if, after opening the peritoneum, they continue as far as the midline and extend downwards. Whenever exposure is adequate for mesenteric artery reconstruction, opening of the peritoneum should be avoided, to simplify surgical exposure. In some cases, control of the reconstruction by an intraperitoneal approach could be done by a limited opening of the peritoneum at the end of the procedure.

The thoracoabdominal incision is performed in the 8th intercostal space, from the posterior axillary line to the lateral edge of the rectus muscle. The left half of the diaphragm is opened 2 cm from its insertion in the ribs. The left crus of the diaphragm is opened longitudinally, close to where it is attached to

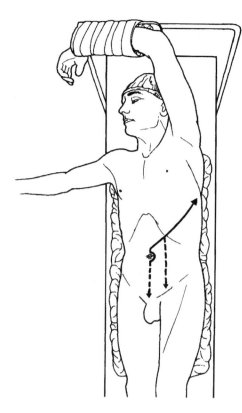

Figure 12. Thoracophreno-laparotomy, intra- or extraperitoneal.

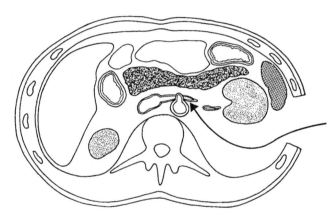

Figure 13. Dissection pathway during an extraperitoneal thoracophreno-laparotomy. The aorta is accessed at the level of the origin of the SMA.

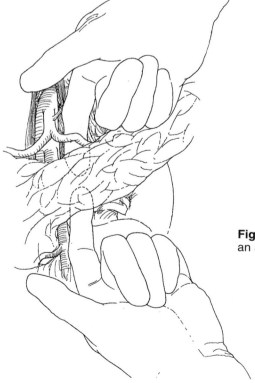

Figure 14. Retropancreatic tunneling for an anterograde aortomesenteric bypass.

the spine, and the inferior diaphragmatic artery is divided. The retroperitoneal space is opened and the peritoneal sac is retracted intact. The spleen and the caudal pancreas are retracted to the right with the foregut. The kidney may be left in its fossa or pulled forward depending on the lesions to be treated. The aorta may then be freed around its circumference in order to clamp it at the level of the diaphragm or in its descending intrathoracic segment (Fig. 13). The origin of the splanchnic arteries is revealed little by little by following the aorta and dividing the nerve plexi that surround them.

Access to the intrarenal aorta and the iliac arteries can be obtained by extending the incision downwards by following the lateral edge of the rectus muscle or by a subumbilical laparotomy.

Choice of Approach

The multiple approaches, the different techniques available, and variations in the topography of the aortic lesions should all be considered when deciding on the type of approach.[13] The midline laparotomy with access to the supraceliac aorta dissecting the crus of the diaphragm is the most frequently employed in our practice. It allows performing anterograde or retrograde bypasses because of the ease of access to the infrarenal aorta (Fig. 14). This access is also recommended for emergency mesenteric embolectomy: it allows direct and effective control of the revascularization performed. The thoracophreno-lumbotomy/laparotomy allows a complete view of the distal thoracic aorta and the entire abdominal aorta. This gives the technique flexibility, and it is equally satisfactory for endarterectomy or bypasses. The disadvantage of this approach is in its opening of the thorax and the complications that may result from it. The midline laparotomy with mediovisceral rotation[7] is a reasonable compromise combining the same view of the aorta and its branches as the thoracophreno-lumbotomy with less morbidity. This technique is adapted to anterograde reconstruction and endarterectomies. Concomitant aortic and renal surgery is feasible using this approach where

the surgeon may choose to combine a retroperitoneal and an intraperitoneal approach to the aorta and its branches. Postoperative pancreatitis has been mentioned by Stoney[7]; this complication should be minimized if the retroperitoneal detachment passes behind the kidney, thus avoiding working too close to the pancreas.

References

1. Kieny R, Cinqualbre J. Chirurgie des artères digestives. *Encycl Med Chir,* Paris, techniques chirurgicales, chirurgie vasculaire, 4.7.12, 43-105.
2. Cormier JM, Uhl JF. Revascularisation antérograde des artères digestives par pontage implanté sur l'aorte sus-rénale. *Nouv Presse Med* 1979; 8: 2195-2197.
3. Goeau Brissonnière O, Coggia M, Leschi JP. Revascularisation rénale à partir des artères digestives. In: Kieffer E, ed. *Chirurgie des Artères Rénales.* Paris, AERCV, 1993, pp 189-204.
4. Bergan JJ. Surgical treatment of chronic visceral arterial insufficiency. In: Bergan JJ, Yao ST, eds. *Operative Techniques in Vascular Surgery.* New York, Grune & Stratton, 1980, pp 109-113.
5. Bonnichon P, Rossat-Mignod JC, Corlieu P, et al. Abord de l'artère mésentérique supérieure par décollement duodéno-pancréatique. Etude anatomique et applications cliniques. *Ann Chir Vasc* 1986; 1: 505-508.
6. Mattox KL, Whisenannd HH, Espada R, Beall AC Jr. Management of acute combined injuries to the aorta and inferior vena cava. *Am J Surg* 1975; 130:720-724.
7. Reilly LM, Ramos TK, Murray SP, et al. Optimal exposure of the proximal abdominal aorta: A critical appraisal of transabdominal medial visceral rotation. *J Vasc Surg* 1994; 19: 375-390.
8. Rob C. Extraperitoneal approach to the abdominal aorta. *Surgery* 1963; 53: 87-89.
9. Ricotta JJ, Williams GM. Endarterectomy of the upper abdominal aorta and visceral arteries through an extraperitoneal approach. *Ann Surg* 1980; 192: 633-638.
10. Kieffer E. Chirurgie des anévrysmes de l'aorte thoraco-abdominale (I). *Encycl Med Chir,* Paris, techniques chirurgicales, chirurgie vasculaire, 43-150, 1993, 18 p.
11. Saifi J, Shah DM, Chang BB, et al. Left retroperitoneal exposure for distal mesenteric artery repair. *J Cardiovasc Surg* 1990; 31: 629-633.
12. Pokrovsky AV, Karimov SI, Yermolyuk RS, et al. Thoracophrenolombotomy as an approach of choice in reconstruction of the proximal abdominal aorta and visceral branches. *J Vasc Surg* 1991; 13: 892-896.
13. Courbier R, Jausseran JM. Les techniques de revascularisation de l'artère mésentérique supérieure. Etude critique et résultats. *Chirurgie* 1983; 109: 523-527.

22

Renal Arteries

Michel Lacombe

Despite the introduction of transluminal angioplasty, reconstructive vascular surgery continues to be indispensable in the treatment of renal arterial lesions due to contraindications, unfeasibility, or failures of angioplasty. Surgeons are required to operate on complex lesions more often than previously and in these circumstances good exposure is essential. The quality of the surgical exposure determines the ease with which the repairs can be performed: exposure should be ample, adapted to the lesions, whether the latter are uni- or bilateral, and finally, adapted to the morphology of the patient.

Anatomic Review

The renal arteries lie deep within the abdomen, practically in contact with the posterior abdominal wall, which explains the potential difficulties in their surgical exposure. Usually there is an artery on each side with its origin on the lateral wall of the abdominal aorta. Each artery runs obliquely posterolateral and downwards towards the renal hilum. At the level of each hilum, the artery is the most posterior element. It is covered, in front, by the renal vein but because of its oblique trajectory it may course higher or lower than the renal vein. The renal pelvis is in close relationship only with the branches of the artery. On the right side, the renal artery before joining the renal hilum has a long main segment covered by the inferior vena cava and, at a more superficial level, by the second segment of the duodenum and the head of the pancreas. The latter can be retracted to the side during the transabdominal approach. On the left side, the renal artery forms part of the renal hilum for its entire length. It is covered in front by the renal vein and by the body and tail of the pancreas, the omental bursa, and the stomach. Because of these factors, its transabdominal approach is more difficult.

The level of origin of the renal artery determines the choice of approach. The renal artery originates on both sides at the level of L1-L2 with some individual variations. If its

From Vascular Surgical Approaches, edited by Alain Branchereau and Ramon Berguer. ©1999, Futura Publishing Co., Inc., Armonk, NY.

origin is higher, its surgical exposure is more difficult. Conversely, a lower origin greatly facilitates exposure. In the case of a pelvic kidney, the transabdominal access to the artery is much easier. Anatomic variations in the number of renal arteries are encountered in 25-30% of cases[1] and they influence the type of vascular reconstruction, but not the choice of approach.

Transperitoneal Approaches

There are several techniques for the transperitoneal approach to the renal arteries (Fig. 1). Some provide limited exposure for selective unilateral renal artery reconstruction; others provide extended exposure for bilateral access and for simultaneous renal and aortic reconstruction. The intraabdominal procedure

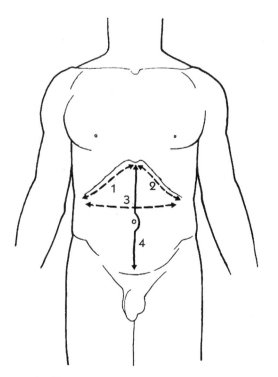

Figure 1. Transperitoneal approach to the renal arteries.
1. Right subcostal approach.
2. Left subcostal approach.
1 + 2. Bisubcostal approach.
3. Transverse abdominal approach.
4. Midline xiphoid-to-pubis.

is the same with the different techniques and only varies in the length of the abdominal incision. The patient is in the supine position. A roll is placed below the 11th and 12th ribs to raise the renal arteries. A costal retractor is needed to lift the rib edges. The table is slightly tilted towards the nonoperated side to facilitate the exposure. The surgeon is on the side to be operated if one renal artery is to be exposed, and to the right if exposure of both is needed. The first assistant and the nurse are opposite the surgeon with a second assistant at his/her side next to the head.

Unilateral Exposure

The left and right subcostal approaches are used for unilateral exposure. On either side, they give direct access to the renal artery and guarantee good exposure of the artery and surrounding structures. This minimizes dissection and manipulation of the viscera and facilitates postoperative recovery and a rapid return of bowel activity. The skin incision is parallel to the edge of the rib cage, 2 cm below. It begins at the tip of the 11th rib and extends as far as the midline by dividing the rectus muscle of the abdomen. The three layers of abdominal wall musculature and the peritoneum are divided. The subcostal approach has the advantage of lessening the disturbance of the respiratory function and allowing a reliable abdominal wall closure with little risk of incisional hernia. This approach, however, is a bit more tedious to perform and requires the division of the large muscles and the terminal branches of several intercostal nerves which supply the rectus muscle. Only isolated repairs of the renal artery are possible using this approach which should not be used for renal autotransplantation or simultaneous aortic surgery.

Extended Exposure

The transverse approaches (bisubcostal and transverse abdominal) and the midline xiphopubic approach are used for extended exposure.

The bisubcostal approach combines in one single incision, the right and left subcostal approaches. The exposure obtained is substantial when the incision extends between the tips of both 11th ribs. It provides access to the renal arteries and to the abdominal aorta and permits simultaneous surgery of the aorta and of the renal arteries. The drawbacks are the lengthiness of the procedure and the extent of muscle and nerves that need to be divided.

The transverse abdominal approach[2] differs from the preceding method in its skin incision, which is approximately parallel to the route followed by the intercostal nerves and crosses the midline above the umbilicus. It is less traumatic from a muscular and peripheral nerve point of view.

The median xiphoid to pubis approach is, in our opinion, a better choice. It follows an anatomic line and requires no muscular or peripheral division. It is simple and quick to perform and close. It gives excellent access to the abdominal aorta and allows all types of renal arterial repair with concomitant aortic surgery. In the immediate postoperative period, the respiratory impairment is a little more serious than in the transverse approach. The risk of postoperative eventration is low if the closure is performed with care. The drawbacks of this approach are fewer than its advantages.

Intraabdominal Dissection

Approach to the Right Renal Artery

This is performed at the submesocolic level. The posterior parietal peritoneum is divided at the external edge of the second portion of the duodenum and the duodeno-pancreatic detachment is extended as far as the infrarenal aorta (Figs. 2 and 3). The peritoneum

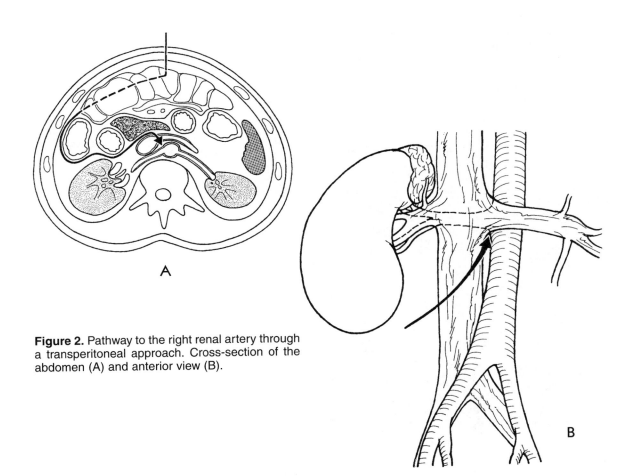

Figure 2. Pathway to the right renal artery through a transperitoneal approach. Cross-section of the abdomen (A) and anterior view (B).

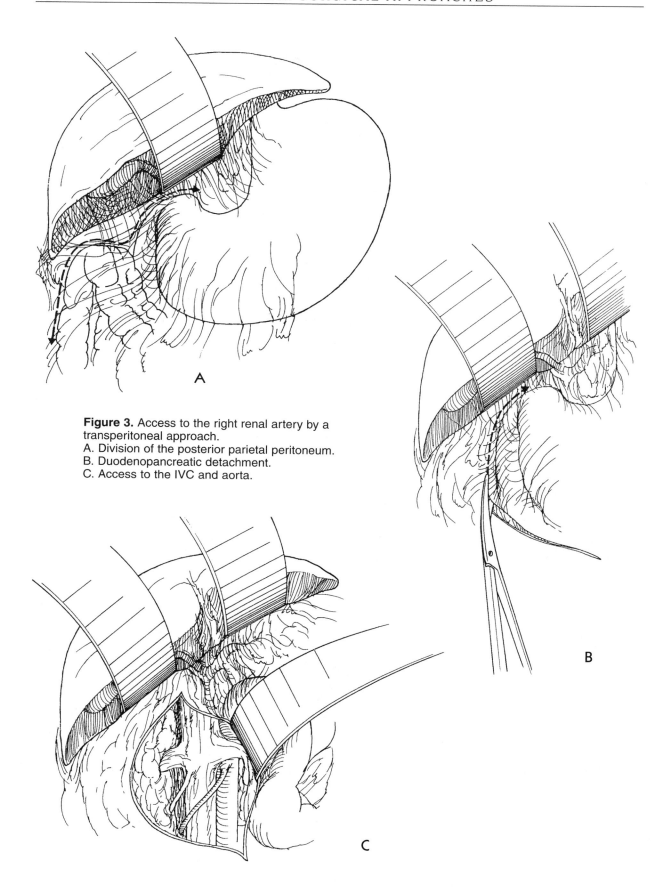

Figure 3. Access to the right renal artery by a transperitoneal approach.
A. Division of the posterior parietal peritoneum.
B. Duodenopancreatic detachment.
C. Access to the IVC and aorta.

is divided upwards as far as the foramen of Winslow, the lower wall of which must be opened to expose the anterior part of the cavorenal venous junction. Downwards, the peritoneum is opened in the direction of the right colic flexure which is retracted inferiorly. The cavorenal venous junction is freed before exposing the renal artery. After freeing the inferior vena cava (IVC), the latter is pulled back with a loop below the renal veins. Occasionally it is necessary to ligate and divide a lumbar vein to free the posterior wall of the vena cava. The left renal vein is also dissected from where it joins the vena cava along its preaortic segment. The renal artery is found behind the renal vein in the angle between the vena cava and the left renal vein. It is covered by lymphatics and nerve fibers which are sometimes thick due to the presence of an aortorenal parasympathetic ganglion; this tissue is cauterized and cut. The renal artery can be raised by traction on a loop. Proximally, dissection is continued up to its origin (Fig. 4). The infrarenal aorta is now freed and encircled with a loop if revascularization using the aorta is planned. Distally, exposure of the right renal artery is gained by traction on the IVC towards the right. By lifting the IVC with a loop and retracting it to the right, the entire length of the retrocaval segment of the artery up to its bifurcation can be isolated. If there are distal renal artery lesions, the dissection is continued to the right of the IVC as far as the hilum of the kidney. Temporary division of the left renal vein, between two clamps, helps in difficult cases, when dissecting the origin and main trunk of the right renal artery. The IVC may then be pulled even further to the right. This division has no effect on the kidney if it is performed preaortically, to the right of the branches of the left renal vein. The latter provide venous drainage of the kidney while the main renal vein is clamped. Once the arterial procedure is finished, the vein is reanastomosed.

Approach to the Left Renal Artery

This approach is more difficult than for the right renal artery because of the anterior relationship of the artery with the viscera located on the posterior mesogastrium. In obese patients, the depth of the operative field may

make a retoperitoneal approach preferable. Several approaches are possible (Fig. 5).

Submesocolic Approach

The transverse colon is pulled upwards, and the small bowel and its mesentery are pulled to the right. The posterior parietal peritoneum is cut along the length of the fourth portion of the duodenum and the ligament of Treitz (Fig. 6). The duodenum is retracted from left to right as far as the aorta. Division of the inferior mesenteric vein is optional. The abdominal aorta is separated from the inferior edge of the left renal vein; this procedure is identical to that performed for controlling the aorta above an infrarenal aortic aneurysm. The left renal vein is raised and retracted upwards. This requires ligature and division of the gonadal vein and other inferior branches of the left renal vein. Occasionally, the venous branch draining the ren-oazygo-lumbar system which joins the posterior wall of the renal vein needs to be divided. The origin of the renal artery can be seen on the left wall of the aorta. The trunk of the artery is dissected towards the periphery (Fig. 6). This approach gives sufficient access to both the trunk and the ostium of the renal artery. Access to the distal lesions on the left side is difficult while the kidney is in place. If one needs access to the distal segment of the left renal artery, it is often preferable to use another approach. In this situation and in difficult cases, the temporary division of the left renal vein facilitates the access to the left renal artery and allows extended exposure of the artery towards the periphery.

Access by Detachment of the Left Colon and the Posterior Mesogastrium

The posterior parietal peritoneum is divided at the external edge of the descending colon, from the flexure of the left colon and the spleen as far as the esophageal hiatus. Dissection follows the retrocolic and retrosplenopancreatic planes. This dissection, which is performed in the prerenal plane, is extended as far as the abdominal aorta. This freeing of the spleen requires particular care and should

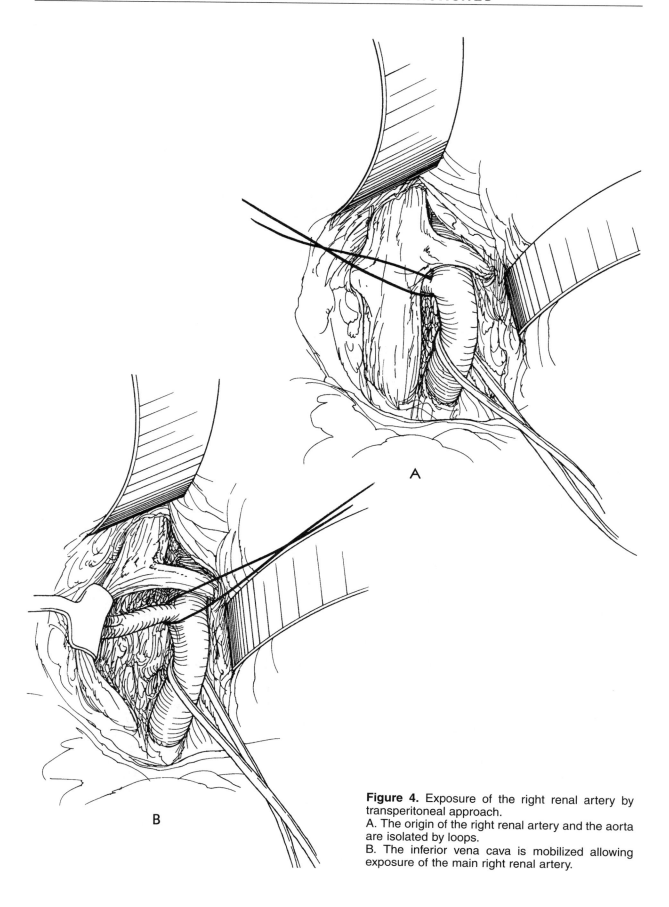

Figure 4. Exposure of the right renal artery by transperitoneal approach.
A. The origin of the right renal artery and the aorta are isolated by loops.
B. The inferior vena cava is mobilized allowing exposure of the main right renal artery.

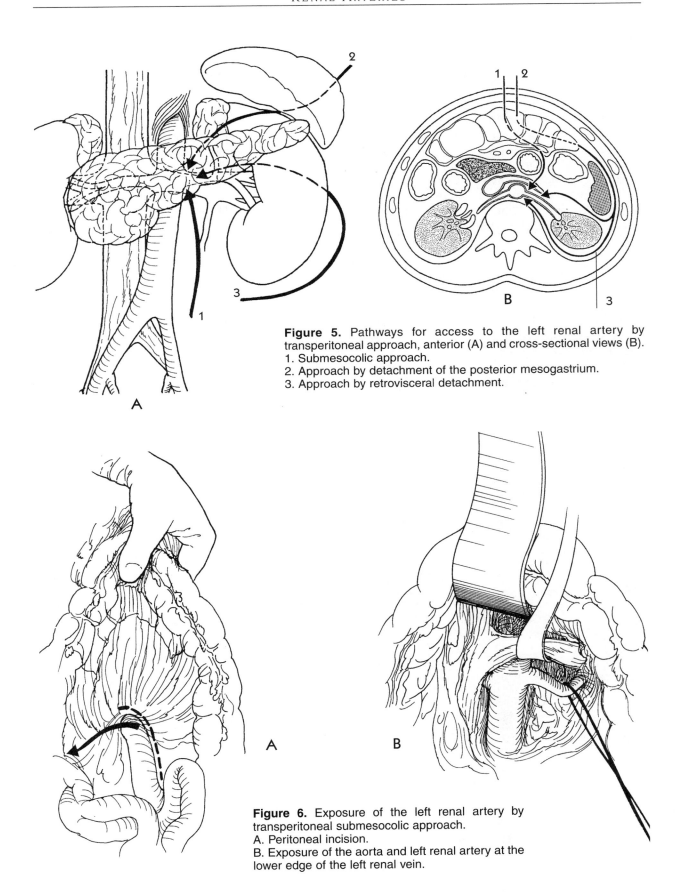

Figure 5. Pathways for access to the left renal artery by transperitoneal approach, anterior (A) and cross-sectional views (B).
1. Submesocolic approach.
2. Approach by detachment of the posterior mesogastrium.
3. Approach by retrovisceral detachment.

Figure 6. Exposure of the left renal artery by transperitoneal submesocolic approach.
A. Peritoneal incision.
B. Exposure of the aorta and left renal artery at the lower edge of the left renal vein.

avoid any traction that may result in bleeding. The spleen, the left hemipancreas, the left colon, and the stomach are rotated to the right and protected by moist laps (Fig. 7). This procedure exposes the anterior face of the kidney and its vascular pedicle. The renal vein covers the artery. This latter is revealed after mobilization of the vein and division of its collaterals. It is often useful to mobilize the kidney by detaching its posterior surface from the lumbar fossa. Surgical drapes are packed behind the kidney and its vessels which are thus raised to facilitate their vascular repair.

Access by Right Visceral Rotation

The dissection is begun as above but passes behind the left kidney. The entire visceral block is completely freed from the posterior abdominal wall and is pulled to the right. The kidney is then almost completely exteriorized (Fig. 8). The renal artery is approached behind

the hilum. The entire length of the abdominal aorta is accessible using this approach. It is preferable for the surgeon to move to the left of the patient and the assistants, who are opposite, to retain the visceral block to the right. Freeing the prerenal plane permits use of both sides of the renal pedicle and facilitates left renal artery reconstruction.

Retroperitoneal Approaches

The retroperitoneal approach allows direct access to the kidney and its vessels without visceral dissection. Its advantages are a simpler postoperative course with fewer respiratory and gastrointestinal problems. The patient is placed in the supine position. The costoiliac space is enlarged by placing a roll under the 11th rib. The ipsilateral leg is placed in abduction to allow access to the greater saphenous vein (Fig. 9). Tilting of the table

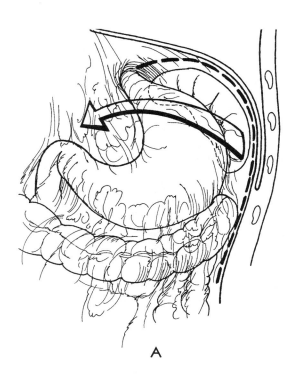

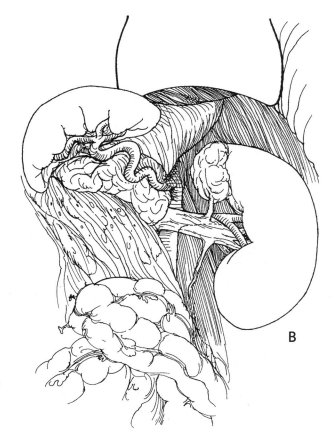

Figure 7. Transperitoneal access to the left renal artery by detachment of the posterior mesogastrium.
A. Peritoneal incision.
B. The exposed left kidney and its vessels.

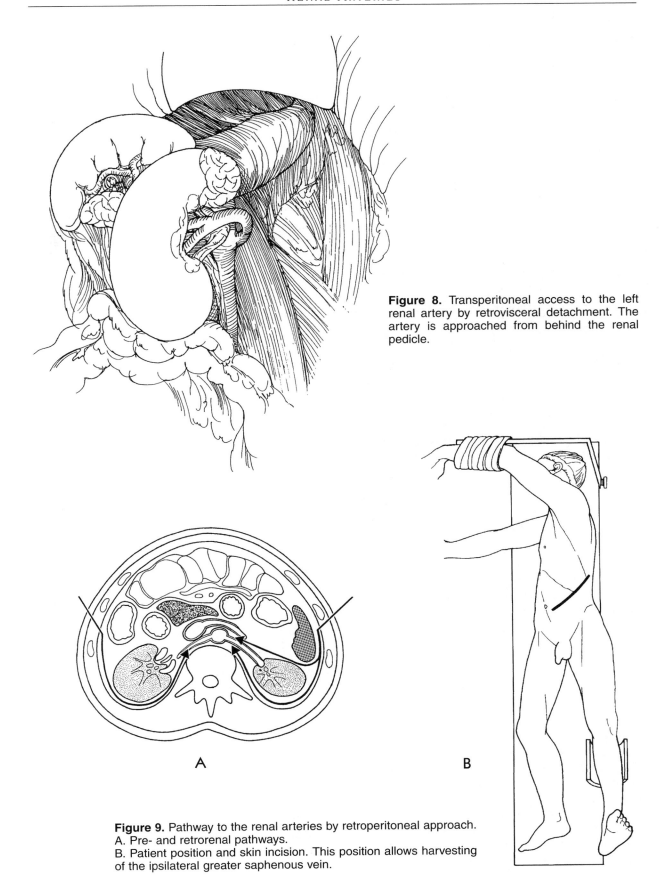

Figure 8. Transperitoneal access to the left renal artery by retrovisceral detachment. The artery is approached from behind the renal pedicle.

Figure 9. Pathway to the renal arteries by retroperitoneal approach.
A. Pre- and retrorenal pathways.
B. Patient position and skin incision. This position allows harvesting of the ipsilateral greater saphenous vein.

A

B

tends to lower the kidney and to improve exposure. The surgeon is behind the patient with the first assistant and the nurse opposite and the second assistant next to the surgeon at the head of the patient.

Incisions

Different incisions are possible but the need for good exposure requires a relatively large incision. Locating the position of the kidney from the preoperative x-ray is important in the choice of the incision. In fact, there are individual variations in the height of the organ depending on the side being operated on and the morphology of the patient. In the case of a high lying kidney, the line of the incision should be displaced upwards. The classic lumbar incision parallel to the ribs gives poor access for reconstruction of the renal artery. It may be necessary in some instances to resort to thoracolumbar or thoracoabdominal incisions. The site of the skin incision depends on the height and size of the kidney.

An incision over the 12th rib and prolonged along its trajectory is sufficient if the kidney is low, especially when operating on the right side.

An incision in the 10th intercostal space, at the upper edge of the 11th rib (Fig. 9B) and continued anteriorly along its trajectory,[3] is in our opinion the best choice in all cases, and it allows management of every eventuality that may arise. It is particularly suited for exposure of the left renal artery. The incision is made over the 11th rib. Behind, it reaches as far as the midaxillary line and, occassionaly, as far as the external edge of the sacrolumbar muscular mass if the celiac aorta needs to be exposed. Anteriorly, the incision extends across the abdomen in the direction of the iliac fossa. The incision need not be longer than 10 cm if used for a renal artery reconstruction in situ.

If autotransplanation of the kidney is necessary after ex situ surgery, the incision should extend obliquely towards the anterosuperior iliac spine, following the fibers of the external oblique muscle towards the pubis spine, to open the iliac fossa. At the level of the thorax, the incision runs along the upper edge of the rib which should not be resected. After detaching the endothoracic fascia, the insertions of the diaphragm are cut close to the ribs, taking special care to stay below the pleural reflection. At the level of the abdomen, after dividing the large muscles the peritoneum is freed and pushed towards the midline. This approach remains totally extrapleural and extraperitoneal. If the pleural cavity is accidentally entered, a small drain is placed in the pleural cavity and removed at the end of the procedure after full lung reexpansion. The access described by Risberg[4] is a variation of the above: its abdominal part runs along the lateral edge of the rectus muscle of the abdomen for almost its complete height, passes four fingerbreadths within the iliac spine, and ends a little above the pubis. It has the drawback of severing most of the nerve supply to the rectus muscle and results in muscular weakness of the abdominal wall. For this reason we do not use this approach. Once the abdominal wall has been opened the renal artery may be accessed by passing behind or in front of the kidney (Fig. 9A).

Retrorenal Approach

The dissection plane follows the posterior abdominal wall, without opening the renal space. This dissection is facilitated by opening the perirenal fascia of Zuckerkandl which allows mobilization of the kidney and the surrounding tissues. The detachment is extended as far as the aorta or IVC. The kidney is retracted forward, along with the abdominal viscera covered by peritoneum. The renal artery is exposed behind the kidney after identifying its position by finger palpation. At this level the artery is surrounded only by a fine fibrofatty tissue. The artery is occasionally crossed behind by a small transversal vein, a branch of the ren-oazygo-lumbar vein which is tied and cut. An anomalous renal venous system, notably a left retroaortic renal vein, may be identified during this dissection, as well as the rare existence of a left IVC. If such anomalies exist the surgical approach should be adapted accordingly. These venous anomalies exist in only 1-3% of cases.[5] The artery can be dissected along its entire length, from its origin to the level of its primary branches (Fig. 10).

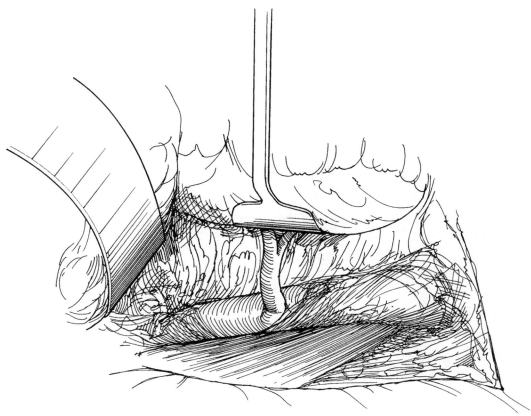

Figure 10. Access to the left renal artery and infrarenal aorta by a retroperitoneal retrorenal approach.

On the left, this approach allows exposure of the infrarenal aorta for its entire height and of the initial segment of the common iliac arteries. It is also possible to expose the suprarenal aorta after dividing the left crux of the diaphragm.

On the right, access to the abdominal aorta is more difficult as the access is blocked by the IVC. By retracting the latter, a limited segment of the aorta can be freed for implantation of a bypass. On the right side, we prefer the transperitoneal approach.

Prerenal Approach

In this variation, the kidney is left in its anatomic position and is not detached from its posterior attachments. Opening the renal space at the lateral edge of the kidney leads to the anterior suface of the organ which is freed in its entire length. The renal pedicle is exposed at the medial edge of the kidney. The first vascular element visible anteriorly is the renal vein. After isolation of the renal vein, the renal artery is exposed by dividing the lymphatics and nerves that surround it. This is achieved by working behind the vein and displacing it downwards or upwards as may be the case (Fig. 11).

On the left side, the dissection continues medially by following the plane of detachment of the posterior mesogastrium. In addition to the renal artery that is exposed posteriorly, this dissection gives access also to the splenic artery in front as it courses along the posterior surface of the pancreas. The division of the parietal mesocolic attachment, after locating the pulse of the splenic artery with a finger, gives access to the latter. This prerenal access

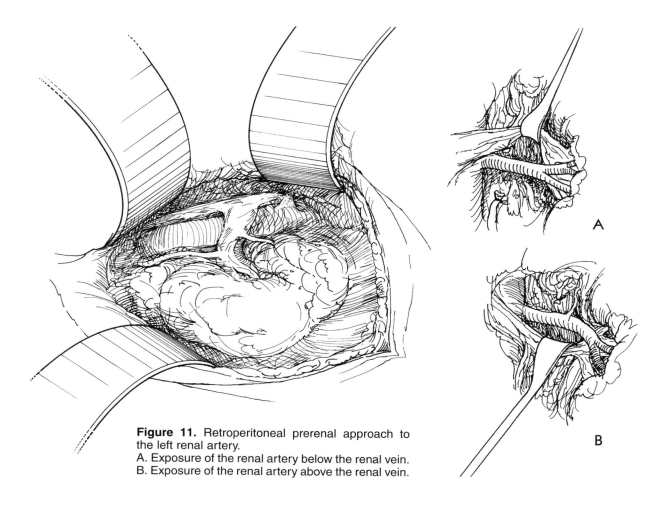

Figure 11. Retroperitoneal prerenal approach to the left renal artery.
A. Exposure of the renal artery below the renal vein.
B. Exposure of the renal artery above the renal vein.

permits freeing the entire length of the renal artery from its origin and allows exposure of the abdominal aorta, after mobilizing the left renal vein. This maneuver may be needed if one chooses to perform a splenorenal anastomosis.

On the right side, the prerenal approach gives easy access to the branches of the artery. Access to the trunk of the artery is more limited due to the venous structures; the IVC and the right renal vein need to be mobilized in order to expose the artery. The field of exposure of the origin of the right renal artery and aorta is in a deep and narrow field.

Thoracophrenolaparotomy

This approach is rarely used in renal artery surgery. Its main indication is in extensive reconstructive surgery of the aorta associated with mesenteric and renal revascularization and it is used only on the left side.

Patient Position

The patient is placed with the thorax lifted 30 degrees towards the right. The left upper extremity is abducted and fixed to the anesthesiologist's frame. The pelvis is flat on the table to facilitate the abdominal part of the operation. The surgeon is to the left for the thoracic part and may possibly change sides for the abdominal part of the procedure. The first assistant and the nurse are opposite the surgeon with the second assistant at his/her side.

Technique

The thoracotomy is performed in the 9th left intercostal space, cutting the condrocostal edge. A higher thoracotomy may be performed depending on the height at which the thoracic aorta needs to be controlled. This latter is exposed after opening the mediastinal pleura. The abdominal part of the incision that prolongs inferiorly the thoracotomy, allows access to the renal artery. This is either an incision that prolongs the thoracotomy downwards or a transversal incision up to the midline after dividing the rectus muscle of the abdomen. The transverse incision may be enlarged by extending from the opposite side (performing a transverse laparotomy) or by extending via a midline laparotomy down to the pubis using a technique similar to that described by Bernard[6] for the right side (Fig. 12).

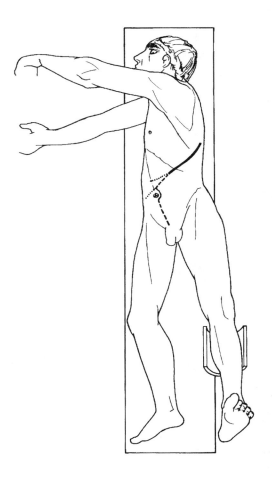

Figure 12. Left thoracophrenolaparotomy. Variations in the extension of the thoracic incision into the abdominal level.

Choice of Approach

The choice of approach for renal artery repairs should be tailored to each individual case. It should take into account the site of the renal artery lesion, its possible bilateral nature, the type of repair technique that is planned, the presence of associated lesions which may require more complex procedures (e.g. simultaneous aortic repairs), the morphology, and the weight of the patient.[7,8]

Side to Be Operated

The choice is simple when the renal artery lesion is isolated and unilateral. For repairs of the left renal artery, a retroperitoneal approach, such as we have described, is the preferred choice as it provides the easiest and most direct access to the renal artery and easier postoperative recovery.

For repair of the right renal artery, when treating distal lesions which can be repaired by simple clamping of the artery, the retroperitoneal approach is again preferred. When treating proximal lesions that require revascularization from the aorta, the midline transperitoneal approach is recommended as it gives the best exposure of the aorta and IVC. The subcostal approach may be considered if a hepatorenal revascularization is planned.

Bilateral Lesions

A transperitoneal approach is required when a bilateral renal artery repair is planned. We prefer the midline xiphopubic approach which is simpler and quicker than transversal approaches. A submesocolic approach to the two renal arteries is preferred (see above). This is achieved after complete mobilization of the left renal vein and separation of the infrarenal aorta. The two arteries are exposed from their origin to their primary branching.

Temporary division of the left renal vein is particularly useful in difficult cases and is extremely helpful in that it facilitates access to the aorta and permits extended exposure of both renal arteries.

Technique

Splenorenal Anastomosis

The subcostal and retroperitoneal approaches can be used. We prefer the retroperitoneal approach. Access to the splenic and renal arteries is by a prerenal approach (see above) which allows access to the splenic artery in front and to the renal artery behind within a limited dissection. The splenic artery should be exposed close to its origin from the celiac trunk and not near the hilum of the spleen so that the revascularization is supported by a large diameter vessel. After ligature and division of the pancreatic branches, the artery needs only to be freed for a length of 4 cm. The anastomosis should preferably be end-to-end to the renal artery.

Hepatorenal Anastomosis

For this, the transperitoneal approach is required and depending on the preference of the surgical team, the right subcostal or the midline approach is used. Dissection of the hepatic artery and its branches at the level of the hepatic pedicle must take into account the different techniques available for repair.[9,10] The renal artery is exposed as described. The entire retrocaval segment of the artery must be mobilized. During reconstruction the renal artery, which has been tied and cut in its healthy segment, is transposed in front of the IVC. It then runs along the right side of the vena cava, above the junction of the right renal vein and IVC towards the hepatic hilum. This maneuver results in a substantial gain in the length of the renal artery.

Ex Situ Surgery with Autotransplantation

This type of repair requires ample exposure of the iliac arteries. It may be necessary to harvest the hypogastric artery to be used as an arterial autograft, or to reimplant the kidney in the iliac vessels. The incision along the 10th rib described above facilitates the latter perfectly as long as it is extended downwards in the direction of the iliac fossa. We do not use Risberg's technique because of the resulting denervation of the rectus muscle. When the anatomic conditions permit, notably when the renal vessels are long, it is sometimes possible to reimplant the kidney in an orthotopic position in the renal fossa which reduces the size of the abdominal wall incision.

Associated Lesions

The most complex possibility is the combination of a renal vascular lesion with an aortic aneurysm requiring simultaneous surgery.

Aortic Aneurysm and Bilateral Renal Artery Lesions

The midline transperitoneal incision is the preferred approach. The renal arteries are accessed via a submesocolic approach described above. If it appears that renal artery repair will be reconstructed using a prosthetic graft, two branches are sutured to the body of the aortic prosthesis before beginning the vascular repair. After the proximal aortic anastomosis is performed each of the renal arteries is tied, cut in a healthy segment, and anastomosed to the corresponding prosthetic branch. The ischemic time for each kidney should be 10 to 20 minutes for each side. Rarely, the renal arteries are sufficiently long to allow their direct implantation to the aortic prosthesis.

Aortic Aneurysm and Right Renal Artery Lesion

After a midline xiphopubic incision, the right renal artery is separated and dissected as described at the beginning of this chapter. To access the aorta, the right colon and the cecum are dissected and retracted towards the midline.

Aortic Aneurysm and Left Renal Artery Aortic Lesion

If the aortic aneurysm extends through the common iliac arteries, a midline xyphoid to pubis incision is preferred. If the aneurysm is limited to the infrarenal aorta or to the initial segment of the common iliac arteries, a left retroperitoneal approach is the best choice.[11]

References

1. Merklin RP, Mitchels NA. The variant renal and supra-renal blood supply with data on the inferior phrenic, ureteral and gonadal arteries. *J Int Coll Surg* 1958; 29: 41-76.

2. Branchereau A, Rosset E, Magnan PE, et al. Revascularisation rénale au cours de la chirurgie de l'aorte sous-rénale. In: Kieffer E, éd. *Chirurgie des Artères Rénales.* Paris, AERCV, 1993, pp 267-304.

3. Fey B, Dossot R, Quenu L. Les voies d'abord du rein. In: *Traité de Technique Chirurgicale,* tome VIII Paris, Masson et Cie, 1956, pp 9-58.

4. Risberg B, Seeman T, Ortenwall P. A new incision for retroperitoneal approach to the aorta. *Acta Chir Scand* 1989; 155: 89-91.

5. Royal SA, Callen PW. CT evaluation of anomalies of the inferior vena cava and left renal vein. *Am J Roentgenol* 1979; 132: 759-763.

6. Bernard R. Une modification de l'incision habituelle des grandes thoraco-phréno-laparotomies droites. *Mém Acad Chir* 1957; 83: 697-701.

7. Ricco JB, Barral X. Voies d'abord de l'artère rénale. In: Kieffer E, éd. *Chirurgie des Artères Rénales.* Paris, AERCV, 1993, pp 133-153.

8. Lacombe M, Maillard C. Chirurgie de l'artère rénale. *Encycl Méd Chir,* Paris, France, Techniques chirurgicales, Chirurgie Vasculaire. 43110, 9-1988, 28 p.

9. Libertino JA, Lagneau P. A new method of revascularization of the right renal artery by the gastroduodenal artery. *Surg Gynecol Obstet* 1983; 156: 220-223.

10. Chibaro EA, Libertino JA, Novick AC. Use of the hepatic circulation for renal revascularization. *Ann Surg* 1984; 199: 406-411.

11. O'Mara CS, Williams GM. Extended retroperitoneal approach for abdominal aortic aneurysm repair. In: Bergan JJ, Yao JST, eds. *Aneurysm: Diagnosis and Treatment.* New York, Grune & Stratton, 1982, pp 327-343.

23

Inferior Vena Cava

Andris Kazmers

Open exposure of the inferior vena cava (IVC) has been required with decreasing frequency since endovascular vena cava filter placement has superceded external vena cava clipping.[1] The need for direct inferior vena cava thrombectomy has also been obviated in most patients by transfemoral venous thrombectomy, thrombolytic therapy, endovascular therapy, or combinations thereof.[2-4] Open exposure of the inferior vena cava is most often required for management of vena cava injuries or malignancies, primarily or secondarily involving the vena cava.[5-12]

The IVC originates at the confluence of the paired common iliac veins on the right side of the 5th lumbar vertebra (Fig. 1). As the IVC ascends to the right of the intraabdominal aorta, it receives lumbar, gonadal, renal, right adrenal, minor and major hepatic branches, and phrenic branches before penetrating the central tendon of the diaphragm to the right of midline at the level of the 8th thoracic vertebra.[13] After leaving the abdomen, the IVC travels superiorly and has a short intrathoracic segment which opens into the posterior, inferior aspect of the right atrium. The IVC has many important anatomic relationships. At its

origin, the IVC may be covered by the aortic bifurcation and right common iliac artery. In some cases, the right common iliac artery may cover the origin of the left common iliac vein. More cephalad, the IVC is covered by the mesentery of the small and large intestine, pancreas and first, second, and third portions of the duodenum. At the level of the renal veins, the IVC covers the right renal artery. As it ascends further cephalad, the IVC is separated from the portal structures by the gastroepiploic foramen and then is covered anterolaterally by the liver.

Renal vein and vena cava anomalies may pose hazards during aortic surgery.[14-15] A circumaortic renal vein or retroaortic left renal vein can be injured during aortic cross-clamping or periaortic dissection. Left-sided or double IVC may be encountered and may mandate alterations of surgical technique for those undergoing aortic surgery or vena cava interruption.

Until relatively recently, survival after IVC injuries was poor. The typical approach to management of IVC and other venous injuries had been ligation. Prior studies indicate that

---

From Vascular Surgical Approaches, edited by Alain Branchereau and Ramon Berguer. ©1999, Futura Publishing Co., Inc., Armonk, NY.

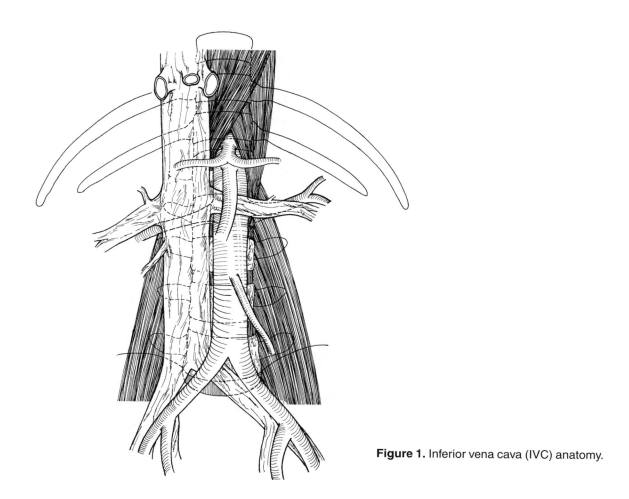

Figure 1. Inferior vena cava (IVC) anatomy.

ligation of the IVC after injury was associated with significant mortality and morbidity. Ligation above the renal veins was associated with a greater mortality rate compared with ligation below the renal veins, but there was a comparable rate of lower extremity edema.[16-17] Because of the precipitous reduction in venous return and profound venous stasis after IVC ligation, techniques were developed to avoid IVC ligation such as lateral venous repair, patch venoplasty, and IVC replacement.

Because of the resulting acute hemodynamic instability and chronic venous stasis in survivors, IVC ligation for prevention of pulmonary emboli was replaced by the application of external caval clips or other methods which theoretically permitted ongoing caval blood flow. The ease of insertion and noninvasive nature of transluminal inferior vena

cava filter placement and the higher incidence of caval patency, however, have eliminated the need for direct caval exposure and IVC plication or external vena cava clip insertion. Even in patients who face laparotomy, it is preferable to insert a transvenous vena cava filter at or prior to the time of laparotomy rather than to place an external caval clip at laparotomy; this is because of the greater likelihood of caval occlusion and worsening venous symptoms in those undergoing external clipping versus insertion of an IVC filter. Transvenous IVC filter insertion is not difficult, does not add to the blood loss of open abdominal surgery, and is more likely to permit ongoing caval patency with resultant reductions in venous stasis. It is likely that few general and vascular surgeons who have trained in the United States during the last decade have placed an external vena cava clip during their training, whereas most surgeons are familiar with transvenous vena cava filter insertion.

Iliofemoral venous thrombectomy has been an infrequently used approach to the management of deep venous thrombosis.[2,4] Though some are more apt to perform iliofemoral venous thrombectomy, with or without subsequent creation of a femoral arteriovenous fistula, surgeons in the United States have reserved venous thrombectomy for patients with phlegmasia cerulea dolens or impending venous gangrene when nonoperative therapy is unsuccessful or lytic therapy is contraindicated. Cavotomy and direct thrombectomy of the inferior vena cava, although still in use, are unlikely to be required for management of patients with deep venous thrombosis and caval involvement. With the availability of thrombectomy catheters designed for use in the venous system, and intraoperative fluoroscopy to guide iliac and caval thrombectomy, direct cavotomy should rarely be required for removal of iliocaval venous thrombus. Use of bilateral femoral venous thrombectomy with placement of an occlusive balloon into the IVC from one groin while performing thrombectomy from the other is one way of clearing the IVC safely without cavotomy. Others have recommended insertion of an IVC filter prior to transfemoral IVC thrombectomy to prevent pulmonary embolism during venous thrombectomy.

Unlike venous thrombosis involving the IVC, removal of tumor thrombus may require cavotomy. Endovenous tumor extension in the IVC most commonly originates from renal tumors, and the right kidney is more commonly the source than the left. About one-half of such tumor thrombi remain within the renal vein, and two-thirds remain infrahepatic in location. The remaining tumor thrombi ascend into the retrohepatic or suprahepatic IVC, and a small number continue into the heart. Venous endothelium tends to prevent tumor invasion. As a result, tumor thrombi have been removed by cavotomy, partial or circumferential cavectomy, atriotomy, or combinations thereof. The use of extracorporeal circulatory support is sometimes required. The complexities and nature of such procedures are beyond the scope

of this brief description of surgical exposure of the IVC.

Primary tumors of the IVC are rare. Secondary malignant involvement of the IVC may result from invasion from adjacent structures such as lymph nodes or from transvenous spread. IVC resection has been performed both for primary and secondary caval malignancy.[6-11,18] Suitable substitutes for replacement of the IVC have yet to be developed. Spiral vein grafts have been used to replace IVC segments, but some centers report no better results with such autogenous grafts than with prosthetic grafts made of externally supported polytetrafluoroethylene (PTFE) in reconstruction of the inferior vena cava. Recent reports of successful IVC replacement using such prosthetic grafts are encouraging.[8]

Access to the IVC may be transperitoneal or retroperitoneal. Transperitoneal exposure of the IVC can be achieved with either paramedian, midline, transverse, or oblique abdominal incisions (Fig. 2). General anesthesia with satisfactory muscle relaxation facilitates IVC exposure regardless of which route or incision is chosen. With transabdominal exposure, the small intestine is reflected to the patient's left and the right colon is mobilized laterally to medially after incising the peritoneum along the right colic gutter (Fig. 3). In some cases the entire right colon can be mobilized superiomedially for excellent caval exposure. An extended Kocher maneuver mobilizing the duodenum and head of pancreas completes exposure of the infrahepatic IVC to the iliac vein bifurcation (Figs. 3 and 4). In selected cases, the suspensory ligaments of the liver can be divided for mobilization of the liver permitting access to the suprahepatic and retrohepatic vena cava.

Historically, access to the infrarenal IVC for placement of external clips was achieved via the retroperitoneal route (Figs. 5 and 6). For such procedures, the right flank is slightly elevated using sheets or a bean bag and a skin incision is made lateral to the rectus muscle at the level of the umbilicus. The incision can be carried onto the flank transversely or obliquely. The external and internal oblique muscles and transversus abdominis muscles can be divided in the direction of their fibers or in the direction of the incision. The retroperitoneum

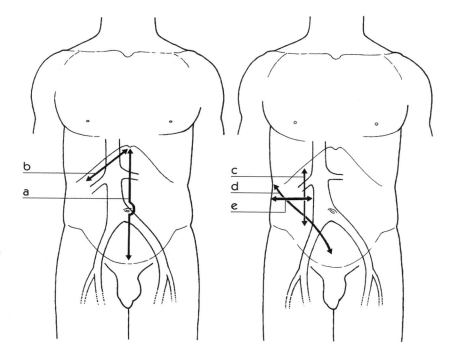

Figure 2. Potential incisions to provide access to the IVC.
a. Midline laparotomy.
b. Right subcostal incision.
c. Right paramedian incision.
d. Right retroperitoneal incision.
e. Transverse flank incision.

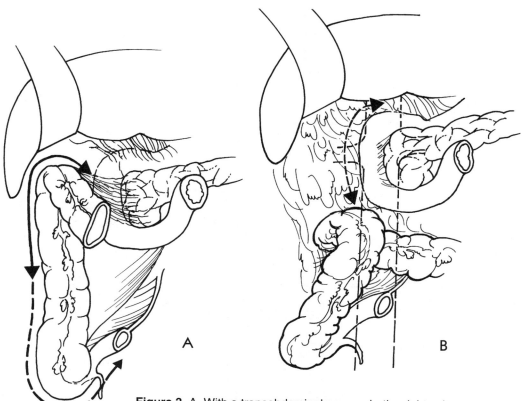

Figure 3. A. With a transabdominal approach, the right colon is reflected medially after dividing the retroperitoneal tissue along the right colic gutter. The entire right colon can be mobilized superomedially. B. The disclosure is mobilized using a Kocher maneuver.

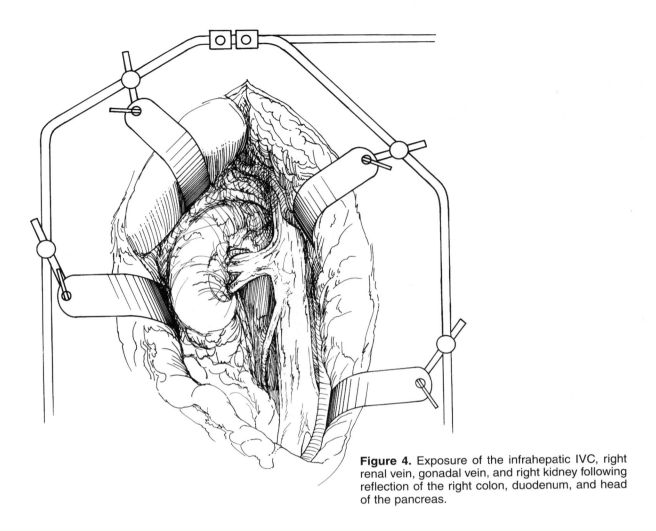

Figure 4. Exposure of the infrahepatic IVC, right renal vein, gonadal vein, and right kidney following reflection of the right colon, duodenum, and head of the pancreas.

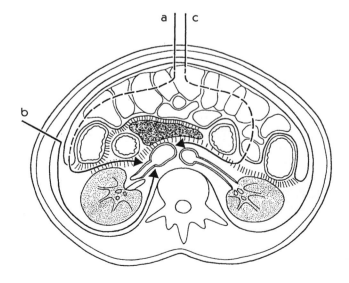

Figure 5. Cross-sectional view from above revealing:

a. Right retrocolic and retroduodenal approach defined in Figures 3 and 4.

b. Right retrorenal approach, which may be useful during a right nephrectomy and resection of the right renal vein tumor thrombus.

c. Transperitoneal approach by detachment of the duodenojejunal angle.

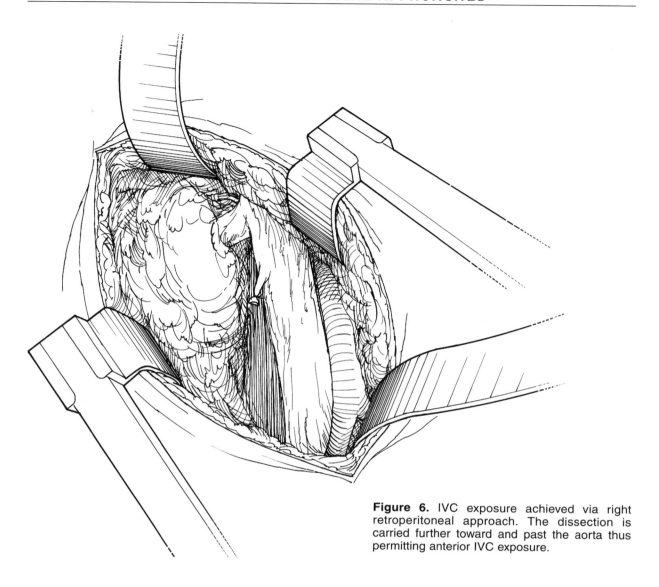

Figure 6. IVC exposure achieved via right retroperitoneal approach. The dissection is carried further toward and past the aorta thus permitting anterior IVC exposure.

is most easily entered laterally after dividing the transversus abdominis and transversalis fascia. The peritoneal contents and ureter are then swept upward. The IVC can be exposed through this right retroperitoneal approach much like exposure of the aorta via the left retroperitoneal approach (Fig. 6).

Some have advocated resection of the IVC obstructed by tumor without reconstruction. This is feasible when the infrarenal IVC is obstructed by the malignant process and adequate venous collateral has already been demonstrated. Otherwise such resection and oversewing of the infrarenal IVC and iliac vein

confluence may be associated with significant venous stasis. When the renal veins are involved with such a malignant process, renal dysfunction and even renal failure may result from renal venous hypertension if reconstruction is not performed. Even more complex reconstructions may be necessary which may require a great deal of planning. Use of circulatory support, including venovenous bypass, cardiopulmonary bypass, and even circulatory arrest has been anecdotally reported.[10,11,18]

Low venous pressures facilitate external compression and failure of such major venous reconstructions. Spiral saphenous vein grafts, composite vein grafts, and superficial femoral veins have been used for vena cava replacements. Ringed expanded PTFE has been a satisfactory conduit for replacement of the suprarenal or infrarenal IVC. It appears one of the newer horizons in vascular surgery may include reconstructive surgery of the vena cava. More aggressive management of tumors involving the vena cava may prompt a revolutionary surge in such major venous surgery.

References

1. Pollak EW, Sparks FC, Baker WF. Inferior vena cava interruption: Indications and results with caval ligation, clips and intracaval devices. *J Cardiovasc Surg* (Torino) 1974; 15: 629.
2. Neglen P, Nazzal MMS, Al-Hassan HKh, et al. Surgical removal of an inferior vena cava thrombus. *Eur J Vasc Surg* 1992; 6: 78-82.
3. Donohue JP, Thornhi JA, Foster RS, et al. Resection of the inferior vena cava or intraluminal vena caval tumor thrombectomy during retroperitoneal lymph node dissection for metastatic germ cell cancer: Indications and results. *J Urol* 1991; 146: 346-349.
4. Eklof B, Einarsson E, Plate G. Role of thrombectomy and temporary arteriovenous fistula in acute iliofemoral venous thrombosis. In: Bergan JJ, Yao JST, eds. *Surgery of the Veins*. New York, Grune & Stratton, 1985, pp 131-144.
5. Bower TC, Nagorney DM, Toomey BJ, et al. Vena cava replacement for malignant disease: Is there a role? *Ann Vasc Surg* 1993; 7: 51-62.
6. Huguet C, Ferri M, Gavelli A. Resection of the suprarenal inferior vena cava: The role of prosthetic replacement. *Arch Surg* 1995; 130: 793-797.
7. Kieffer E, Berrod JL, Chomette G. Primary tumors of the inferior vena cava. In: Bergan JJ, Yao JST, eds. *Surgery of the Veins*. New York, Grune & Stratton, 1985, pp 423-443.
8. Okada Y, Kumada K, Terachi T, et al. Long-term followup of patients with tumor thrombi from renal cell carcinoma and total replacement of the inferior vena cava using an expanded polytetrafluoroethylene tubular graft. *J Urol* 1996; 155: 444-447.
9. Schecter DC. Cardiovascular surgery in the management of exogenous tumors involving the vena cava. In: Bergan JJ, Yao JST, eds. *Surgery of the Veins*. New York, Grune & Stratton, 1985, pp 393-412.
10. Sener SF, Arentzen CE, O'Connor B, et al. Hepatic and vena cava resection using cardiopulmonary bypass with hypothermic circulatory arrest. *Am Surg* 1996; 62: 525-529.
11. Yanaga K, Okadome K, Ito H, et al. Graft replacement of pararenal inferior vena cava for leiomyosarcoma with the use of venous bypass. *Surgery* 1993;113:109-112.
12. Degiannis E, Velmahos GC, Levy RD, et al. Penetrating injuries of the abdominal inferior vena cava. *Ann Rev Coll Surg Engl* 1996; 78: 485-489.
13. Wind GG, Valentine RJ. *Anatomic Exposures in Vascular Surgery*. Baltimore, Williams & Wilkins, 1991, pp 294-307.
14. Brener BJ, Darling RC, Frederick PL, Linton RR. Major venous anomalies complicating abdominal aortic surgery. *Arch Surg* 1974; 108: 159.
15. Miles RM, Flowers BF, Parson HL, Benitone JD. Some surgical implications of the anatomy of the caviliofemoral system. *Ann Surg* 1973; 177: 740-747.
16. Ehrichs E. Major vascular ligations. In: Eiseman B, ed. *Prognosis of Surgical Disease*. Philadelphia, WB Saunders, 1980, pp 102-105.
17. Nesbit RM, Wear JB. Ligation of the inferior vena cava above the renal veins. *Ann Surg* 1964; 154: 332.
18. Baumgartner F, Milliken J, Scudamore C, Nair C, Gelman J, Scott R, Rajfer J, Klein S. Extracorporeal methods of vascular control for difficult IVC procedures. *Ann Surg* 1996; 62: 246-248.

24

Suprarenal Inferior Vena Cava

Jean-Georges Kretz, Nabil Chafke, Philippe Nicolini

Surgical reconstruction of the inferior vena cava (IVC) is rare. The most frequent indications relate almost exclusively to the infrarenal segment of the vessel. Access to the latter is easily accomplished because of its very close relationship to the abdominal aorta. Access to the suprarenal vena cava (suprarenal tumors, leiomyosarcomas of the IVC, complex traumatisms) is more complex, and infrequently performed by vascular surgeons.

Anatomic Review

The IVC originates at the confluence of two common iliac veins, right anterolateral to the fifth lumbar vertebra. From there, the single venous trunk rises vertically on the right face of the spine as far as L1. There, the IVC bends to the right and passes behind the liver to reach the diaphragm, where it crosses the right part of its tendinous center at the level of T9. It then reaches the inferior face of the right atrium by curving slightly forward and to the left.

Branches

The renal veins join the IVC at the level of L1. The left renal vein is a little higher than the right. After a trajectory of 4-8 cm, it crosses over the aorta at the angle formed by the latter and the first segment of the superior mesenteric artery. The right renal vein is short and goes directly from the renal hilum to the right wall of the IVC. The right middle adrenal vein is always present and fairly large; it is usually situated 3-4 cm above the right renal vein, but this can vary greatly. It may be very close, almost attached to the right renal vein, in which case surgical control may be difficult. The right retrohepatic veins are frequently double: the right inferior and right middle retrohepatic veins (the larger of the two). The left retrohepatic veins are more variable both in number and size; they drain the caudate lobe of the liver towards the anterior surface of the IVC. These retrohepatic veins make direct access to the anterior face of the retrohepatic IVC difficult and when this exposure is needed

From Vascular Surgical Approaches, edited by Alain Branchereau and Ramon Berguer. ©1999, Futura Publishing Co., Inc., Armonk, NY.

it is best to perform vascular exclusion of the liver. Generally there are two diaphragmatic veins; they join the IVC at the level of the orifice of the diaphragm. Control of the interhepato-diaphragmatic segment of the IVC is easier when these veins are divided and ligated. There are usually three suprahepatic veins: the right, left, and middle (Fig. 1).

the IVC is surrounded by the duodenopancreatic complex, the portal vein, and the common bile duct. In front of the pancreas we find the root of the transverse mesocolon, the vertical part of the root of the mesentery, and the superior mesenteric artery and vein. The duodenopancreatic complex is mobilized to the left to distance these elements from the IVC. The hepatic pedicle is contained in the right edge of the lesser omentum and constitutes the anterior limit of the foramen of Winslow. The IVC covered by the posterior parietal peritoneum constitutes the posterior limit. In its retrohepatic segment, the IVC runs in the groove situated between the right and the caudate lobes of the liver close to the hepatic parenchyma to which it is tightly attached by the retrohepatic veins. The close proximity between the liver and the IVC constitutes the main difficulty of the surgical approach to this segment of the IVC.

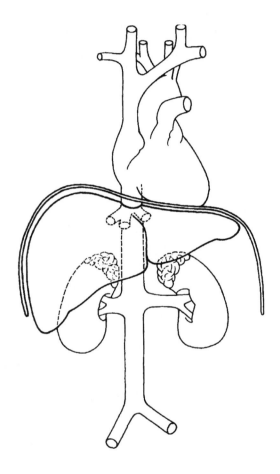

Figure 1. Topographic anatomy of the IVC.

Indications and Considerations

A basic principle is the need to control the upper and lower adjacent venous segments before exposing the suprarenal segment of the IVC. Operations on the suprarenal IVC always require control of the suprahepatic IVC, and possibly the intrapericardial segment, as well as control of the infrarenal IVC. This surgical approach should not be undertaken except in conditions that allow management of large blood losses. Venous access permitting large volume flow infusion and a system for intraoperative blood recovery should be available.[1-3]

The patient is supine. The arms are placed along the body. Monitoring of arterial pressure with a catheter in the radial artery is mandatory. The surgeon is to the right of the patient with an assistant opposite and a second assistant to his/her left. The instrument nurse is at the foot of the patient, on the left side. Temperature monitoring is done via an esophageal probe, and generally supplemented by a urinary bladder thermometer incorporated in the Foley catheter.

Anterior Relationships

We discuss only those relationships relevant to the surgical approach to the suprarenal segment of the IVC. From L1 to L3,

Incisions

A median laparotomy, xiphoid to pubis, is the basic approach used for all types of traumatic lesions. It allows access to all intraabdominal viscera and treatment of associated lesions. It may easily be extended upwards using a sternotomy to control the intrapericardiac IVC, to place the patient on cardiopulmonary bypass, if necessary, or to insert an intracaval shunt.

Bilateral subcostal access can also be obtained by a chevron incision which passes 4 cm or 5 cm above the umbilicus and provides access to the entire abdominal cavity. When accessing the IVC, the incision must be extended to the sides as far as the midaxillary line in the lumbar area. This large incision is better tolerated, from a respiratory point of view, and it rarely results in an incisional hernia. Where necessary it can be enlarged upwards by an additional midline prolongation extending as far as the xiphoid process (Fig. 2).

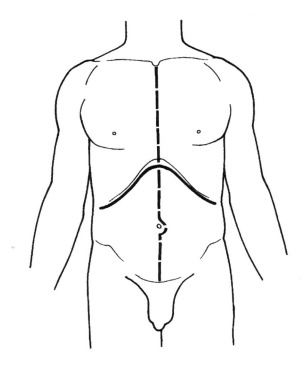

Figure 2. Different incisions.

Whichever incision is used, orthostatic retractors are needed. Towards the top, the canopy of the ribs must be retracted and the diaphragm stretched upwards. A subcostal retractor is used for this purpose and ensures excellent exposure. Widening the edges of the wound is performed using any of the fixed-frame retractors available (Bookwalters, Omni).

Infrarenal and Juxtarenal Vena Cava

After opening the peritoneum, the greater omentum and transverse mesocolon are exteriorized over the rib cage. The right colon is pulled forward and to the left, and the right gutter is opened from top to bottom. The colonic detachment is performed cutting the parietal mesocolic attachment as far up as the wall of the second portion of the duodenum. This detachment is followed upwards by cutting the hepatocolic ligament which frees the right colic angle. The dissection is followed by complete detachment of the duodenopancreatic complex following its posterior attachment fascia (Kocher's maneuver). This detachment allows the ascending colon and the mass of the duodenopancreatic block to be displaced to the left exposing the anterior surface of the suprarenal IVC (Fig. 3). Division of the posterior peritoneum, following the left edge of the root of the mesenterium and of the inferior mesenteric vein near the duodenojejunal angle, allows the right colon and small bowel to be exteriorized and laid over the rib margin. A retractor is placed over the inferior surface of the liver, and another retracts the duodenopancreatic block to the left allowing excellent exposure of the entire IVC from its origin as far as the lower edge of the liver. The dissection is made over the anterior face of the IVC to avoid its collaterals. Once the anterior face is freed, the renal veins are controlled by soft loops and freed for a length of 2 cm.

Gentle traction on the loops placed around the renal veins allows separation of the IVC from the posterior plane. In this way a blunt instrument may be passed behind the IVC under visual control. This maneuver should be performed very gently and on no account

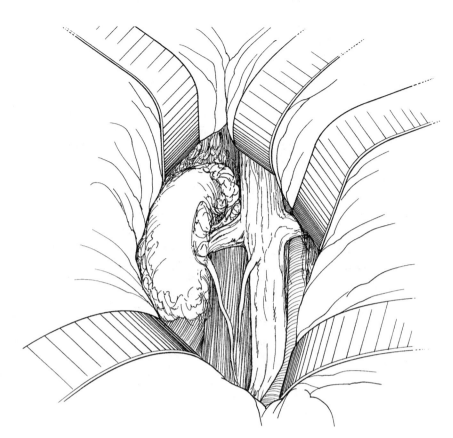

Figure 3. Abdominal access to the infra- and juxtarenal IVC.

should an instrument be forced or used to overcome any resistance in order to surround the IVC. If there is any resistance, the instrument should be removed and the same procedure attempted 2 cm above or below the level where the attempt was made. Exposure above the renal veins may be continued as far as the lower edge of the caudate lobe of the liver where the dissection stops because of the potential danger of injury to the left retrohepatic veins, which are always difficult to control. At this point attention is directed to control of the suprahepatic IVC.

Suprahepatic Vena Cava

Abdominal Approach

Control of the IVC between the liver and the diaphragm can be achieved using an abdominal approach, especially a bisubcostal incision extending to the sides. The round ligament is divided and the hepatic dome is lowered with the palm of the hand. This maneuver puts the falciforme ligament under tension and facilitates its division using an electric cautery. Close to the anterior face of the IVC, the falciforme ligament divides into two leaves. Between them there is some fat tissue covering the anterior wall of the IVC (Fig. 4). Towards the top the vein joins the orifice of the diaphragm, recognizable by some muscular fibers that pass across. A dissection plane between the IVC and the orifice of the diaphragm allows freeing the foramen for a few centimeters (Fig. 5).

It is then possible to cut, in sequence, the right and left coronary ligaments. This is done by pushing down each lobe of the liver and placing the ligament under tension before dividing them with cautery up to the lateral border of the IVC. If the veins of the diaphragm hinder the freeing of the IVC, they are divided between ligatures.

Once the IVC is freed from the front and sides a soft loop is passed around it. The IVC is

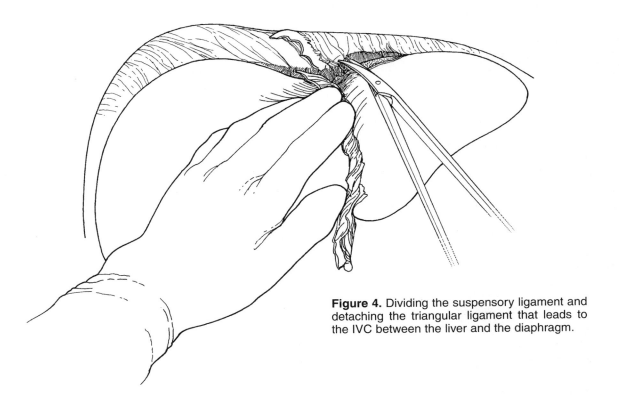

Figure 4. Dividing the suspensory ligament and detaching the triangular ligament that leads to the IVC between the liver and the diaphragm.

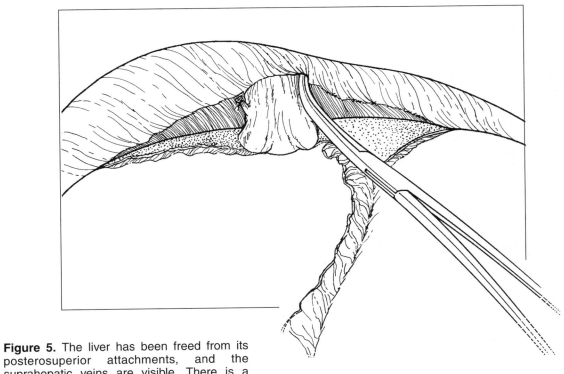

Figure 5. The liver has been freed from its posterosuperior attachments, and the suprahepatic veins are visible. There is a plane for dissection between the IVC and the orifice of the diaphragm.

surrounded using a crooked left index finger to collar the posterior face of the IVC while passing the loop away from the venous wall and in contact with the crus of the diaphragm.[4]

Thoracic Approach

In the case of a mixed approach using a sternolaparotomy, control of the intrapericardiac IVC is simple. After opening the pericardium, the right atrium is pushed back using a sponge on a stick and the space between the IVC below and the inferior pulmonary vein to the right is opened with the scissors. A large, curved, soft blunt dissector is passed below the right atrium in contact with the left wall of the IVC. It then surrounds the IVC in order to exit from the space that has been previously opened (Fig. 6). In this area the IVC can be exposed for a length of 2-3 cm.[5]

Retrohepatic Vena Cava

As already discussed, the retrohepatic IVC can only be exposed after obtaining separate control of the suprarenal-infrahepatic and the suprahepatic segments of the IVC. To expose the retrohepatic IVC, it is sufficient to keep one hand on the right lobe of the liver and to progressively pull it from right to left and back to front following division of the triangular and right coronary ligaments as far as possible. The IVC is thus exposed and freed from bottom to top, while the right lobe is progressively luxated to the left (Fig. 7). At this point the posterior peritoneum still needs to be incised. Its line of reflection crosses the anterior surface of the superior pole of the right kidney. The anterior surface of the right adrenal gland and the middle adrenal vein are dissected free. After the latter is tied and cut the surgeon has access to the entire right wall of the retrohepatic IVC. During these maneuvers it is important to check the hemodynamic tolerance to the

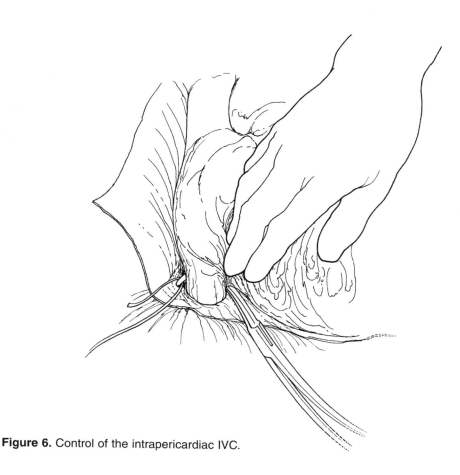

Figure 6. Control of the intrapericardiac IVC.

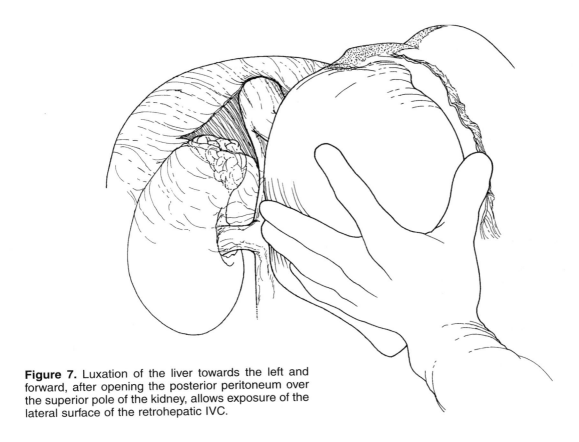

Figure 7. Luxation of the liver towards the left and forward, after opening the posterior peritoneum over the superior pole of the kidney, allows exposure of the lateral surface of the retrohepatic IVC.

luxation of the right hepatic lobe and, if required, release the traction. At the end of the dissection, the entire right lateral and posterior surfaces of the retrohepatic IVC are free. It is then possible to pass a hand behind it.[4]

Thoracoabdominal Approach

Access to the IVC was classically described via a right thoracoabdominal approach. This is a more aggressive approach, more difficult to close and with more postoperative complications, and thus it has been almost completely abandoned. Nevertheless, this technique may still be used if a previous retrohepatic approach to the IVC has already been performed using a midline or subcostal approach (such as in a tumor recurrence), or if a right thoracotomy is formally indicated at the same time, as may be the case when confronted with a penetrating wound or right thoracic trauma. Access to the IVC itself is identical to the

technique previously described and consists of first controlling the juxtarenal IVC and the suprahepatic IVC. The retrohepatic segment may be accessed after luxation of the right lobe of the liver.

References

1. Berguer R, Wilson RF, Wiencek RG Jr. Traumatismes aigus de la veine cave inférieure. In: Kieffer E, ed. *Chirurgie de la veine cave inférieure et de ses branches*. Paris, Expansion Scientifique française, 1985 pp 101-104.
2. Howell HS, Ingram CH. Techniques for controlling hemorrhage after injuries of the lower inferior vena cava and iliac veins. *Am Surg* 1981; 47: 507-508.
3. Misra B, Wagner R, Boneval H. Injuries of hepatic veins and retrohepatic vena cava. *Am Surg* 1983; 49: 55-60.
4. Wolf P, Mattox K, Cinqualbre J. Chirurgie de la veine cave inférieure. *Encycl Méd Chir*. Paris, Techniques chirurgicales, Chirurgie Vasculaire, 43172, 4.9, 12, 24p.
5. Pouyet M, Perrin JP. Réflexions sur le traitement des lésions veineuses sus-hépato-caves traumatiques. A propos de 53 cas. *J Chir* 1980; 117: 305-311.

25

Portal Vein and Branches

Charles E. Lucas

Anatomic Review

The portal vein (PV) lies posterior in the right upper quadrant and passes obliquely from medial to lateral as it ascends superiorly. The PV arises at the confluence of the splenic vein (SV) and superior mesenteric vein (SMV) behind the neck of the pancreas. This point is anterior and to the right of the second lumbar vertebra. As the PV ascends, it passes posterior to the proximal duodenum where it becomes part of the portal triad; it lies posterior to the more medial hepatic artery and the more lateral common bile duct. The length from the confluence of the SMV and SV to the PV bifurcation into the right and left branches ranges from 7-9 cm in adults with a diameter of 1-2 cm.

The main tributaries of the PV are the SV and the SMV. The SV is formed by the confluence of 4-8 splenic hilar veins which join along the posterosuperior border of the pancreatic tail. The SV passes medially just posterior to the body and tail of the pancreas from which it receives many short pancreatic veins. Along the superior border, the proximal SV receives the short gastric veins and the left

gastroepiploic vein, whereas the inferior mesenteric vein enters its inferior border where the SV joins with the SMV to form the PV. Thus, access to the proximal PV requires exposure and control of the SV and its more distal tributaries.

The SMV is fed by the right gastroepiploic vein which joins the SMV just inferior to the pancreatic head and the posterior pancreatico-duodenal vein which joins the SMV or PV near the superior margin of the pancreas. One or more of the pyloric veins, the prepyloric vein, and right gastric vein will enter the proximal PV on the anterior medial border as one or two separate, small, but potentially treacherous veins, especially in patients with portal hypertension. The left gastric vein, commonly known as the coronary vein, drains the proximal lesser curvature of the stomach, passes through the lesser omentum near the inferior margin of the liver, and enters the PV along the medial or anteromedial wall close to the bifurcation into the right and left PV branches.

One or more smaller cystic veins, after receiving the venous drainage of the

From Vascular Surgical Approaches, edited by Alain Branchereau and Ramon Berguer. ©1999, Futura Publishing Co., Inc., Armonk, NY.

gallbladder, enter the PV laterally near the bifurcation or after the bifurcation into the right branch of the PV. The umbilical vein passes through the round ligament between the lateral and medial segments of the left lobe of the liver and joins the left branch of the PV intrahepatically.

Positioning and Incisions

Anterior Right Subcostal Approach

The most common incision used for exposing the PV is the right subcostal incision which provides optimal exposure for performing most portal systemic shunts in patients with portal hypertension, typically seen with Laennec's cirrhosis or schistosomiasis (Fig. 1).[1] Although fewer shunts are being performed since the widespread accept-

ance of the transjugular intrahepatic portal shunt (TIPS), sclerotherapy, and liver transplantation, portal decompression is still needed in patients for whom sclerotherapy and/or TIPS are not successful.[2,3] The patient is positioned supine with the right lower rib cage and right upper abdomen elevated approximately 2 inches with sheets or blankets. The right arm is elevated on an ether screen to help retract the enlarged liver. The incision is made two fingerbreadths below the right rib margin and extends from the left costal margin medially to the anterior axillary line or midaxillary line laterally (Fig. 1). Upon entering the abdomen, the round ligament is divided. After completing the intraabdominal examination, the filmy adhesions between the gallbladder and both the hepatic flexure of the colon and/or the proximal duodenum are divided (Fig. 2). Normally, these filmy adhesions are avascular, but in patients with portal hypertension, they have multiple collateral lymphatics and veins thus mandating careful hemostasis.

The hepatic flexure of the colon is mobilized by dividing the retroperitoneal attachments which extend up to the inferior posterior margin of the liver and to the right retroperitoneal white line of Told (Fig. 2). Careful hemostasis of the multiple unnamed collateral vessels is necessary. A formal Kocher maneuver is now performed as the proximal and lateral duodenum are mobilized inferiorly and medially, thereby unroofing the distal common bile duct. These tissues contain many unnamed vessels with portal hypertension. The portal triad now is widely exposed (Fig. 3). The distal common bile duct can now be dissected along the anterior and lateral margins. As this dissection is carried out, the surgeon must be careful to avoid inadvertent division of an anomalous cystic duct that may enter inferiorly into the common duct and may be mistaken for one of the thickened sclerotic lymphatic channels typically seen in patients with portal hypertension. Once identified and dissected free, the common bile duct is retracted medially, thereby identifying the lymphatic tissues between the common bile duct and PV. These tissues are divided and ligated down to the periadventitial plain. Once this plain is identified, the PV can be dissected circumferentially at its mid-portion without fear of

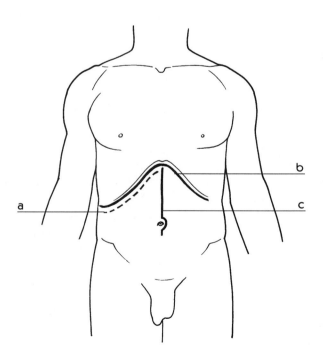

Figure 1. Common incisions used for exposure of the portal vein and branches.
a. Anterior right subcostal approach.
b. Chevron incision.
c. Upper midline approach.

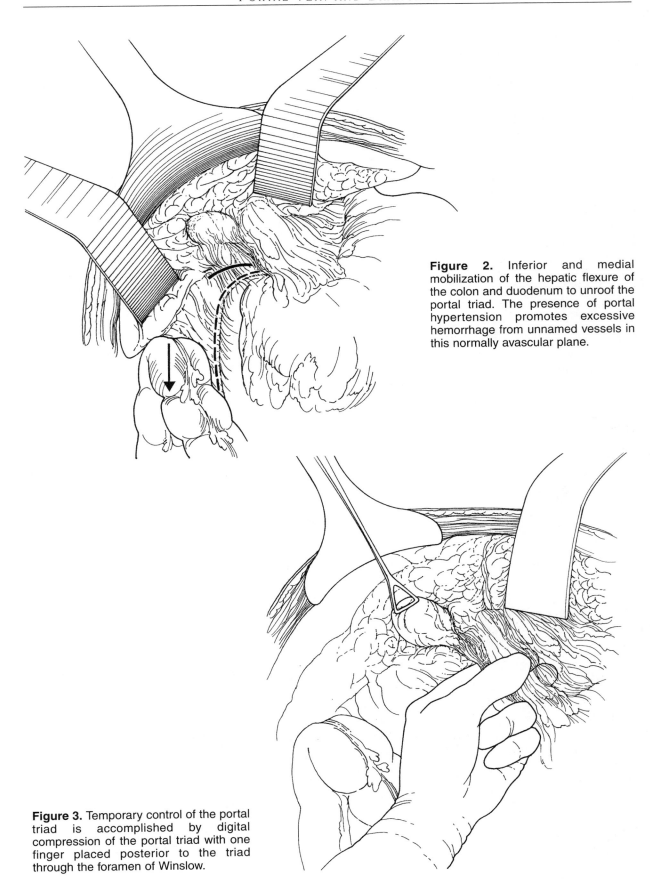

Figure 2. Inferior and medial mobilization of the hepatic flexure of the colon and duodenum to unroof the portal triad. The presence of portal hypertension promotes excessive hemorrhage from unnamed vessels in this normally avascular plane.

Figure 3. Temporary control of the portal triad is accomplished by digital compression of the portal triad with one finger placed posterior to the triad through the foramen of Winslow.

injuring venous branches (Fig. 4). Careful excision of this lymph node followed by ligation of these veins circumvents significant hemorrhage. A branch of the pyloric vein or right gastric vein entering along the anteromedial wall of the proximal PV may require division and ligation but usually can be left undissected while freeing up enough of the PV to accomplish most portal systemic shunts. After the PV has been circumferentially dissected, gentle lateral traction allows for the distal vein to be dissected. The right gastric vein enters into the PV along the medial margin closer to the origin of the left branch of the PV. When necessary to obtain adequate length, this vein can be doubly clamped, divided, and ligated. This approach allows for a 5-6 cm segment of PV mobilization. This length of PV is enough to perform an easy end-to-side portal caval shunt, interposition graft between the PV and vena cava, and side-to-side portal caval shunt (Fig. 5). Some patients with hepatomegaly will have a large caudate lobe which compromises a tension-free side-to-side anastomosis between the PV and vena cava. This problem can be obviated by resection of the inferior portion of the caudate lobe using electrocoagulation to obtain hemostasis. The small veins between the caudate lobe and the anterior wall of the vena cava usually do not have to be divided when performing this maneuver.

Upper Abdominal Chevron Incision

The combined bilateral subcostal incision, often known as the chevron incision,[1] is convenient for performing a distal splenorenal shunt which requires mobilization of the SV to its junction with the PV (Fig. 1A). This approach is also frequently used for pancreaticoduodenectomy which, in some patients, may require venous resection due to adherence of tumor into the junction of the SMV with the proximal PV.[4,5] The patient is in the supine position. Following the chevron incision, the round ligament is divided and the lesser sac is entered through the greater omentum between the arcades of the gastroepiploic vessels and the transverse colon. The attachments between the posterior gastric wall and the pancreas are divided in the avascular plane adjacent to the pancreas. The transverse mesocolon is followed proximally to where the superior leaf inserts along the inferior border of the pancreas (Fig. 6). This relatively avascular plane may have unnamed collaterals in patients with portal hypertension or in patients with tumor invading the SMV-PV junction. Once the inferior and posterior surfaces of the pancreas have been mobilized, the surgeon can expose the inferior mesenteric vein, the small pancreatic veins draining into the SV, and the right gastroepiploic vein which drains into the SMV (Fig. 6). Each of these structures needs to be carefully freed up, divided, and ligated. After the distal SV has been freed to the PV, the junction can be divided followed by suture ligation of the PV side and mobilization of the splanchnic vein for subsequent anastomosis to the left renal vein (Fig. 7).

In patients with pancreatic tumors, the superior margin of the pancreas should be freed up in its avascular plane. This allows the hepatic artery to be identified and mobilized after which the right gastric artery and gastroduodenal artery can be individually dissected and ligated. The hepatic artery is then retracted superiorly in order to expose the PV which runs through the posterior portion of a triangle formed by the hepatic artery, distal common bile duct, and superior border of the pancreas. Typically, one can dissect the PV-SMV junction posterior to the pancreas. When tumor involves the PV-SMV junction, an extended pancreaticoduodenectomy with venous resection may be performed.[5] The SMV and PV are divided and the tumor removed. An end-to-end venovenous anastomosis is then performed; when the gap is excessive, an interposition vein graft is placed. During pancreaticoduodenectomy, the lymph node that lies lateral and posterior to PV is exposed when the distal bile duct is mobilized inferiorly. This node which is resected has one or two veins that drain into the PV; they must be doubly clamped, divided, and ligated. Separation of the uncinate process from the distal SMV is best accomplished by dividing the tissues along the SMV margin with clamps followed by suture ligatures.

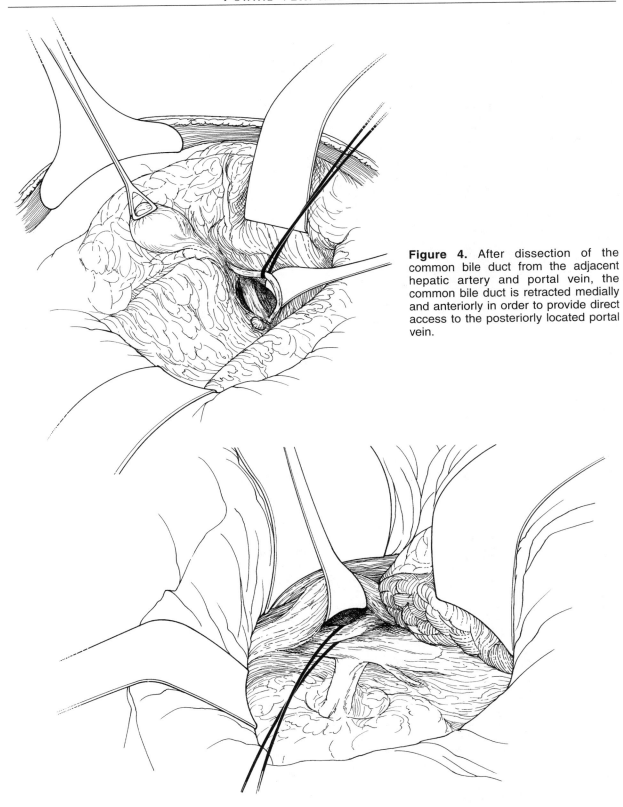

Figure 4. After dissection of the common bile duct from the adjacent hepatic artery and portal vein, the common bile duct is retracted medially and anteriorly in order to provide direct access to the posteriorly located portal vein.

Figure 5. Once the adventitial plane surrounding the portal vein has been entered laterally and anteriorly, the vein can be circumferentially dissected free in the mid-portion. More proximal and distal dissection can then be carried out while looking for branches which are carefully dissected free and ligated.

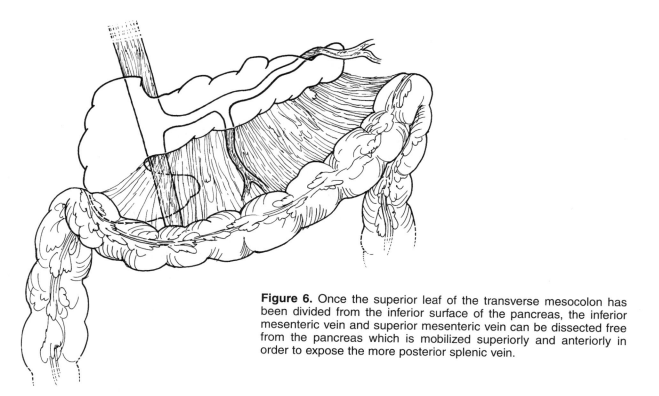

Figure 6. Once the superior leaf of the transverse mesocolon has been divided from the inferior surface of the pancreas, the inferior mesenteric vein and superior mesenteric vein can be dissected free from the pancreas which is mobilized superiorly and anteriorly in order to expose the more posterior splenic vein.

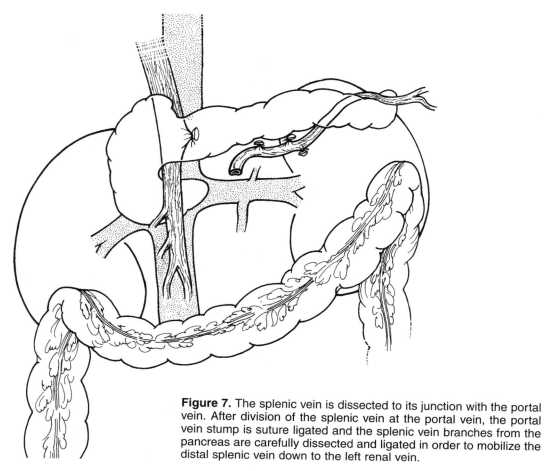

Figure 7. The splenic vein is dissected to its junction with the portal vein. After division of the splenic vein at the portal vein, the portal vein stump is suture ligated and the splenic vein branches from the pancreas are carefully dissected and ligated in order to mobilize the distal splenic vein down to the left renal vein.

Upper Midline Approach

The upper midline incision is sometimes used for performance of the distal splenorenal shunt, pancreatic resection, and trauma.[6] The incision typically extends from xiphoid to umbilicus or slightly below (Fig. 1). When the injured patient is bleeding from the PV, the injury is exposed by the same techniques outlined above, taking care to prevent injury to the adjacent common bile duct and hepatic artery. When the injury involves the proximal PV or retropancreatic portion of the SMV, control of hemorrhage during mobilization is extraordinarily difficult. The most expeditious way to approach these injuries is by division of the pancreas anterior to the PV-SMV junction. This facilitates either primary repair or vein graft interposition.

Left Subcostal Incision

The left subcostal incision provides excellent exposure in patients with segmental portal hypertension involving the proximal stomach. Segmental portal hypertension may be due to SV thrombosis in association with pancreatitis or pancreatic pseudocyst. Pseudoaneurysm of the splenic artery in association with pancreatic pseudocyst or splenic arteriovenous fistula may result from a splenic artery aneurysm which erodes into the SV or from severe pancreatitis with peripancreatic phlegmon. Once the incision is made and the abdominal cavity is entered, the left transverse colon, ascending colon, and splenic flexure are carefully mobilized inferiorly and medially. This allows for the undersurfaces of both the pancreas and spleen to be fully identified and mobilized with the same technique that was described earlier (Fig. 7).

The stomach is freed by dividing the greater omentum, the left gastroepiploic vessels, and short gastric vessels. The stomach is retracted anteriorly and medially, thereby allowing the operator to free up the retroperitoneal attachments of the spleen. The spleen with distal pancreas is then mobilized anteriorly and medially. Usually, the inflammatory reaction along the peripancreatic plane precludes safe proximal ligation of the splenic vessels; when the peripancreatic inflammation is not excessive, the proximal splenic artery adjacent to the distal SV can be doubly clamped, divided, and ligated in preparation for a distal pancreatectomy with splenectomy. The remainder of the operation is performed according to the operator's preferences for dealing with the pancreatic stump.

Summary

The portal vein courses through the right upper quadrant from the union of the superior mesenteric and splenic veins to the bifurcation into the right and left hepatic veins at the liver hilum. Multiple branches entering into these veins create potential danger during portal vein dissection. Knowledge of the anatomy and careful dissection will help circumvent these dangers when performing: (1) any of the portal systemic shunts; (2) distal splenorenal shunt; (3) extended pancreatectomy with portal venous resection for cancer; and (4) rapid exposure of the portal vein in patients with penetrating injuries. This chapter has reviewed the exposure of the portal vein and branches during performance of these technical procedures.

References

1. Bismuth H. Les anastomoses porto-caves tronculaires. Encyl Med Chir Paris. Techniques chirurgicales, Appareil digestif 408, 4.4.06.

2. Franco D. Existe t-il encore une place pour la chirurgie dans le traitement de l'hypertension portale de la cirrhose? *Gastroenterol Clin Biol* 1988; 12; 229-233.

3. Rikkers LF, Jin G. Surgical management of acute variceal hemorrhage. *World J Surg* 1994; 18: 193-201.

4. Henderson JM, Warren WD, Millikan WJ, et al. Distal splenorenal shunt with splenopancreatic disconnection: A 4-year assessment. *Ann Surg* 1989; 210: 332-339.

5. Yeo CJ, Cameron JL, Lillemore KD, et al. Pancreaticoduodenectomy for cancer of the head of the pancreas: 201 patients. *Ann Surg* 1995; 221: 721-729.

6. Feliciano D, Martin T, Cruse P, et al: Management of combined pancreatoduodenal injuries. *Ann Surg* 1991; 215: 503-509.

26

Access to the Femoral Artery

Keith D. Calligaro, Matthew J. Dougherty

Knowledge of techniques to gain access to the femoral artery is critical to all surgeons dealing with complex revascularization procedures. The common femoral and proximal superficial femoral arteries are the most common sites for proximal anastomoses of distal bypasses. The common, superficial, and deep femoral arteries are the most common sites for the distal anastomosis of bypasses originating from the infrarenal aorta and iliac and axillary arteries. For these reasons, the femoral artery in the groin is the most common location for repeat arterial surgery because of failed previous bypasses. Dense scar tissue in this area can render reexplorations extremely challenging and tedious. The groin is also the most common location for wound and arterial graft infections. The abundant lymphatic supply and proximity to the perineum make the groin more susceptible to wound and arterial graft infection, particularly in repeat dissections. Gaining access to the arterial tree proximal and distal to this site is essential to achieve successful revascularization and limb salvage. For these reasons, all surgeons performing vascular surgery should have an in-depth understanding of various approaches to the common, superficial, and deep femoral arteries. Familiarity with adjacent nerves, veins, and lymphatics is essential to prevent complications unrelated to the femoral artery itself. Additionally, knowledge of routes to tunnel bypasses through appropriate sterile or unscarred fields around the groin is also critical.

Anatomic Review

The femoral triangle containing the femoral artery is defined by the inguinal ligament superiorly, the sartorius muscle laterally, and the adductor longus muscle medially. The skin, subcutaneous tissue, and fascia overlie the femoral triangle anteriorly. The adductor longus, pectineus, and iliopsoas muscles form the posterior boundary. A mnemonic that aids medical students and residents (and frequently experienced surgeons) to identify nerves and blood vessels in the femoral triangle is NAVEL: located laterally to medially in the femoral triangle are the femoral Nerve, Artery, Vein, and *Empty* space (where femoral hernias

From Vascular Surgical Approaches, edited by Alain Branchereau and Ramon Berguer. ©1999, Futura Publishing Co., Inc., Armonk, NY.

occur), and Lymphatic channels (Fig. 1). Important points concerning each of these structures will be reviewed.

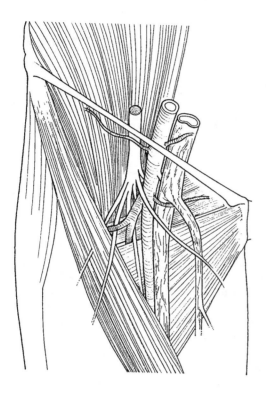

Figure 1. Relationship of the femoral arteries within the femoral triangle.

The femoral nerve can be injured during repeat groin dissections with extensive scarring, particularly when the femoral artery pulse is absent. This error usually results from dissection lateral to the artery and can result in disabling nerve injuries.

The common femoral artery begins at the inguinal ligament as a continuation of the external iliac artery. The femoral bifurcation is generally located 5 cm inferior to the inguinal ligament.[1] The artery divides into the superficial femoral artery, which has a slightly smaller diameter and continues in a straight course, and the deep (profundus) femoral artery, which originates posterolaterally and continues parallel, deep, and slightly lateral to the superficial femoral artery. The deep femoral artery travels anteromedially to the femur throughout its course. It is conveniently divided into a proximal, mid- and distal third by its main branches (Fig. 2).[2] The lateral circumflex femoral artery arises from the proximal part of the deep femoral artery, the first and second perforation branches from the middle part, and the third perforating branch from the distal segment. The most distal segment of the deep femoral artery lies between the adductors longus and magnus. When dissecting the femoral artery bifurcation, the lateral circumflex femoral vein is located between the origins of the superficial and deep femoral arteries; inadvertent injury to this venous branch is not

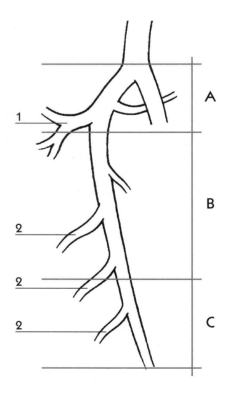

Figure 2. Division of the deep femoral artery. A, B, C: 3 segments of the deep femoral artery.
1. Circumflex artery.
2. Perforating arteries.

uncommon in repeated groin dissections unless the surgeon is particularly careful.

The greater saphenous vein joins the common femoral vein in the femoral triangle as the saphenofemoral junction. The deep femoral vein empties into the common femoral vein several centimeters distally, not in the femoral triangle. This is an important point to remember if the superficial femoral vein is excised for use as an in-situ conduit to replace an infected arterial bypass.[3] The superficial femoral vein should not be excised proximal to the junction of the deep femoral vein and the common femoral vein or severe limb swelling can result.

If the inguinal ligament is disrupted during proximal groin exposures, it should be repaired to prevent the development of femoral hernias. Repair is accomplished with interrupted absorbable sutures.

Finally, great care must be taken not to disrupt lymph nodes or lymphatic channels in the groin. The superficial lymphatic system comprises lymphatic vessels that follow the greater saphenous vein and superficial inguinal lymph nodes that lie anterior to the femoral artery. These superficial nodes consist of an upper group located immediately below the inguinal ligament and a lower group distributed vertically along the most proximal part of the greater saphenous vein. The deep lymphatics follow the femoral artery and pass through the deep inguinal lymph nodes that are located deep and medial to the femoral vein. Lymphatic disruption is probably the leading cause of postoperative edema following lower extremity revascularization. Lymph nodes should not be transected. Dissections should be performed adjacent to the nodes, preferably on the lateral aspect. If it proves necessary to divide lymphatic channels, larger ones should be divided between ligatures, and smaller ones should be coagulated. If careful attention is not paid to lymphatic vessels, a common and disturbing complication is a lymphocele. These collections, may require repeated needle aspirations and, not infrequently, require a repeat groin exploration to identify the leaking lymphatic vessel or node. Groin lymphatic complications have been reported to occur in 1-2% of incisions and more commonly in previously operated groins.[4,5]

Approaches to the Common Femoral Artery

Access to the common femoral artery can be gained through either a vertical or transverse groin incision. A vertical skin incision should begin 1 cm or 2 cm proximal to the inguinal crease and continue distally 3 cm or 4 cm directly over the femoral artery pulse. If the pulse is absent, the common femoral artery is usually located about two fingerbreadths lateral to the pubic tubercle. Once the bifurcation is identified, the incision can be extended proximally or if exposure of the distal external iliac artery is required, the skin incision can be carried proximally and the inguinal ligament partially transected. However, another helpful technique that we use to gain more proximal exposure of the external iliac artery and avoid division of the entire ligament is to mobilize the inferior border of the inguinal ligament for approximately 1 cm medial and 2-3 cm lateral to the common femoral artery. The tissues posterior to the ligament can be bluntly dissected exposing the distal external iliac artery. Use of a self-retaining retractor with the blade positioned slightly under the lower edge of the inguinal ligament and retracted proximally enables the surgeon to gain exposure of the distal, and occasionally the middle, segment of the external iliac artery (Fig. 3). If proximal control of the external iliac artery is required for trauma or a large pseudoaneurysm of the common femoral artery, a small transverse suprainguinal incision is made and the external iliac artery can be exposed through a retroperitoneal approach.

If the surgeon knows preoperatively that an anastomosis will be performed to the common femoral artery and a preoperative arteriogram demonstrates a normally located femoral artery bifurcation, a transverse or oblique skin incision may be performed. This approach is especially useful in obese patients with a large pannus. The skin incision should be made in the skin crease below the inguinal ligament.

As the dissection continues deeper, the femoral arteries should be exposed longitudinally to avoid lymphatic disruption. The plane of dissection should be slightly lateral to the

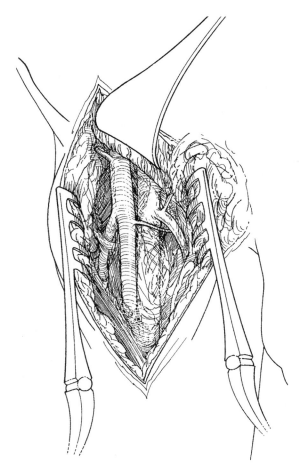

Figure 3. Medial retraction of the lymph nodes during the femoral artery approach.

artery to avoid lymphatic tissue and the femoral nerve and its branches. Constant palpation of the underlying femoral artery pulse is essential to avoid traumatizing adjacent soft tissues, which helps to prevent postoperative limb swelling or neuropathy. If the pulse is absent, the artery will frequently be calcified and this finding can help to identify the femoral artery.

Proper clamping of the femoral artery is essential to vascular procedures in the groin. Although we generally use a vertical angled clamp to occlude the common femoral artery, we find that clamping the more proximal common femoral or distal external iliac artery is best accomplished using a Satinsky clamp,

especially in obese patients with an overhanging pannus. A calcified posterior plaque may require similar clamping techniques. The handles of this horizontal clamp lie to the side of the artery allowing unencumbered exposure of the vessel. If the origins of the superficial and deep femoral arteries are soft and noncalcified, securing vessel loops around these vessels is preferred because the operative field is not crowded with obtrusive clamps. However, if the vessels are calcified, angled clamps can be placed in a way to allow adequate arterial exposure.

Approaches to the Superficial Femoral Artery

Previous reports have documented the usefulness of the superficial femoral artery as an inflow source for lower extremity bypasses.[6] Exposure of the superficial femoral artery varies depending on whether the proximal or distal portion of the vessel needs to be exposed. The sartorius muscle, which originates from the anterior superior iliac spine, courses anteriomedially, and inserts on the medial femoral condyle, is the important landmark. This muscle can be visualized in thin patients, or palpated in heavier patients, by flexing the knee and externally rotating the hip. In the groin and upper thigh, the superficial femoral artery is best approached medial to the sartorius muscle. If this approach is prohibited by localized infection in the groin, the superficial femoral artery can be approached lateral to the sartorius even in the proximal thigh. The distal half of the artery is best approached by reflecting the sartorius muscle posteromedially.

Approaches to the Deep Femoral Artery

The deep femoral artery in the groin is most easily approached medial to the sartorius muscle (Fig.4). The superficial femoral neurovascular bundle is identified and the dissection continues laterally with avoidance of any

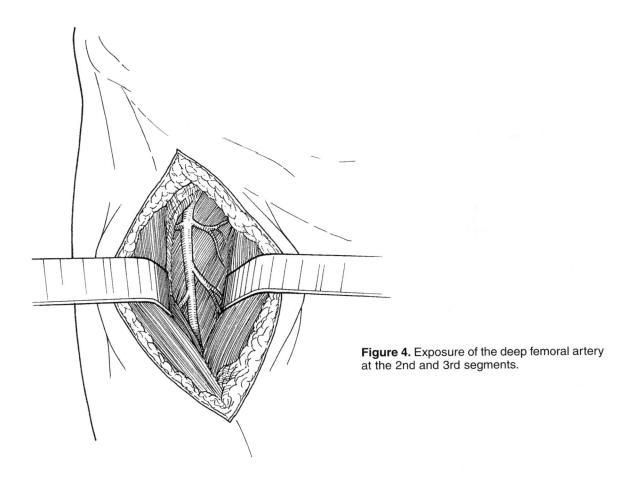

Figure 4. Exposure of the deep femoral artery at the 2nd and 3rd segments.

crossing branches of the femoral nerve. When the proximal part of the deep femoral artery requires exposure, the overlying lateral circumflex femoral vein must be divided between ligatures. The deep femoral artery continues posterolateral to the superficial femoral artery and anteromedial to the femur. The distal deep femoral artery can be approached in three ways. It can be exposed between the sartorius and adductor longus muscles (just medial to the superficial femoral neurovascular bundle) (Fig. 5A). A more medial approach is possible between the adductor longus and gracilis muscles, which does not necessitate exposure of the superficial femoral neurovascular bundle (Fig. 5B). Our preferred approach, however, is lateral between the sartorius and rectus femoris/vastus medialis muscles (lateral to the superficial femoral neurovascular bundle).[2] The fascia between the adductor longus and vastus medialis is incised. The deep femoral artery pulse may not be palpable until this fascia is divided. Use of vessel loops

will elevate the artery more superficially into the wound. Graft length must be adjusted to allow for retraction of the vessel into the normal deep position in the thigh. Self-retaining retractors are essential to provide adequate exposure of the distal deep femoral artery (Fig. 5).

Nunez et al. reported 37 patients who required repeat revascularizations for severely ischemic lower extremities in whom the deep femoral artery was used as an inflow or outflow source.[2] The type of bypass performed (axillofemoral or aortofemoral) affected the patency rate of reconstructions, but use of the deep femoral artery rather than the common or superficial femoral artery did not adversely affect patency rates.[2] More recently, Darling et al. reported 563 revascularization procedures using the deep femoral artery as an inflow source and noted similar patency rates compared to use of the common femoral artery.[7] Mills et al. also noted similar patency results and recommended use of the deep femoral

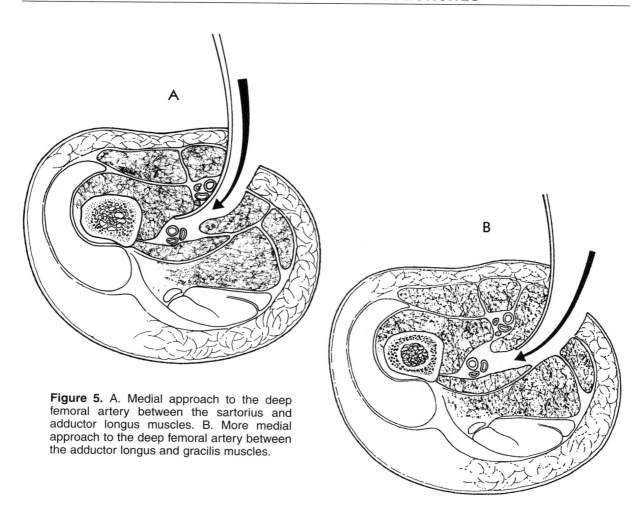

Figure 5. A. Medial approach to the deep femoral artery between the sartorius and adductor longus muscles. B. More medial approach to the deep femoral artery between the adductor longus and gracilis muscles.

artery as an inflow artery if the length of vein is limited or in the case of a severely scarred groin.[8]

Tunneling Bypasses to and from the Femoral Arteries

Tunneling a graft to or from the femoral arteries is an extremely important aspect of lower extremity revascularization especially for scarred or infected groins.[9] First-time aortobifemoral or iliofemoral bypasses are relatively straightforward. When tunneling these grafts, the surgeon's finger and clamp used to pass the graft should be directly anterior to the external iliac artery to avoid injury to adjacent veins and to ensure that the

graft is positioned deep to the ureter, which can be obstructed by a graft tunneled anterior to it. We prefer to ligate and divide the small vein that crosses anterior to the distal external iliac artery to avoid unnecessary and troublesome venous bleeding. Axillofemoral grafts are tunneled subcutaneously medial to the anterior superior iliac spine. Bypasses originating from the femoral arteries in the groin are tunneled deep to the sartorius muscle if an anatomic plane is desired. However, if a bypass is performed to the anterior tibial artery, or if a lateral approach to the popliteal artery is required, we generally pass the graft anterolaterally and subcutaneously across the thigh.

In cases where the graft needs to be tunneled away from the groin because of infection or dense scar tissue from previous operation, we prefer an approach lateral to the common femoral artery, preferably medial to the anterior superior iliac spine.[9] However, if a groin infection extends far laterally, the graft can be tunneled lateral to the iliac spine. We find these routes simpler and less traumatic than an obturator bypass. The new graft is tunneled deep to the inguinal ligament, carried to the subcutaneous tissue, and then down to the superficial or deep femoral arteries lateral to the sartorius muscle.

Summary

A thorough knowledge of the anatomy of the femoral arteries and surrounding structures, along with a detailed understanding of various ways to tunnel arterial grafts to and from these vessels is mandatory for the surgeon performing complex revascularization procedures. The superficial and deep femoral arteries can be an excellent inflow or outflow source for lower extremity revascularization when the common femoral artery is encased in scar tissue or involved with infection.

References

1. Fleming JFR, Levy LF. Lower extremity. In: Grant JCV, ed. *An Atlas of Anatomy.* Baltimore, Williams & Wilkins, 1972, pp 257.
2. Nunez AA, Veith FJ, Collier P, et al. Direct approaches to the distal portions of the deep femoral artery for limb salvage bypasses. *J Vasc Surg* 1988; 8: 576-581.
3. Clagett GP, Valentine RJ, Hagino RT. Autogenous aortoiliac/femoral reconstruction from superficial femoral-popliteal veins: Feasibility and durability. *J Vasc Surg* 1997; 25: 255-270.
4. Tyndall SH, Shepard AD, Wilczewski JM, et al. Groin lymphatic complications after arterial reconstruction. *J Vasc Surg* 1994; 19: 858-864.
5. Roberts JR, Walters GK, Zenilman ME, Jones CE. Groin lymphorrhea complicating revascularization involving the femoral vessels. *Am J Surg* 1993; 165: 341-346.
6. Veith FJ, Gupta SK, Samson RH, et al. Superficial femoral and popliteal arteries as inflow sites for distal bypasses. *Surgery* 1981; 90: 980-990.
7. Darling RC, III Shah DM, Chang BB, et al. Can the deep femoral artery be used reliably as an inflow source for infrainguinal reconstruction? Long-term results in 563 procedures. *J Vasc Surg* 1994; 20: 889-895.
8. Mills JS, Taylor SM, Fujitani RM. The role of the deep femoral artery as an inflow site for infrainguinal revascularization. *J Vasc Surg* 1993; 18: 416-423.
9. Calligaro KD, Veith FJ, Gupta SK, et al. A modified method for management of prosthetic graft infections involving an anastomosis to the common femoral artery. *J Vasc Surg* 1990; 11: 485-492.

27

Popliteal Artery

Jean-Michel Chevalier, Patrick Feugier

The popliteal artery which may be spared from atheroma is readily available for proximal or distal bypass anastomosis. It has its own particular pathology: popliteal entrapment, adventitial cyst, arterial dissection. When the popliteal artery is involved in knee trauma or when it is aneurysmal, the approach that is chosen determines the technical difficulties that may be encountered during the operation and even the outcome of the procedure.

Anatomic Review (Fig. 1)

The popliteal artery is the continuation of the superficial femoral artery after the latter crosses the adductor canal; it begins at the level of the ring of the great adductor muscle behind its tendon and it terminates at the level of the soleus muscle. Between these two levels it has three surgical segments: the upper or proximal popliteal artery which runs from the ring of the great adductor muscle to the insertions of the medial and lateral heads of the gastrocnemius muscle; the middle popliteal or retroarticular segment situated between the condylar insertions of the gastrocnemius muscle in the intercondylar fossa; and the distal popliteal artery which runs from the level of the interarticular line to the upper edge of the soleus muscle. The flexion point of the popliteal artery in the crease of the knee is situated above the interarticular line.

Medial Approach

Patient Position (Fig. 2)

The patient is placed in the supine position, the thigh slightly abducted and flexed and the knee half-flexed. The surgeon is seated opposite the operation site. The first assistant is opposite the surgeon at the outside of the leg to be operated and the nurse is at the side of the surgeon towards the foot of the patient. The table is slightly inclined towards the first assistant.

From Vascular Surgical Approaches, edited by Alain Branchereau and Ramon Berguer. ©1999, Futura Publishing Co., Inc., Armonk, NY.

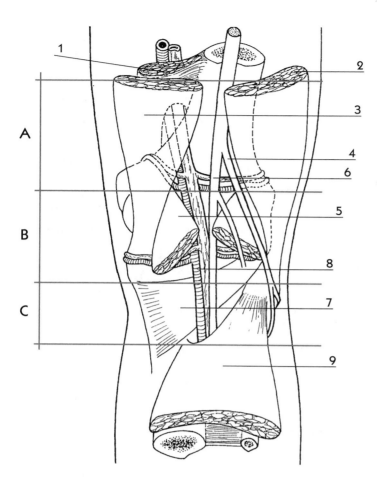

Figure 1. Anatomy of the popliteal fossa and segments of the popliteal artery.
A. Proximal popliteal artery.
B. Middle popliteal artery.
C. Distal popliteal artery.
1. Adductor magnus muscle.
2. Biceps muscle.
3. Semimembranous muscle.
4. Common peroneal nerve.
5. Gastrocnemius muscle.
6. Tibial nerve.
7. Popliteal muscle.
8. Popliteal artery and vein.
9. Soleus muscle.

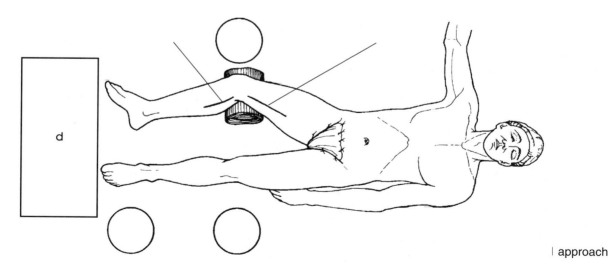

approach
1. Skin incision for distal popliteal exposure. 2. Skin incision for proximal popliteal exposure. Position of:
a. Surgeon.
b. Assistant.
c. Nurse.
d. Instrument table.

Distal Popliteal Artery

This is the segment most frequently exposed and is the quickest and easiest approach to the popliteal artery. The skin incision which is slightly arched begins 1 cm behind the medial femoral condyle and runs for 1-2 cm behind the posterior edge of the tibia (Fig. 2); it then descends as far as the meeting point of the upper and middle third of the leg and may be enlarged as required either upwards or downwards. The subcutaneous tissue is divided down to the subcutaneous fascia where the greater saphenous vein lies and which must be avoided. Depending on the location of the greater saphenous vein, its anterior or posterior collaterals are tied. The superficial fascia is opened at the bottom of the incision and the medial head of the gastrocnemius muscle is detached from the posterior face of the tibia and retracted posteriorly. The opening of the fascia continues upwards behind the sartorius, gracilis and semitendinous muscles, whose tendons are cut. During this maneuver the descending arteries of the knee (arteria anastomostica magna) and its satellites, and the branches of saphenous nerve should be avoided. The first is a large collateral which anastomoses to the peroneal or posterior tibial arteries. The branches of the saphenous nerve, if traumatized, may cause anesthesia of the knee and of the anterior face of the leg. A self-retaining Beckman retractor holds the edges of the wound. The lower popliteal artery lies in front, at the far end of the detachment of the medial head of the gastrocnemius muscle, and is usually accompanied by two popliteal veins, one medial, the other lateral. The tibial nerve lies posterolaterally and generally is not seen. The popliteal artery is isolated for 5-6 cm and is separated from its satellite vein(s). In this segment, the popliteal artery has only a small posterior articular branch which may be tied. Two to seven centimeters below the articular interline, just before or at the level of the upper edge of the soleus muscle, the popliteal artery bifurcates into the anterior tibial artery and the tibioperoneal trunk. The anterior tibial artery takes off in an oblique angle and runs towards the upper edge of the interosseous space between the tibia and fibula to enter the anterior compartment of the leg. This artery gives rise to the first recurrent collateral branch

which should be preserved. The tibioperoneal trunk runs in front of the soleus muscle and may be exposed by dividing the arcade of this latter and then cutting the muscle fibers; this may be continued as far as its bifurcation into the peroneal and posterior tibial arteries. Meticulous hemostasis of the venous network surrounding the artery should be performed. Using this low medial access a total of 7-8 cm of the lower popliteal artery may be isolated, from the interarticular line to the bifurcation of the tibioperoneal trunk (Fig. 3).

Proximal Popliteal Artery

The skin and subcutaneous incision begins on the thigh at the level where the middle and lower third meet in front of the outline of the sartorius muscle. It then curves slightly backwards towards a point situated 1-2 cm behind the medial femoral condyle (Fig. 2). The greater saphenous vein should be preserved; it is mobilized forward or backwards depending on its relation to the incision line. Cutting the superficial fascia allows entry into the sheath of the sartorius muscle, the edge of which is isolated. A Beckman retractor retracts the muscle posteriorly. Opening the deep fascia of the compartment of the sartorius muscle exposes the semitendinous, semimembranosus, and gracilis muscles. The semitendinous and gracilis muscles are retracted posteriorly with the sartorius muscle. Cutting their recurrent fibers in front opens the fat space where the vascular pedicle is situated and where the popliteal artery is exposed. The artery can be located by palpation of its pulse or by feeling the calcification of its wall. This space is limited at the top by the tendon of the great adductor muscle under which the artery passes. Distally, the limit is the insertion of the medial head of the gastrocnemius muscle into the femoral condyle. The artery then drops into the intercondylar fossa between the medial and lateral heads of the gastrocnemius muscle. The artery may be located in one of two ways: either below the tendon of the great adductor muscle within the loose fat of the upper part of the popliteal fossa or, after dividing the tendon of the great adductor muscle, the artery can be found immediately below. In both cases, once the artery is isolated and separated from its adjacent veins, it is easy to extend the exposure as required either upwards or downwards while remaining in contact with the artery, with or without dividing the tendon of the great adductor muscle (Fig. 4). Unlike the lower popliteal artery, the upper popliteal artery gives rise to collaterals which must be

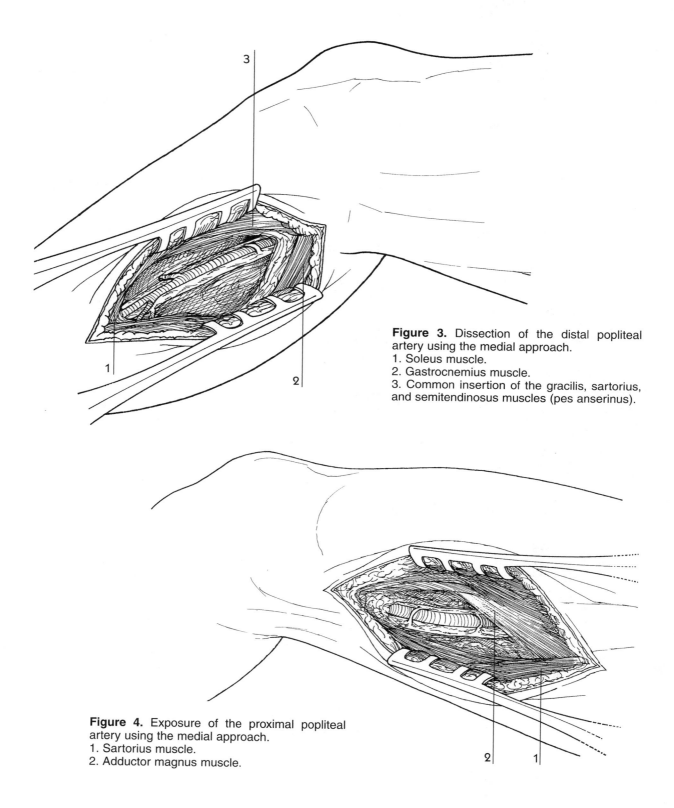

Figure 3. Dissection of the distal popliteal artery using the medial approach.
1. Soleus muscle.
2. Gastrocnemius muscle.
3. Common insertion of the gracilis, sartorius, and semitendinosus muscles (pes anserinus).

Figure 4. Exposure of the proximal popliteal artery using the medial approach.
1. Sartorius muscle.
2. Adductor magnus muscle.

preserved during its dissection as they are an important part of the periarticular arterial circle of the knee. Proximal and anteriorly is the origin of the fourth perforating anastomosis to the deep femoral artery. Proximal and posteriorly is the origin of the genicular descending artery which contributes to the supply of the leg, joined by branches of the saphenous nerve. More distally below is the origin of two to four infragenicular arteries. This proximal medial approach allows exposure of 10-12 cm of the popliteal artery.

Extended Medial Approach

The midpopliteal artery is rarely approached medially; the posterior approach gives better access without the need to divide muscles. Combined with the described approaches to the proximal and distal popliteal artery, the medial approach to the popliteal artery allows extensive access to the popliteal artery at the expense of extensive muscular division. The cutaneous and subcutaneous incisions combine the cutting lines of the proximal and distal approach previously described. The middle popliteal artery runs through the intercondylar fossa and is surrounded by the tendons of the sartorius, gracilis, and semitendinous muscles, by the semimembranous muscle, and by the medial head of the gastrocnemius muscle as the latter inserts on the medial condyle of the femur. Classically, these muscles can be divided through their distal tendinous portion and their ends can be marked by ties in order to identify them at the end of the procedure for reconstruction (Fig. 5). The middle popliteal artery may be exposed for 5-6 cm. The

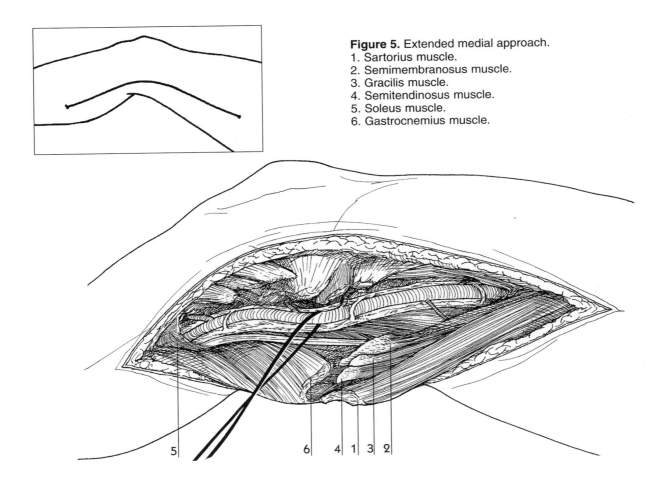

Figure 5. Extended medial approach.
1. Sartorius muscle.
2. Semimembranosus muscle.
3. Gracilis muscle.
4. Semitendinosus muscle.
5. Soleus muscle.
6. Gastrocnemius muscle.

collateral arteries should be preserved. Branchereau[1] has suggested a technique for exposing the middle popliteal artery by isolating the sartorius, gracilis, semitendinosus and semimembranous muscles with a loop dividing the recurrent fibers of the latter muscle. The block of tendon and periostium formed by the insertions of the sartorius, semitendinosus, gracilis, and semimembranosus muscles is lifted with a periosteal elevator as far as the anterior edge of the tibia and cut. The medial head of the gastrocnemius muscle is either mobilized or cut to expose the middle popliteal artery. At the end of the operation, the block of periostium and tendon is reattached using a Blount stapler. After repair of the tendons it is advisable to immobilize the knee with a splint in the postoperative period.

Posterior Approach

The posterior approach allows access to the entire popliteal artery but is specifically used for the middle popliteal artery. Its downward extension is easy but its proximal extension is limited. The patient is placed in ventral decubitus with a roll under the ankle to allow slight flexion of the knee which relaxes the muscles surrounding the popliteal fossa. The leg is prepped as far as the upper third of the thigh. This position does not permit extended harvesting of the greater saphenous vein or proximal extension of the exposure. The lateral decubitus position resting on the contralateral extremity and combining abduction of the hip and rotation of the table towards the back of the patient allows harvesting of the entire greater saphenous vein as well as exposure of the femoral artery at the adductor canal. Rob has suggested putting the operated leg in extension and raising it on a platform in order to allow changes in its position. The posterior approach to the popliteal artery is performed with the knee in extension while the contralateral member is flexed at the hip and knee (Fig. 6).

The incision is S-shaped in order to avoid contraction of the scar (Fig. 7). The horizontal portion which is 2-3 cm long is at the popliteal crease. The distal vertical portion which is 8-10 cm long is centered between the outline of the medial and lateral heads of the gastrocnemius muscle. The proximal vertical portion lies more medially and runs upwards following the lateral edge of the semimembranous muscle and is 8-10 cm long. The superficial fascia is opened following the same line. At the calf level the lesser saphenous vein and its satellite nerve, which run in a fascial fold, are retracted laterally. A medial nerve branch, which innervates the medial head of the gastrocnemius muscle, often needs to be cut. The saphenopopliteal junction allows identification of the popliteal vein. This junction may lie at a variable height in the popliteal cavity but is usually 2 cm below the crease of the knee. The popliteal artery runs deep through the diamond-shaped fossa framed above the articular line by the bulge of the semimembraneous muscles inside, and the biceps outside. Below the articular line, the diamond shape is bordered by the medial and lateral heads of the gastrocnemius muscles. The popliteal artery descends behind the popliteal muscle which is inserted into the posterior surface of the tibia. It passes in front of the arcade of the soleus muscle where it gives origin to the anterior tibial artery; the latter crosses the interosseous space to reach the anterior compartment of the leg. Behind the upper part of the soleus muscle is the tibioperoneal trunk that continues the distal popliteal artery. Below the superficial fascia, the tibial nerve is the most superficial element of the neurovascular bundle, as the latter crosses the diamond-shaped popliteal fossa. The tibial nerve is retracted laterally after sectioning the nerve to the medial head of the gastrocnemius muscle. The artery is found within the fat accompanied by its two satellite veins. A number of collateral branches arise from the proximal and middle segments of the popliteal artery. Generally, retracting the medial and lateral heads of the gastrocnemius muscle allows the preservation of these collaterals. Two Beckman self-retaining retractors pull back respectively the supra- and infraarticular muscle elements of the popliteal fossa giving excellent exposure of the entire popliteal artery. If necessary, the distal segment of the lesser saphenous vein as it joins the popliteal vein is tied and cut as well as the vascular pedicle supplying the medial head of the gastrocnemius muscle. Cutting the arcade

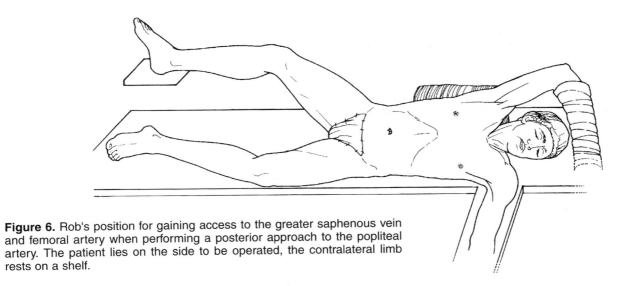

Figure 6. Rob's position for gaining access to the greater saphenous vein and femoral artery when performing a posterior approach to the popliteal artery. The patient lies on the side to be operated, the contralateral limb rests on a shelf.

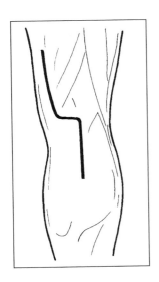

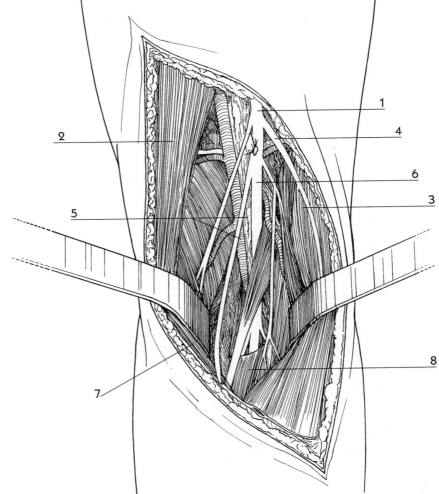

Figure 7. Posterior approach to the popliteal artery. (Inset: skin incision).
1. Sciatic nerve.
2. Semimembranosus muscle.
3. Biceps muscle.
4. Common peroneal nerve.
5. Popliteal artery and vein.
6. Tibial nerve.
7. Gastrocnemius muscle.
8. Soleus muscle.

of the soleus muscle and dividing its muscle fibers allow exposure of the trunk of the tibioperoneal artery. The periarterial venous plexus may cause some bleeding and it should be dissected with care. The first few centimeters of the anterior tibial artery may be exposed if required after cutting the upper edge of the interosseous membrane.

Combined Posterior and Medial Approaches[3]

Described in 1949 by Arnulf and Benichoux, this approach combines the medial approach to the upper popliteal artery with the posterior approach to the distal popliteal artery. The patient is placed in the lateral position resting on the limb to be operated (Fig. 6). This allows harvesting of the great saphenous vein and proximal extension of the exposure. The skin incision is at the level of the lower third of the thigh, the same as for the standard medial approach. It then curves backward from the medial condyle of the femur, slightly above the crease of the knee to join the midline (Fig. 8). Access to the midpopliteal artery is gained as in the extended medial approach by dividing the sartorius, gracilis, semitendinous, and semimembranous tendons. The medial head of the gastrocnemius muscle may be preserved by mobilizing it after surrounding it with loops.

Lateral Approach

The lateral approach to the popliteal artery is a procedure that is easily performed and is similar to the usual medial approach. The upper lateral approach (Figs. 9 and 10) described by Henry[4] and revived by Veith[5,6] allows access to the proximal popliteal artery. There are two possible routes depending on whether the skin incision is located in front of or behind the biceps muscle. The lower lateral approach (Figs. 9 and 11) described by Elkin and Kelly[7] permits exposure of the lower popliteal artery. The technique is described in detail in the chapter on unusual approaches (see Chapter 30). This extended

lateral approach combining the two previous incisions allows the entire popliteal artery to be exposed.

Discussion

Knowledge of these different approaches is essential to the successful outcome of infrainguinal revascularization. The treatment of certain lesions may require the preferential use of one method. The medial approach has the advantage of being performed with the patient in the supine position. It may be associated with all other types of vascular exposure in the lower extremity and with abdominal, thoracic, neck, and upper extremity vessels. This approach is routinely used when treating occlusions of the superficial femoral artery. It is also the best for treatment of long aneurysms of the popliteal artery where one wishes to obtain access to the superficial femoral artery in the thigh or groin. The lower medial approach is preferred for the treatment of popliteal or infrapopliteal embolisms. In the case of popliteal traumatism the choice between

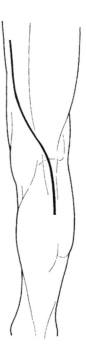

Figure 8. Incision for the combined posterior and medial approaches. The patient is in the lateral position resting on the side to be operated.

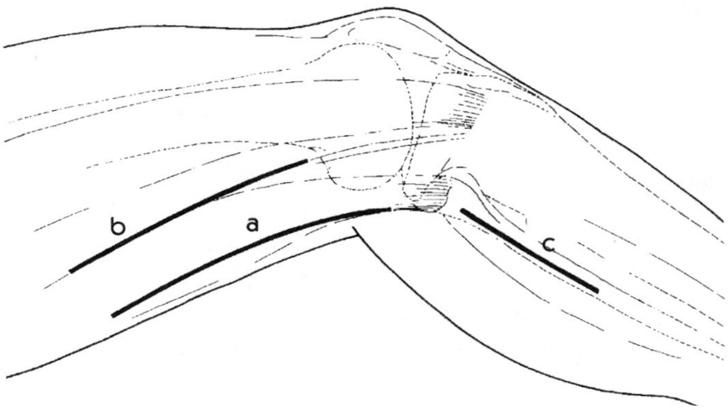

Figure 9. Lateral approach to the popliteal artery.
a. Incision posterior to the outline of the biceps muscle.
b. Incision posterior to the fascia lata.
c. Incision over the bony prominence of the upper fourth of the fibula.

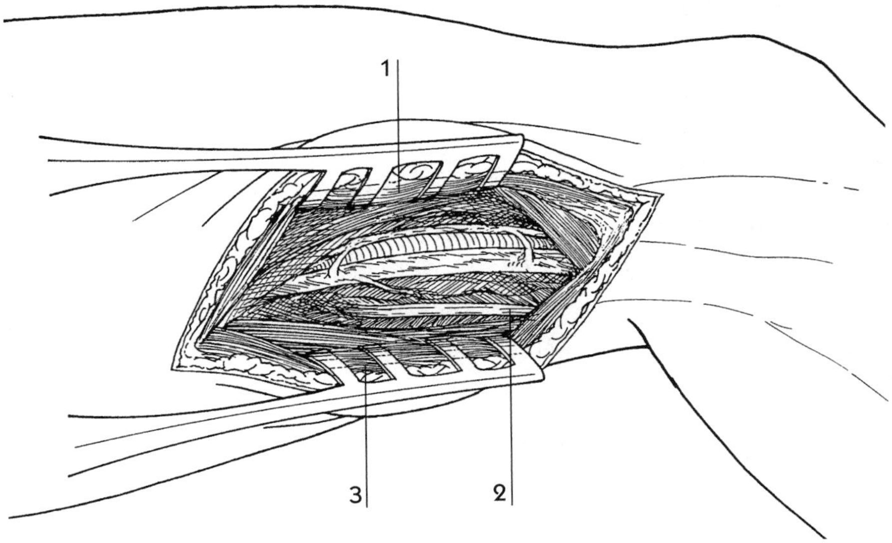

Figure 10. Access to the proximal popliteal artery using a lateral approach.
1. Vastus lateralis muscle.
2. Common peroneal nerve.
3. Biceps muscle.

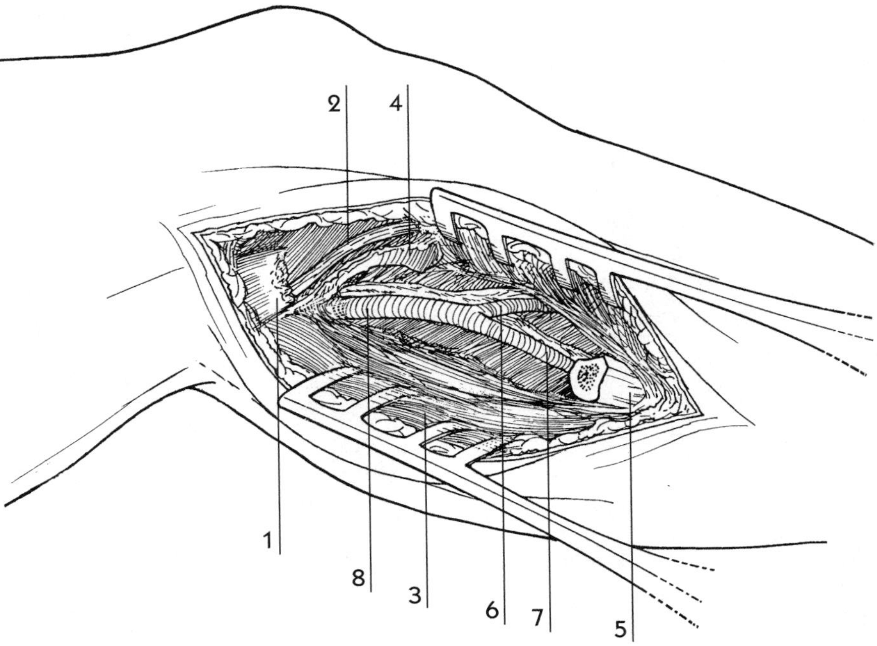

Figure 11. Distal lower approach.
1. Biceps muscle.
2. Common peroneal nerve.
3. Gastrocnemius muscle.
4. Tibial surface of the upper peroneal joint.
5. Fibula.
6. Anterior tibial artery.
7. Tibioperoneal trunk.
8. Distal popliteal artery.

the medial, posterior, or lateral access depends on the associated bone and soft tissue injuries.

The posterior approach to the popliteal artery when performed in the usual manner, with the patient prone, does not permit access to the pelvic/abdominal arteries. It is possible, however, to expose the posterior tibial and the peroneal arteries in this approach. The posterior approach has drawbacks when performed on elderly patients and in those with lung problems. We use the posterior approach for large popliteal aneurysms, especially when associated with arteriomegaly. This position permits harvesting the greater saphenous vein from the thigh where it has the largest diameter. We use the lateral position with the patient lying on the nonoperated side rather than use the Rob technique. The combined posterior and medial approach is rarely used, but may facilitate the surgical treatment of an extensive aneurysm of the lower third of the superficial femoral artery if a prosthetic or an arterial allograft replacement is planned. The posterior approach is our choice for the treatment of small or medium caliber aneurysms. This often permits removal of the sac which reduces the risk of postoperative hemorrhage and of compression of the bypass by the aneurysmal sac.

The posterior approach is preferred when the entire popliteal artery needs to be explored, e.g. when a popliteal artery entrapment syndrome is suspected. We recommend this approach for all popliteal thromboses where the etiology is unclear. In the case of an adventitial cyst of the middle popliteal artery the posterior approach is less traumatic and permits identification of a possible communication between the cyst and the knee joint.

The lateral approach to the popliteal artery should be used more frequently because it is simple, nontraumatic, and gives excellent exposure of the distal popliteal artery and of the origin of the anterior tibial artery. After their identification, the arteries are easily pulled towards the surface with loops. The position of the patient has the same advantage as the medial approach and it may also be associated with other proximal or distal approaches. In redo operations of the popliteal artery it is the preferred technique for exposing previously operated areas. In the case of infection of the groin or of the adductor canal, the lateral approach allows popliteal access in an uninfected area and provides an external route for the bypass through the lateral aspect of the thigh. These lateral routes are an alternative to bypasses which pass via the obturator foramen or the perineum. The lateral approach is also indicated when simultaneous access to the popliteal artery and to the anterior proximal tibial artery is required. The risk of palsy of the common peroneal nerve is minimal if it is dissected with care. Finally, some patients have major internal collaterals from the descending artery of the knee, the periarticular circle, and the sural arteries; the lateral approach allows preservation of these collaterals.

Conclusion

There are various approaches to the proximal, middle, and distal popliteal artery. While the medial approach is the most frequently used, a posterior approach facilitates the treatment of the majority of popliteal aneurysms. The posterior approach is also recommended for the treatment of specific lesions of the popliteal artery such as entrapment or popliteal cyst. The lateral approach has some advantages over the medial approach but it is inadequate for the harvesting of the greater saphenous vein.

References

1. Branchereau A, Ondon'Dong F. Extended medial approach to the popliteal artery without muscular division. *Ann Vasc Surg* 1989; 3: 77-80.
2. Cormier JM, Sautot J, Frileux C, Arnulf G. *Nouveau traité de technique chirurgicale: artères, veines, lymphatiques.* Paris, Masson, 1970, pp 166-184.
3. Arnulf G, Benichoux R. Découverte large de la fémoro-poplitée. *Lyon chirurgical* 1949; 44: 203-208.
4. Henry AK. Extensile Exposure: 2nd ed. New York, Churchill-Livingstone, 1957, pp 298-310.
5. Veith FJ, Ascer E, Gupta SK. Lateral approach to the popliteal artery. *J Vasc Surg* 1987; 6: 119-123.
6. Padberg FT. Voie d'abord latérale externe de l'artère poplitée. *Ann Chir Vasc* 1988; 2: 397-401.
7. Elkin DC, Kelly RP. Arteriovenous aneuvrysm: exposure of the tibial and peroneal vessels by resection of the fibula. *Ann Surg* 1945; 122: 529-545.

28

Arteries of the Leg

Jacques Watelet, Didier Plissonnier
Patrick Soury, Jacques Testart

With the general acceptance of in situ venous graft techniques the indications for bypasses of the arteries of the leg have multiplied. The conventional approaches (medial retrotibial incision for the posterior tibial and peroneal arteries, anterior incision for the anterior tibial artery) are still the most frequently employed. However, the topography of some arterial lesions may make other approaches preferable, such as the lateral approach with fibulectomy for distal peroneal bypass, or the posterior approach which may be used for distal popliteal bypass when the lesser saphenous vein is used. The choice of approach, in fact, is based on several factors: the topography of the arterial lesions, the venous graft tissue available, the presence of ulceration/gangrene and, of course, the surgeon's preferences. The postoperative outcome is in part determined by the care exercised in achieving the various exposures and in the meticulous closure of the surgical wound.

Tibioperoneal Trunk

To expose the tibioperoneal trunk (TPT), the patient is placed in the same position as for the standard anterior or anterolateral approach to the arteries of the leg. The patient is supine with the thigh rotated externally and the knee flexed (30-50 degrees) to perform a medial retrotibial approach.

The medial approach to the TPT is simply a distal extension of the approach to the distal popliteal artery. The skin incision is extended downwards by several centimeters while remaining one centimeter anterior to the posterior edge of the tibia or, even better, in front of the previously identified greater saphenous vein (GSV). The fascia is incised close to its tibial insertion. Cutting the arcade of the soleus muscle is helped by exposing the anterior tibial artery and vein. The disinsertion of the muscle is performed parallel to the medial edge of the tibia exposing the TPT, as it

From Vascular Surgical Approaches, edited by Alain Branchereau and Ramon Berguer. ©1999, Futura Publishing Co., Inc., Armonk, NY.

runs alongside a large satellite vein which is often double, and its bifurcation into the posterior tibial and peroneal arteries.

Posterior Tibial Artery

Upper and Middle Thirds (Fig. 1)

The skin incision is made anterior to the GSV which usually lies 1-2 cm behind the posteromedial edge of the tibia. Once the fascia is incised, the medial border of the medial gastrocnemius muscle appears and is freed and retracted posteriorly. The soleus muscle may be disinserted from the tibia or incised perpendicularly to its fibers about one fingerbreadth from its medial border. The deep fascia, once incised, gives access to the neurovascular bundle that includes the posterior tibial nerve and, medially and anterior to it, the posterior tibial artery with its two satellite veins.

Lower Third (Fig. 2)

The soleus muscle joins the gastrocnemius muscle and, at this level, does not have any bony insertions. Incision of the fascia of the leg leads to areolar tissue between the sural triceps posteriorly and the long flexor muscle of the toes and the posterior tibial muscle anteriorly. Within this space lies the neurovascular bundle covered by the deep fascia of the leg.

Retromalleolar Approach (Fig. 3)

To open the retro- and submalleolar space the knee is flexed 60 degrees, the extremity is rotated externally, and the foot is placed on a roll. The skin incision is 6-8 cm long, first vertical and then curved sightly forward around the medial malleolus. The line of incision is equidistant between the Achilles tendon and the posterior border of the medial malleolus. With the foot forcibly flexed, the superficial fascia is cut anterior to the Achilles tendon. The foot is then placed in equinus and the Achilles tendon retracted. The deep fascia

which is pearly and thick is cut and the vascular sheath is opened. The posterior tibial artery, accompanied by one or two satellite veins, is identified.

Routes of the Bypasses

For in situ bypass, the GSV is mobilized for approximately 10 cm. The superficial and deep aponeuroses of the leg should be incised sufficiently high to avoid angulation of the vein. For reversed bypass the tunnel may be subcutaneous or follow the anatomic course of the arteries.

The subcutaneous route runs along the anteromedial surface of the thigh parallel to the superficial femoral artery, and continues along the medial side of the knee and leg. The tunneling instrument should have sufficient diameter to create a tunnel wide enough that the bypass will be protected from any compression.

The anatomic route follows the posterior edge of the sartorius muscle, crosses the popliteal fossa between the two heads of the gastrocnemius muscles, and then passes anterior to the soleus muscle and joins the posterior tibial artery. This route requires exposure of the distal popliteal fossa to guide the tunneler along the vascular axis between both heads of the gastrocnemius muscles. It is generally possible to pass the tunneler from the lower popliteal to the femoral region following the posterior edge of the sartorius muscle without exposing the proximal popliteal region above the joint line.

The subcutaneous tunnel has the advantage of being simple and accessible but it is more susceptible to compression. The anatomic tunnel is not subject to the risk of kinking when the knee is flexed and the bypass is less susceptible to the risk of superficial infection. This route is used in preference to the subcutaneous route for reversed venous bypasses and especially when prosthetic material is employed.

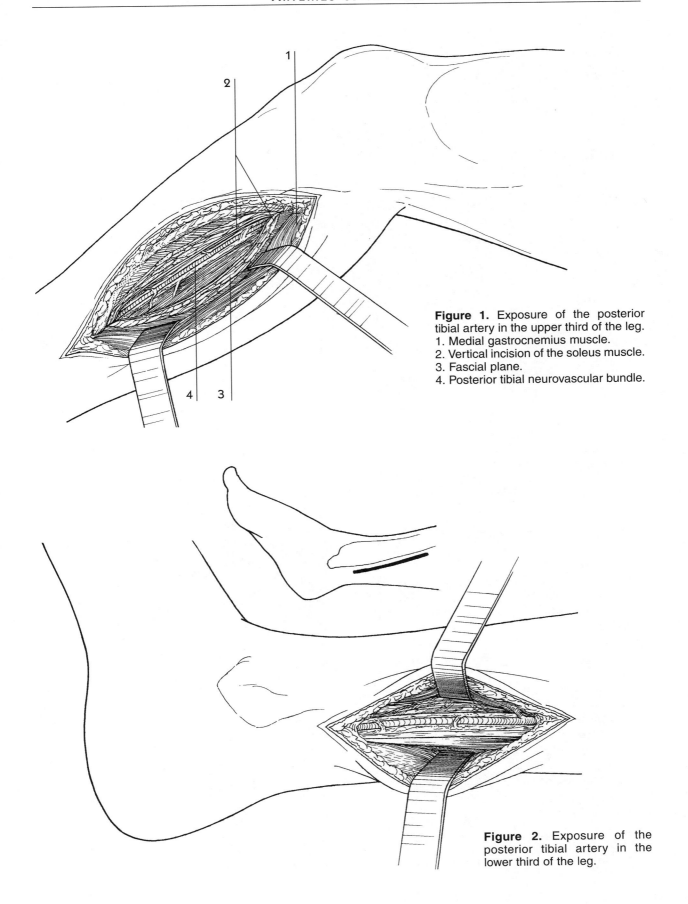

Figure 1. Exposure of the posterior tibial artery in the upper third of the leg.
1. Medial gastrocnemius muscle.
2. Vertical incision of the soleus muscle.
3. Fascial plane.
4. Posterior tibial neurovascular bundle.

Figure 2. Exposure of the posterior tibial artery in the lower third of the leg.

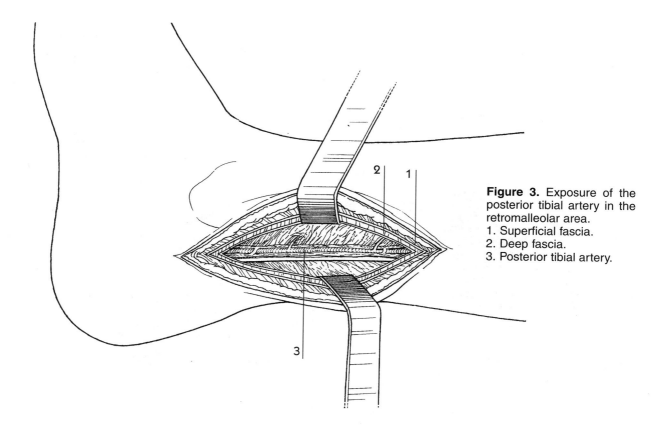

Figure 3. Exposure of the posterior tibial artery in the retromalleolar area.
1. Superficial fascia.
2. Deep fascia.
3. Posterior tibial artery.

Peroneal Artery

Medial Retrotibial Approach (Fig. 4A)

This approach allows access to the proximal half of the artery but the depth of the artery at this level may make it difficult to perform the anastomosis. The first steps for this approach are the same as described for the approach to the posterior tibial artery. Once identified, the posterior tibial pedicle is retracted forward dissecting the plane between the posterior tibial muscle and the flexor hallucis longus. The deep fascia is cut at this level and the medial edge of the flexor hallucis longus is freed and pulled backwards to reveal the peroneal vascular pedicle which lies on the posterior tibial muscle. The artery is surrounded by its satellite veins. The use of an elastic Esmarch bandage allows limiting the dissection of the artery to a minimum.

The relation between the peroneal artery and the flexor hallucis longus muscle varies at different levels. In the upper third of the leg, the artery lies on the posterior tibial muscle and is found at the medial edge of the long flexor muscle. In the middle third of the leg (Fig. 4B), the artery is frequently surrounded by muscular fibers of the flexor hallucis longus as if it were a muscular canal. Isolation of the artery is facilitated by beginning its exposure at a higher level and separating the muscular fibers from this point downwards. In the lower third of the leg, the artery is best approached laterally resecting the fibula.

Lateral Approach with Segmental Resection of the Fibula (Fig. 5)

The skin incision, about 10-12 cm long, is centered on the middle or lower third of the fibula depending on the site chosen for anastomosis. The peroneus longus muscle is

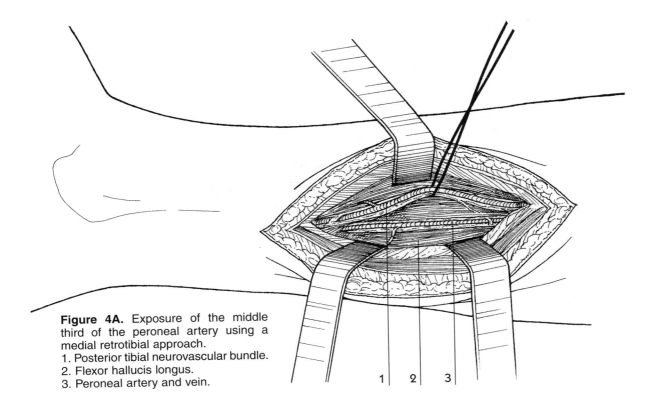

Figure 4A. Exposure of the middle third of the peroneal artery using a medial retrotibial approach.
1. Posterior tibial neurovascular bundle.
2. Flexor hallucis longus.
3. Peroneal artery and vein.

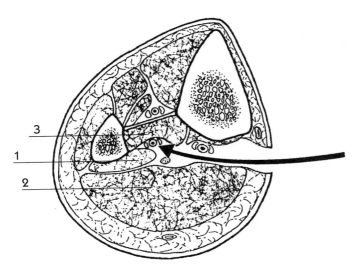

Figure 4B. Cross-section of the middle third of the leg showing the path of the medial retrotibial approach to the peroneal artery.
1. Flexor hallucis longus.
2. Sural triceps muscle.
3. Posterior tibial muscle.

freed at its lateral edge from the bone and retracted posteriorly with the flexor hallucis longus. The lateral and posterior surfaces of the bone are then freed for about 8 cm using an elevator. This is easier in the lower part of the leg where the fibula separates from the muscles that surround it higher up. The tendons of the peroneal muscles remain on the posterior face of the fibula and the third peroneal belly which is the last head of the extensor digitorum longus and inserts only on the anterior surface of the bone. It is then easy to resect a 6-8 cm

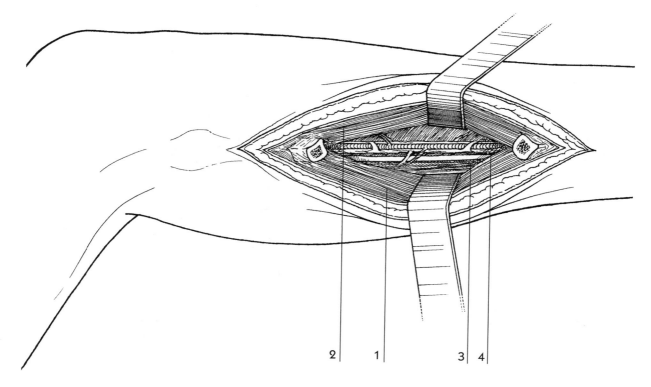

Figure 5. Exposure of the middle third of the peroneal artery using a lateral approach with segmental resection of the fibula.
1. Peroneal muscles.
2. Extensor digitorum longus.
3. Flexor hallucis longus.
4. Peroneal vascular bundle.

segment of the fibula using a Gigli saw after dissecting the interosseous membrane which adheres to the medial surface of the bone. This fibular resection does not reduce the stability of the ankle joint. The vascular pedicle is easily identified lying directly on the flexor digitorum longus.

Posterolateral or Retrofibular Approach

The posterolateral or retrofibular approach to the leg gives only limited access to the peroneal artery in its middle segment.

Routes of the Bypasses

When the artery is accessed via a medial retrotibial approach, the trajectory of the bypass is the same as for the bypasses to the posterior tibial artery. If the artery has been exposed through a lateral approach, the most practical path for the bypass is a lateral one. The bypass follows an extra-anatomic route which crosses obliquely the anterior and the lateral sides of the thigh, and the lateral side of the knee. It then passes in front of the fibula to join the anterolateral compartment of the leg. The lateral route has the advantage of allowing easy monitoring and avoids the risk of kinking during acute flexing of the knee. In the case of a lateral approach and an in situ venous graft, especially in the lower third, there is the alternative of following a transosseous route as described for the anterior tibial artery (see below).

Anterior Tibial Artery

Anterior Access to the Upper and Middle Thirds (Fig. 6A)

The leg is maintained in 30-40 degree flexion by a roll placed below the knee. The skin incision follows a vertical line that starts at the prefibular depression. The fascia is incised over the space which separates the anterior tibial muscles and the long extensor of the toes. This space is more easily located in the lower part of the incision when the foot is in extension. Once the muscles are relaxed by flexion of the foot, the anterior tibial muscle may be easily retracted medially. This muscle covers the long extensor of the toes and the dissection is continued upwards for the entire length of the incision. The neurovascular pedicle is deep. The nerve frequently crosses the artery which is hidden by the fibers emerging from the interosseous membrane or by dilated satellite veins.

Access to the Lower Third (Fig. 6B)

Access to the anterior tibial artery in its lower third is easy as it is less deep and the muscle bellies have been replaced by large tendons. Separation of the two tendons of the anterior tibial and extensor hallucis muscles reveals the neurovascular bundle as it lies against the bone. At the lower part of the incision, the artery runs behind the tendon of the extensor hallucis longus. The latter must be retracted clear of the tendon of the long

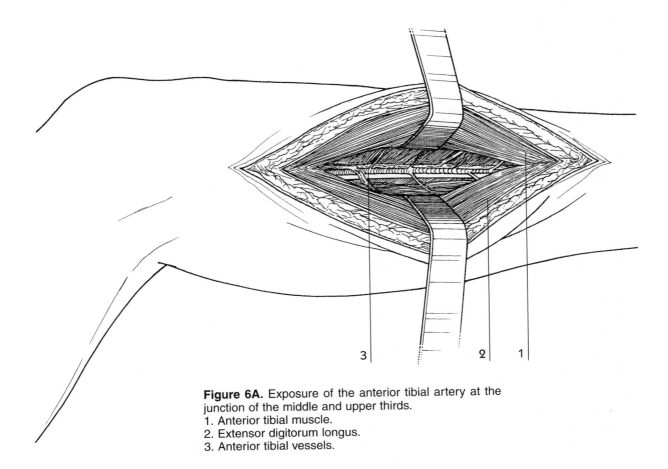

Figure 6A. Exposure of the anterior tibial artery at the junction of the middle and upper thirds.
1. Anterior tibial muscle.
2. Extensor digitorum longus.
3. Anterior tibial vessels.

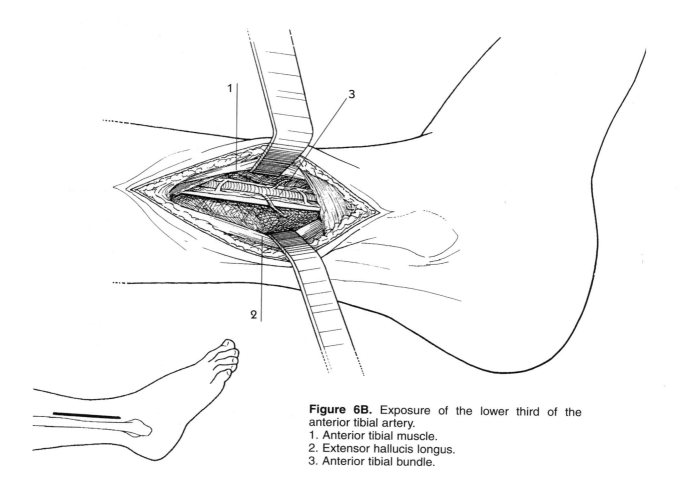

Figure 6B. Exposure of the lower third of the anterior tibial artery.
1. Anterior tibial muscle.
2. Extensor hallucis longus.
3. Anterior tibial bundle.

extensor of the toes to find the vascular bundle as it lies in contact with the lateral edge of the anterior tibial muscle. The downward extension of this exposure requires cutting the retinaculum of the extensor muscles.

Access to the Upper Fourth (Fig. 6C)

This approach may be extended as far as the head of the fibula. Dissection between the anterior tibial and the long extensor muscle of the toes exposes the anterior tibial artery as it becomes deeper up to the point where it penetrates the interosseous membrane. Complete exposure of the artery may be facilitated by cutting the nerve branch that the common peroneal and anterior tibial nerves send to the anterior tibial muscle. Its section

causes only partial paralysis of this muscle as the lower portion receives another motor branch.[1] Using this access, it may be possible to dissect the popliteal bifurcation and the tibioperoneal trunk. This exposure is greatly helped by resection of the head of the fibula.

Posteromedial Approach

The posteromedial approach is rarely used because the location of the anterior tibial artery is deep, which makes the anastomosis difficult (Fig. 7). The incision follows the posteromedial edge of the tibia. The first steps are the same as for the approach to the posterior tibial artery described above. The dissection continues in front of the posterior tibial artery and the deep

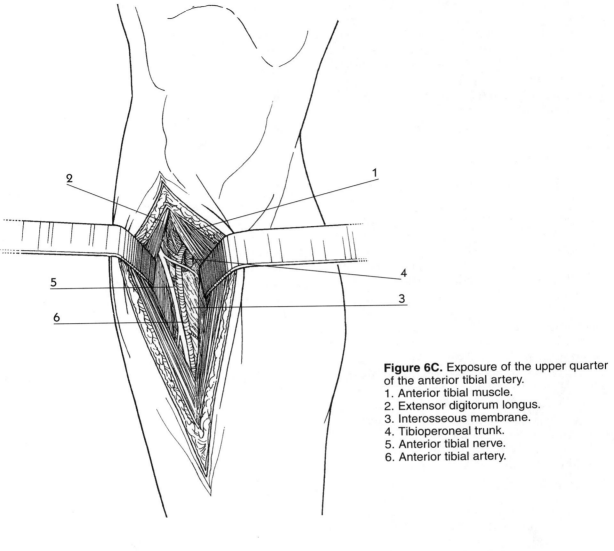

Figure 6C. Exposure of the upper quarter of the anterior tibial artery.
1. Anterior tibial muscle.
2. Extensor digitorum longus.
3. Interosseous membrane.
4. Tibioperoneal trunk.
5. Anterior tibial nerve.
6. Anterior tibial artery.

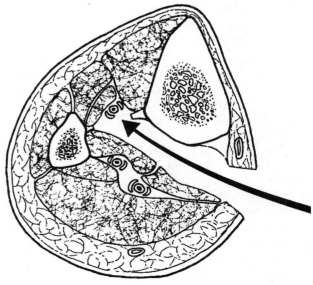

Figure 7. Cross-section of the leg. Pathway of the posterior approach to expose the anterior tibial artery.

muscles until the interosseous membrane is exposed. The membrane is excised, exposing the posterior aspect of the anterior tibial neurovascular bundle. The latter is mobilized and then partially exteriorized using loops to perform the anastomosis. This approach is indicated only when cutaneous lesions prevent an anterior approach.

Routes of the Bypasses

For in situ bypasses, the vein should be mobilized through the leg starting at the interarticular line of the knee. The lower part of the popliteal fossa is dissected with limited exposure of the popliteal bifurcation. The interosseous membrane is freed and then incised longitudinally for 2-3 cm. A blunt instrument is passed, guided by a finger from inside, from the anterior compartment toward the popliteal fossa. The distal anastomosis should be performed far enough from the point where the vein graft crosses the interosseous space. In fact, the vein should be parallel to the artery in order to perform the anastomosis. If the anastomosis is performed too close to the point where the graft crosses the interosseous membrane, there is a risk of compressing it at the level of its heel.[2]

Reversed bypasses follow the anatomic route previously described, behind the sartorius muscle, and between the heads of the gastrocnemius muscles before joining the anterior compartment. The lateral subcutaneous route (see above) is employed preferably when access to the popliteal fossa is contraindicated because of sepsis or severe scarring from previous procedures.

The transosseous tunnel is recommended for in situ bypasses of the lower part of the anterior tibial artery (Fig. 8).[2] Without a tunnel, the vein needs to take a subcutaneous route which crosses the anterior edge of the outline of the tibia to join the anterior tibial artery. The transosseous route is a technically easy procedure and removes the risk of extrinsic compression. The theoretical risk of weakening the bone implies that this technique should be avoided in patients with osteoporosis. For this

technique, an oblique transtibial osseus tunnel allows the bypass to join the anterolateral compartment following a direct route. The tunnel should avoid the edges of the bone. The entry orifice is made on the medial surface of the tibia. From there, the tunnel exits the lateral surface of the tibia following an oblique course at an angle that should not exceed 60 degrees in order to avoid weakening the tibial diaphysis. The site of the exit orifice is selected depending on the level of the anastomosis to the anterior tibial artery. There should be a distance of 2-3 cm between the bone and the site of anastomosis to avoid the risk of kinking. The lateral surface of the bone is freed of its periosteum for one square centimeter and the cortex is pierced with a pneumatic drill. On the lateral surface the orifice should be posterior and close to the medial edge. The entry and exit orifices are smoothed using a fine drill bit or a rongeur to avoid sharp edges.

A variation of this technique consists of creating a simple trough, instead of a tunnel, in the cortex of the anterior edge of the bone.[3] The

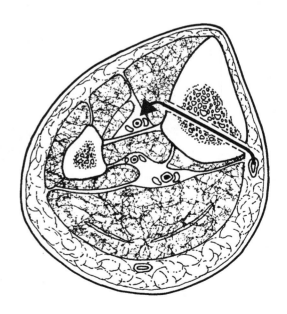

Figure 8. Cross-section of the leg showing the transosseous route of a bypass of the anterior tibial artery.

incisions previously used for venous harvesting to expose the artery permit exposing the medial and lateral surfaces of the bone. The anterior edge of the tibial crest may be superficially drilled and the rough edges are then rounded and smoothed. This technique does not have any advantage over the preceding method. In addition, it is more difficult to perform and carries the risk of weakening the bone.

Posterior Approach

Access to the arteries of the leg using a posterior approach may be indicated when the arterial lesions are infrapopliteal and a popliteal distal bypass is planned. The patient is placed in ventral decubitus position with a roll under the iliac crest. The leg is included in the operating field as far as the upper third of the thigh. Surgical drapes placed under the knee facilitate its extension as well as access to the popliteal artery. Because of the position of the patient and the length of these operations, we prefer general to epidural anesthesia.

The incision (Fig. 9a) is centered over the lesser saphenous vein, begins at the fold of the knee, and extends downwards to the site of the distal anastomosis. If the anastomosis is to the distal posterior tibial artery, a short additional incision is made parallel to the medial edge of the Achilles tendon to avoid extensive subcutaneous dissection which may result in problems with healing. Depending on whether the bypass is in situ or reversed, the lesser saphenous vein is harvested in its entirety or is left in place after mobilizing both ends.

The lesser saphenous vein is considered usable if its external diameter, previously measured by ultrasound, is > 3.0 mm. In its lower half, the lesser saphenous vein is superficial and accompanied by the lateral saphenous nerve. In the middle third of the leg it disappears into a folding of the superficial fascia which leaves the nerve separated in front of the vein. At the level of the popliteal fossa it is situated between the superficial and deep fascia, piercing the latter at the level of the interarticular line to enter the posterior wall of the popliteal vein. The arcade may occur

higher in the interarticular line, providing 5 cm or 6 cm of additional length for a bypass.

The popliteal artery below the knee joint line is exposed after retracting the tibial nerve and the popliteal vein. Access to the popliteal artery requires an upward S-shaped extension of the incision.

The approach to the tibioperoneal trunk and to the origin of the arteries of the leg necessitates cutting the medial fusion of the heads of the gastrocnemius muscles which are retracted aside with their vascular supply. The soleus muscle forms a thick, wide cover on the upper part of the leg (Fig. 9b). In the lower part of the leg, it becomes narrower and may be retracted medially. The soleus muscle may be disinserted from its attachment to the tibia for its entire length, or alternatively, it may be cut close to its insertions. It may also be incised along the median line using the classic access for ligation of the posterior tibial artery (Fig. 9c). The incision extends distally as far as the calcaneus. In this way the TPT is exposed: the posterior tibial arteries are located medially and the peroneal artery outside. The latter is crossed, close to its origin, by the tibial nerve. The TPT and the origin of the arteries of the leg are hidden by a plexus of veins and by nerve branches that should be preserved in order to avoid neuromuscular deficits. The proximal part of the posterior tibial and peroneal arteries can be satisfactorily exposed using this approach. The anterior tibial artery, on the other hand, is only accessible for its first 1.5 cm before reaching the upper edge of the interosseous membrane. Sectioning the latter allows exposure of an additional 1-2 cm of anterior tibial artery.

Distal Approach

Posterior Tibial Artery (Fig. 10)

A vertical incision of 8-10 cm is made following the medial edge of the Achilles tendon. Incision of the superficial fascia gives access to the space between the sural triceps muscle and flexor digitorum longus on which

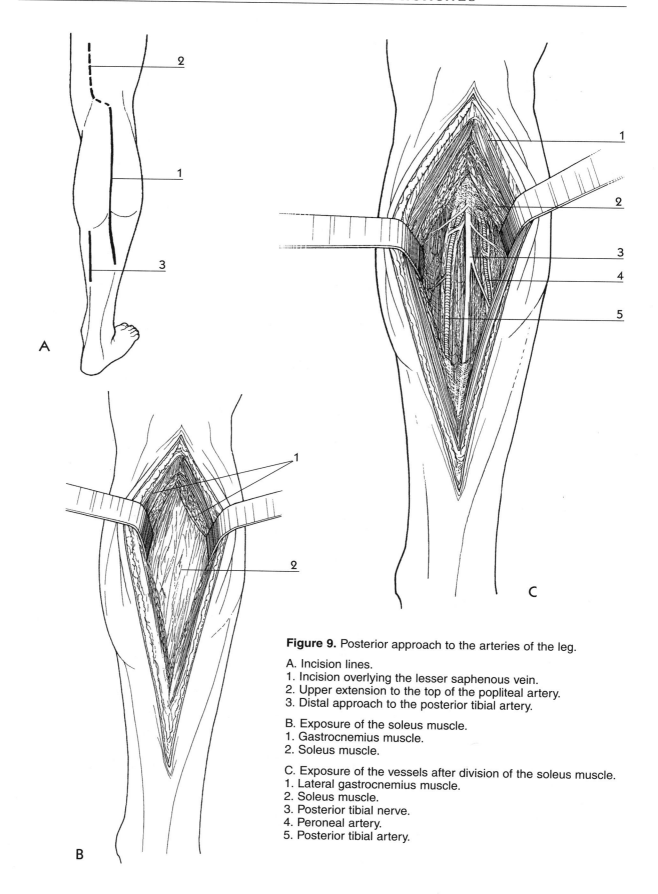

Figure 9. Posterior approach to the arteries of the leg.

A. Incision lines.
1. Incision overlying the lesser saphenous vein.
2. Upper extension to the top of the popliteal artery.
3. Distal approach to the posterior tibial artery.

B. Exposure of the soleus muscle.
1. Gastrocnemius muscle.
2. Soleus muscle.

C. Exposure of the vessels after division of the soleus muscle.
1. Lateral gastrocnemius muscle.
2. Soleus muscle.
3. Posterior tibial nerve.
4. Peroneal artery.
5. Posterior tibial artery.

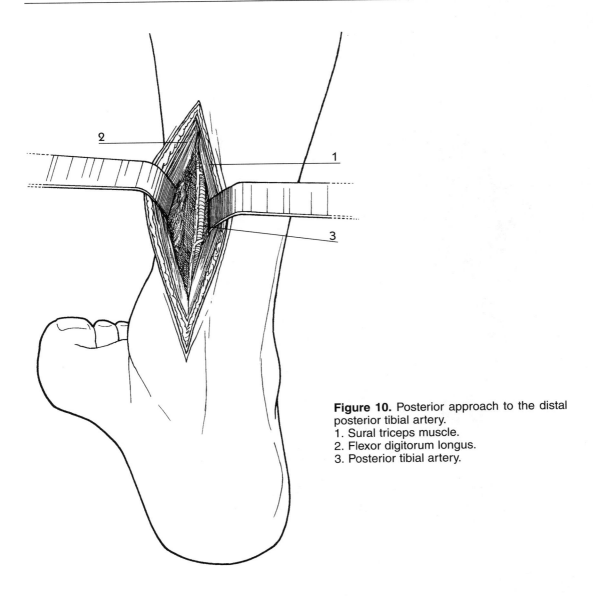

Figure 10. Posterior approach to the distal posterior tibial artery.
1. Sural triceps muscle.
2. Flexor digitorum longus.
3. Posterior tibial artery.

the artery lies and is covered by the deep fascia of the leg. Close to the malleolus, the posterior tibial artery runs behind the flexor digitorum longus, which must be retracted medially in order to expose the distal part of the artery.[4]

Peroneal Artery (Fig. 11)

The superficial and deep fascia of the leg are incised longitudinally outside the calcaneus tendon at the lower end of the incision used for harvesting the lesser saphenous vein. The artery is covered behind by the flexor

hallucis longus which is retracted laterally.[5] At its lower part, the artery lies on the interosseous membrane and divides into its anterolateral and posteromedial branches. The artery may be easily located by palpating the fibula which is just lateral to it.

Discussion

A number of factors determine the outcome of a distal bypass. The availability of a good venous graft and an adequate arterial outflow

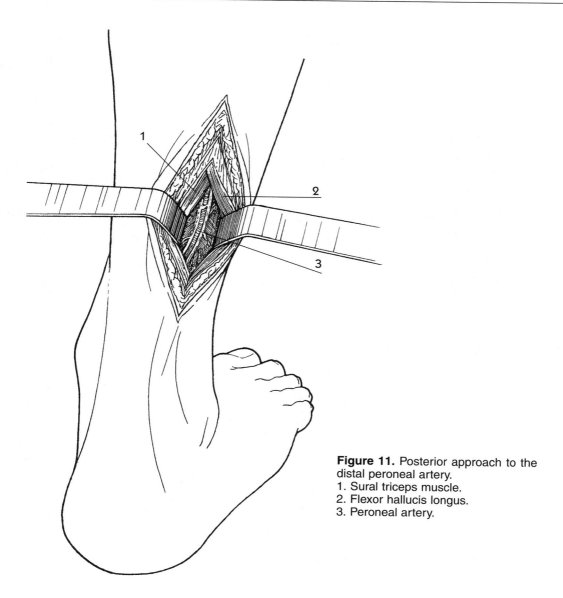

Figure 11. Posterior approach to the distal peroneal artery.
1. Sural triceps muscle.
2. Flexor hallucis longus.
3. Peroneal artery.

are the most important. A smooth postoperative course depends on the appropriate choice of approach and on the quality of its execution. Successful primary healing allows a quick return to ambulation and shortens the period of hospitalization. Inversely, problems with healing and slow rehabilitation can cause pain and prolong the period of hospitalization, even when they do not cause septic complications. Cutaneous complications are reported in 7% to 30% of cases. Their occurrence depends on local and general factors including nutritional state, degree of ischemia, presence of infection, or proximity of ischemic ulcerations. The

choice of incision is important and should be outlined by the surgeon: it should allow access to the vein, exposure of the artery, and permit tunneling. In bypasses with a high risk of thrombosis, the choice of approach and the line of incision should take into account the possibility of failure and the need not to interfere with an amputation later on.

The surgical exposure should be performed with careful attention to the handling of tissue. Skin and the subcutaneous tissue are particularly vulnerable in ischemic conditions. Rough dissection, the use of cautery too close to the skin, and aggressive and excessive retraction should be avoided. Muscular trauma, which often results from poor anatomic knowledge, should also be avoided. Nerves should be handled with care as well; the contusion of superficial nerves, although not always avoidable, may be responsible for troublesome postoperative neuralgia. The muscular vessels that supply the deep nerves should be preserved as much as possible because their division may cause muscular weakness. The deep veins of the leg adhere closely to the adjacent arteries and are occasionally plexiform. Their injury often requires ligation which is a cause of postoperative phlebitis. The use of an Esmarch type elastic bandage to perform the distal anastomosis allows minimizing the amount of exposure of the artery to be revascularized. The artery is exposed but does not need to be freed circumferentially. A segment of only 15-20 mm in length is needed to perform an anastomosis.

Choice of Approach

The choice of approach depends on several factors: the presence of cutaneous lesions, the available venous material, prior surgery, and the morphology of the patient. The topography of the arterial lesions is the determining factor. In severe ischemia, usually one artery provides the conditions required for a suitable outflow, i.e. absence of diffuse distal lesions, direct continuity with the arterial network of the foot, or indirect continuity (via the peroneal artery) by collaterals.

The posterior tibial artery rarely provides these conditions. Revascularization is more frequently done on the anterior tibial artery or in the peroneal artery which is often free of atheroma. At the lower leg level, the long-term outcome of revascularization depends on the quality of the collaterals that connect with the arterial network of the foot. The medial retrotibial approach permits simultaneous exposure of the greater saphenous vein, the posterior tibial artery, and the upper half of the fibular artery. The distal part of the peroneal artery is best exposed using a lateral approach. This approach may be the best choice when access using a medial approach is difficult because of previous operations or the morphology of the patient (large leg). In general the anterior tibial artery is exposed using the anterior approach. The posteromedial approach is used only to extend the exposure provided by a medial retrotibial approach in the first few centimeters of the artery or when a cutaneous lesion prohibits an anterior approach. The posterior access to the posterior tibial and peroneal arteries is rarely used; it is reserved for infrapopliteal lesions when the lesser saphenous vein is to be used. In Ouriel's experience,[4] the latter technique may be used in 72% of patients needing infrapopliteal revascularization. There are numerous advantages to this approach as it preserves the greater saphenous vein and facilitates arterial access for redo operations. Cutaneous complications are rare and edema is unusual.[6] The distal approach to the peroneal artery is easier and less traumatic than the lateral approach. Conversely, this approach provides only limited access to the upper and middle thirds of the arteries of the leg and requires division of the gastrocnemius muscles and of the soleus muscle. The nerves of the muscles of the superficial posterior compartment can be injured using this approach with resulting muscular paresis.

References

1. Cadenat FM. *Les voies de pénétration des membres*. Paris, Doin, 1964.
2. Watelet J, Peillon C. Pontages jambiers et distaux. Paris, *Encycl Med Chir*, Techniques chirurgicales, Chirurgie Vasculaire, 43029H, 1991.
3. Valentine RJ, Blankenship CL, Wind GG. The tibial gutter: a protected route for bypass grafts to the distal anterior tibial artery. *J Vasc Surg* 1989; 10: 465-467.
4. Ouriel K. The posterior approach to popliteal-crural bypass. *J Vasc Surg* 1994; 19: 74-80.
5. Rouvière H. *Anatomie humaine descriptive et topographique* Paris, Masson, 1991, 13° édition, Tome 3 pp 457-458.
6. Mukherjee D. Posterior approach to the peroneal artery. *J Vasc Surg* 1994; 19: 174-178.

29

Arteries of
the Ankle and Foot

Michael Jacobs

Femorocrural and pedal bypasses are effective in patients with limb-threatening ischemic disease. In diabetic patients, pedal revascularization improves limb salvage up to 80% after 3 years. It is generally accepted that grafts to the level of the ankle and foot should consist of autologous material. Preoperative assessment of the distal circulation and bypass possibilities is achieved by selective angiography, duplex scanning, and pulsatility indices. Distal bypass procedures demand surgical skill, careful tissue handling, and patience. Finally, graft surveillance is essential in the field of pedal revascularization.

Anatomic Structure of the Ankle and Foot Arteries[1,2]

The anterior tibial artery (ATA) is a terminal branch of the popliteal artery, passing between the head of the posterior tibial muscle and through the interosseous membrane to the front of the leg. In the lower part it lies on the tibia, and at the level of the ankle it is midway between the malleoli, continuing on the dorsum of the foot as the dorsalis pedis artery.

At the ankle, the ATA is crossed by the tendon of the extensor hallucis longus and continues between it and the first tendon of the extensor digitorum longus (Fig. 1). The upper part of the ATA is covered by the tibialis anterior and extensor digitorum muscles, and the lower part is covered by skin, fascia, and the extensor retinaculum. The artery is accompanied by venae comitantes on each side and there are small crossing connecting veins between the latter.

At the lower part of the leg the following branches are given off from the anterior tibial artery: the anterior medial malleolar artery exits 5 cm above the ankle, passing medially to the tendons of the extensor hallucis longus and

From Vascular Surgical Approaches, edited by Alain Branchereau and Ramon Berguer. ©1999, Futura Publishing Co., Inc., Armonk, NY.

tibialis anterior, and anastomosing with branches of the posterior tibial artery.

The anterolateral malleolar artery passes behind the extensor digitorum longus, and anastomoses with perforating branches of the peroneal artery and collaterals of the lateral tarsal artery. The anterolateral and anteromedial malleolar arteries form an extensive network with the tarsal branches of the dorsalis pedis and the plantar arteries of the posterior tibial artery.

The dorsalis pedis artery is the extension of the ATA distal to the ankle joint. It follows the tibial side of the dorsum of the foot to the proximal end of the first intermetatarsal space where it turns into the foot to complete the plantar arch (Fig. 2). The dorsalis pedis pulse can be felt between the tendon of the extensor hallucis longus and extensor digitorum longus. The dorsalis pedis artery gives off the following branches: lateral tarsal, arcuate and first dorsal metatarsal arteries.

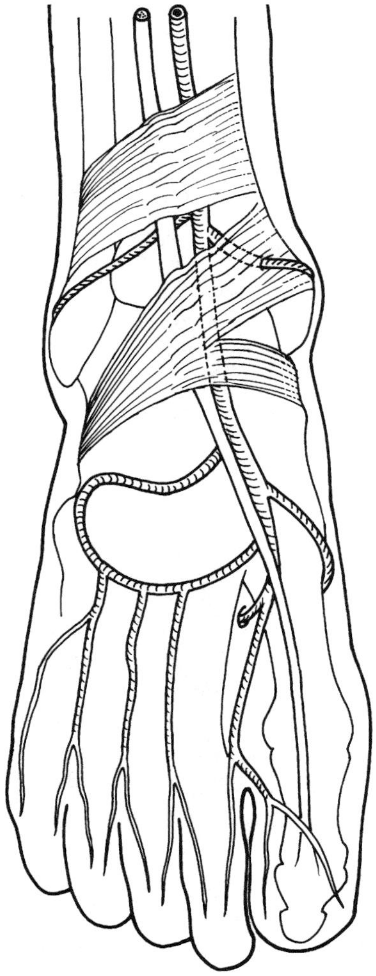

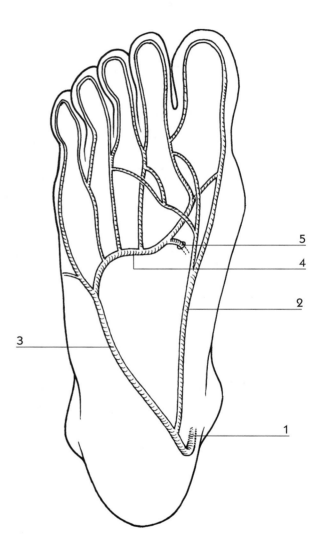

Figure 1. The right anterior tibial and dorsalis pedis arteries.
Note the crossing of the retinaculum and the extensor hallucis longus.

Figure 2. The plantar arteries and arch of the right foot.
1. Posterior tibial artery.
2. Medial plantar artery.
3. Lateral plantar artery.
4. Deep plantar arch.
5. Anastomosis between the deep plantar arch and the dorsalis pedis artery.

The lateral tarsal artery (Fig. 2) arises from the dorsalis pedis as it crosses the navicular bone, and has collateral anastomosis with the arcuate, the anterolateral malleolar and lateral plantar arteries, and with perforating branches of the peroneal artery.

The superficial plantar arch (Figs. 1 and 2) arises from the dorsalis pedis opposite the medial cuneiform bone, then passes laterally over the base of the metatarsal bones, anastomosing with the lateral tarsal and lateral plantar arteries, and giving off the second, third and fourth dorsal metatarsal arteries. These dorsal metatarsal arteries divide into two dorsal digital branches. At the proximal part of the interosseous space the dorsal metatarsal arteries receive the proximal perforating branches from the plantar arch, and at the distal part of the interosseous space they are joined by the distal perforating branches from the plantar metatarsal arteries. The first dorsal intermetatarsal artery arises just before the terminal portion of the dorsalis pedis passes into the sole.

The peroneal artery passes obliquely towards the fibula and descends along its medial crest in a fibrous canal between the tibialis posterior and flexor hallucis longus muscles (Fig. 3). It passes behind the tibiofibular syndesmosis and divides into calcaneal branches. The muscular branches of the peroneal artery supply the soleus, posterior tibialis, and flexor hallucis longus. A perforating branch traverses the interosseous membrane about 5 cm above the lateral malleolus anastomosing with the anterolateral malleolar artery. Its communicating ramus anastomoses with branches of the posterior tibial artery approximately 5 cm above the ankle.

The posterior tibial artery (PTA) passes downwards from the lower border of the popliteus muscle, between the tibia and fibula, finally dividing under the origin of the abductor hallucis into the medial and lateral plantar arteries. At this level the PTA is deep to the flexor retinaculum. Its muscular branches are distributed to the soleus and the deep muscles on the back of the leg. The posteromedial malleolar branch winds around the medial malleolus, and anastomoses with branches of the anteromedial malleolar artery.

The calcanean branches anastomose with the malleolar network and with the calcanean branches of the peroneal arteries. The medial plantar artery (Fig. 2), the smaller terminal branch of the PTA, passes distally along the medial side of the foot between the abductor hallucis and flexor digitorum brevis, finally anastomosing with a branch of the first metatarsal artery, supplying three small superficial digital branches.

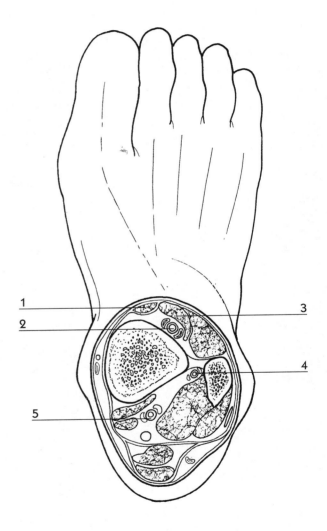

Figure 3. Transverse-section through the right leg, about 6 cm above the tip of the malleolus.
1. Anterior tibial muscle.
2. Anterior tibial artery.
3. Extensor hallucis longus.
4. Peroneal artery.
5. Posterior tibial artery.

The lateral plantar artery (Fig. 2), the larger terminal branch of the PTA, passes laterally and distally to the base of the 5th metatarsal bone with the lateral plantar nerve on its medial side. Turning medially between the bases of the 1st and 2nd metatarsal bones, it anastomoses with the dorsalis pedis artery, completing the plantar arch.

The plantar arch is deeply situated and has three perforating and four plantar metatarsal branches, that supply to the skin, fascia and plantar muscles (Fig. 2). The three perforating branches anastomose with the dorsal metatarsal arteries. The four plantar metatarsal arteries each divide into two plantar digital arteries. Near its division, each plantar metatarsal artery sends dorsally a distal perforating branch to join the corresponding dorsal metatarsal artery.

Surgical Exposure of the Ankle and Foot Arteries

Anterior Tibial Artery

The anterior tibial artery above the ankle is exposed in the anterior compartment through a vertical anterolateral incision, about 1 cm lateral of the crest of the tibia and just lateral to the anterior tibial tendon and medial of the extensor hallucis longus muscle (Fig. 4), which is retracted laterally.

At this level, from 10 cm above the ankle and down, it is necessary to divide the upper extensor retinaculum (Fig. 5). Exposure is limited by the extensor tendons: often it is not

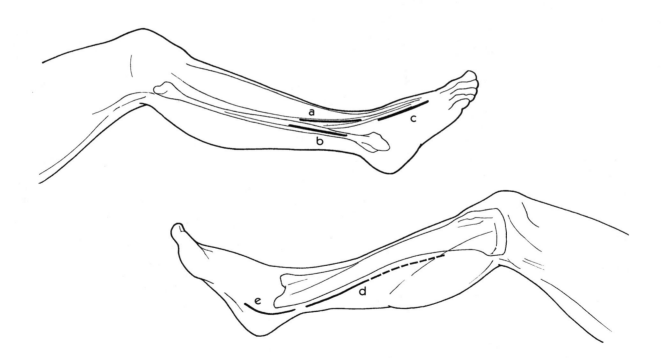

Figure 4. Schematic drawing of incisions for surgical exposure of the:
a. Anterior tibial artery.
b. Peroneal artery (lateral approach).
c. Dorsalis pedis artery.
d. Posterior tibial artery
   Peroneal artery (medial approach)
e. Inframalleolar posterior tibial artery and plantar arteries.

possible to place a self-retaining retractor in this area and hand-held small retractors provide a better view. After careful exposure of the neurovascular bundle, the anterior tibial artery can be seen between its two comitant veins. Normally, an adequate exposure can be obtained by dissecting around the artery only at the place where the small vessel loops will be used. This provides a 3-4 cm segment of anterior tibial artery for the anastomosis.

The arteriotomy is performed on a small portion of the lateral wall of the artery to provide a better lie for the bypass.

The dorsalis pedis artery may be exposed through a longitudinal incision, lateral to the tendon of the extensor hallucis longus (Fig. 4). After incising the skin, subcutaneous tissue, and the superficial fascia, the artery can be easily identified medial to the extensor hallucis brevis muscle (Fig. 6). For more proximal exposure of the dorsalis pedis artery and to allow a compression-free tunnel for the graft, the lower extensor retinaculum must be divided. The retinaculum should always be divided to allow a compression-free tunnel for the graft.

When the dorsalis pedis artery is dissected, care should be taken to avoid damage to the

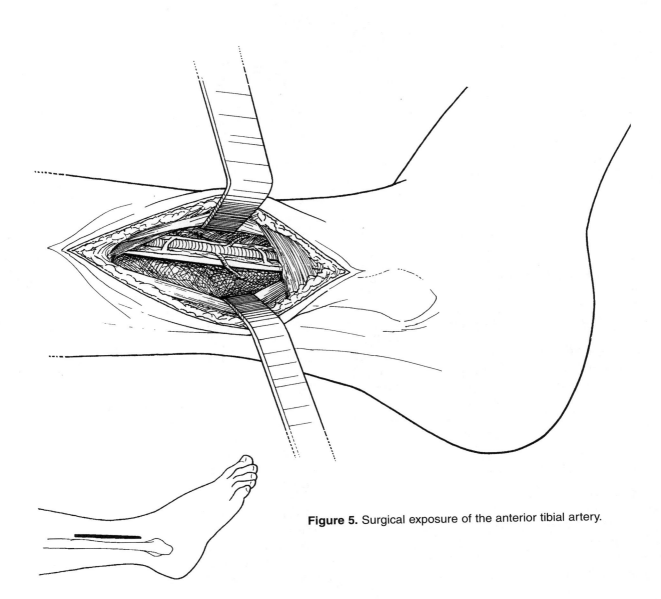

Figure 5. Surgical exposure of the anterior tibial artery.

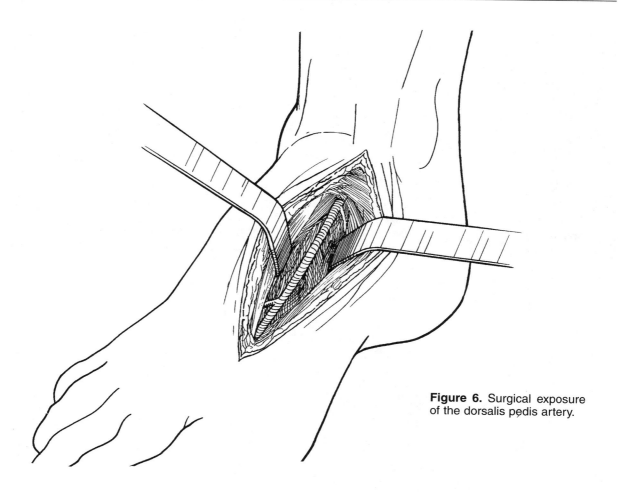

Figure 6. Surgical exposure of the dorsalis pedis artery.

deep peroneal nerve, which runs on its medial side.

If the saphenous vein has to be harvested down to the dorsum of the foot, especially in conjunction with the in situ technique, the skin incision should be made more medially, allowing exposure of the greater saphenous vein and dorsalis pedis artery. The skin and subcutaneous tissue should be handled with extreme care to avoid problems with healing.

Peroneal Artery

The peroneal artery in the lower limb can be used as a recipient vessel in patients with critical limb ischemia. At the level of the ankle, however, the diameter of the peroneal artery is often less than 1 mm. Approximately 10 cm above the lateral malleolus, the peroneal artery may have an acceptable diameter and can be approached by an incision on the lateral aspect of the leg directly over the fibula. The incision is deepened through the fascia and posterior to the peroneal musculature, to expose the fibula. The peroneal neurovascular bundle lies deeper than the fibula (Fig. 4D). By blunt dissection, the third peroneus, the short peroneus, and flexor hallucis longus are cleared from the bone. A 5-7 cm segment of the exposed fibula is resected carefully to provide direct access to an envelope of fascia containing the peroneal artery and its venae comitantes, which lie directly on the belly of the tibialis posterior muscle (Fig. 7). The peroneal artery can also be approached by a medial incision, as discussed below, posterior to the tibia and anterior to the flexor hallucis longus muscle.

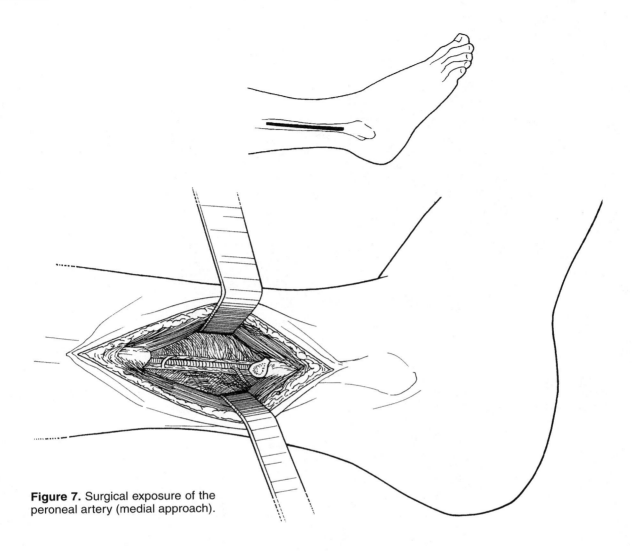

Figure 7. Surgical exposure of the peroneal artery (medial approach).

Posterior Tibial Artery

The posterior tibial artery above the ankle is exposed by making a longitudinal incision, beginning posterior to the medial malleolus and extending proximally 1 cm posterior to the edge of the tibia (Fig. 8)

The superficial fascia is divided and the Achilles tendon is retracted posteriorly. The intermuscular fascial septum, covering the deep muscles and the posterior tibial neurovascular bundle, is incised over the artery. The neurovascular bundle is found between the flexor hallucis longus and flexor digitorum longus muscles. More distal dissection requires division of the flexor retinaculum.

Plantar Arteries

The plantar artery is exposed by a curved incision starting posterior to the medial malleolus (Fig. 9). The posterior tibial artery divides under the origin of the abductor hallucis muscle into the medial and lateral plantar arteries. The neurovascular bundle can be found posterior to the flexor digitorum longus after transection of the flexor retinaculum (Fig. 10). Care should be taken not to

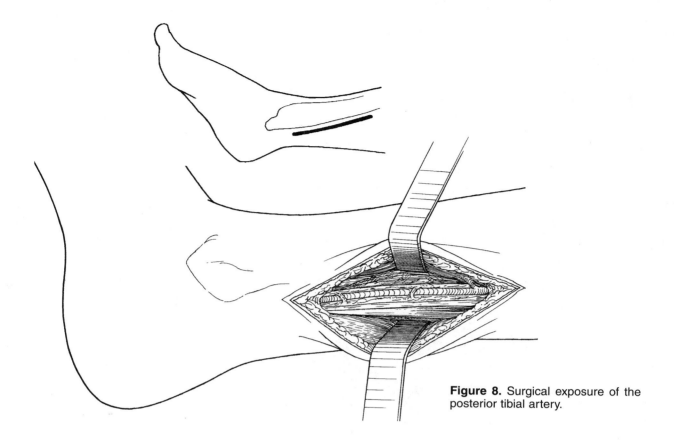

Figure 8. Surgical exposure of the posterior tibial artery.

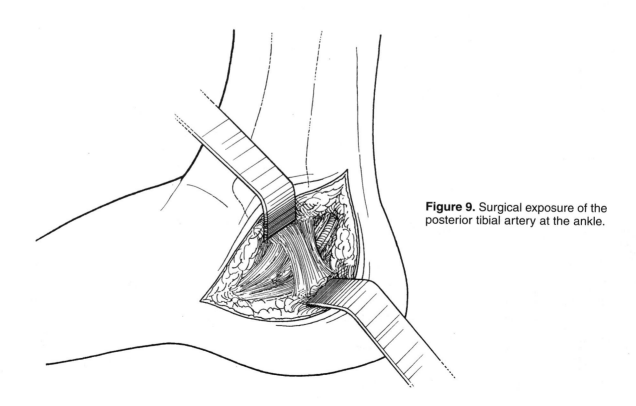

Figure 9. Surgical exposure of the posterior tibial artery at the ankle.

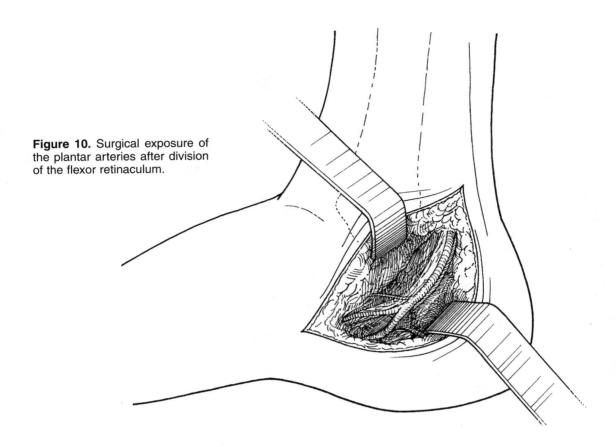

Figure 10. Surgical exposure of the plantar arteries after division of the flexor retinaculum.

injure the tibial nerve, which is close to the distal posterior tibial artery.

Generally, the lateral plantar artery is used as a recipient vessel since its diameter is larger than that of the medial plantar artery. Beyond its bifurcation, the lateral plantar artery can be dissected for approximately 2 cm before it disappears at the level of the 5th metatarsal.

If the most distal part of the posterior tibial artery is calcified and cannot be used as a recipient vessel, a common opening between the medial and lateral plantar arteries can be created. Following spatulation of both arteries, they are sewn to create a single opening which is anastomosed end-to-end to the graft.

References

1. Kamina P, Di Marino V. *Vaisseaux des membres*. 2ème éd. Paris, Maloine, 1993, 176 pages.
2. Sobotta édité par R. Putz et R. Pabst. *Atlas d'anatomie humaine*. Tome 2. Paris, Editions Médicales Internationales, 1994, 400 pages.

30

Unusual Surgical Approaches to the Deep Femoral, Popliteal and Infrapopliteal Arteries

Frank J. Veith

The last decade has witnessed increasingly widespread acceptance of arterial reconstruction surgery to save limbs that are in jeopardy because of infrainguinal arteriosclerosis. Because most bypass conduits that are used below the inguinal ligament are imperfect and because the disease process continues, it is not surprising that an important proportion of infrainguinal arterial reconstruction will fail during the lifetime of patients having them. Moreover, these failures are often, although not always, associated with a renewed threat to the involved limb. Because limb salvage is a desirable goal, there is therefore a real and increasingly common need in many patients for some form of secondary intervention to correct the ischemia and again save the extremity.

We, and others, have shown clearly that secondary interventions, which usually require a surgical operation, are worthwhile; they comprise a very important component of an aggressive approach to saving lower extremities that are threatened because of ischemia from arteriosclerosis.[1,2] These secondary operations are often more difficult to perform, however, because the access routes to the arteries have been previously dissected and the surgeon must perform his secondary operation through scarred, and occasionally infected, tissue planes. An additional problem that is frequently encountered in patients who need arterial reconstruction after one or more of these procedures in the same extremity is the scarcity of good autogenous vein that can be used as an arterial bypass conduit. Finally, the incidence of wound infection is much higher after arterial reconstruction that requires a repeat dissection of an artery than it is after the primary arterial procedure.[3]

From Vascular Surgical Approaches, edited by Alain Branchereau and Ramon Berguer. ©1999, Futura Publishing Co., Inc., Armonk, NY.

For these reasons, we have used increasingly and whenever possible our secondary lower extremity arterial reconstruction. Moreover, when appropriate virginal arterial segments are not available, we have developed a variety of new or unusual anatomic approaches to infrainguinal arteries that permit surgical access to these arteries without the need to traverse the scarred or infected tissue planes of the previously used standard approach. These new or unusual approaches also facilitate the use of shorter grafts and may therefore allow a patient to have a limited segment of lesser saphenous or upper extremity vein rather than a prosthetic graft for his or her arterial reconstruction.

The purpose of this chapter is to detail these new or unusual approaches to infrainguinal arteries. Although these approaches are particularly useful in patients who require a secondary lower extremity arterial reconstruction, they are also valuable in facilitating the use of autogenous vein grafts if the length or quality of this material is inadequate.

Direct Approaches to the Middle and Distal Portions of the Deep Femoral Artery

The deep femoral artery has been widely advocated as an outflow site for aortofemoral or axillofemoral bypasses when disease makes the common femoral artery unsuitable. The deep femoral artery has also been used as a site of origin for more distal bypasses when the common femoral artery is diseased or scarred or when autogenous vein length is limited.[4] The standard surgical technique for exposing the deep femoral artery uses a groin incision to identify its origin from the common femoral artery. After the large crossing veins that are frequently present are divided, the deep femoral artery is then traced distally as far as necessary.[5]

As a result of our experience with a large number of patients who required secondary arterial reconstruction after failure of one or more previous vascular operations, we realized that gaining surgical access to the common femoral artery, and proximal few centimeters of the deep femoral artery, could be extremely difficult or impossible because of scarring or residual infection. Because of this and also because the more distal portions of the deep femoral artery appeared relatively disease-free in many of these patients, we developed methods to approach the distal parts of this artery directly without the use of a groin incision. These techniques are now used to perform a variety of otherwise difficult second-ary bypasses that terminate or originate in the middle or distal portions of the deep femoral artery. They have also been used for sites of origin for primary bypasses to the popliteal or infrapopliteal arteries when available vein length is limited.

Anatomic Review

The deep femoral artery originates from the posterior or posterolateral side of the common femoral artery as one of the two terminal branches of this vessel. The femoral bifurcation can occur from 1-9 cm below the inguinal ligament. From there the deep femoral artery runs distally and posteriorly in a course roughly parallel to the femur, to which it becomes progressively closer. The artery ends in a terminal bifurcation located close to the linea aspera on the posterior surface of the femur near the junction of its middle and lower thirds. The deep femoral artery can be divided into three portions or zones (Figs. 1 and 2). The proximal zone extends from the artery's origin to just beyond the origin of the lateral femoral circumflex artery. The middle zone extends to the second perforation branch, and the distal zone extends from beyond the second perfor-ation branch to the artery's termination.

The anatomic landmark for the location of the distal two zones of the femoral artery is the sartorius muscle, which overlies the second and third portions of this artery (Fig. 2, inset). Between the posterior surface of the sartorius muscle and the deep femoral artery lie the

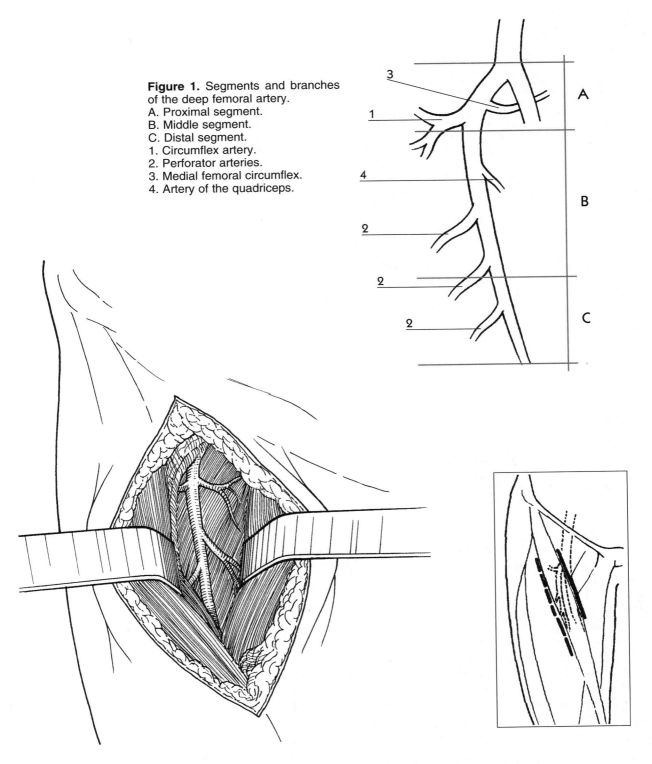

Figure 1. Segments and branches of the deep femoral artery.
A. Proximal segment.
B. Middle segment.
C. Distal segment.
1. Circumflex artery.
2. Perforator arteries.
3. Medial femoral circumflex.
4. Artery of the quadriceps.

Figure 2. Direct approach to the middle and distal thirds of the deep femoral artery. Following an anteromedial incision, the sartorius muscle and the superficial femoral artery are retracted laterally. The fascia that binds the vastus medialis and abductor longus muscles has been incised to expose the distal portion of the deep femoral artery. Insert: Anteromedial incision (solid line) along the medial edge of the sartorius muscle and anterior incision (dashed line) over the external border of the sartorius muscle. Both incisions are placed below the femoral triangle.

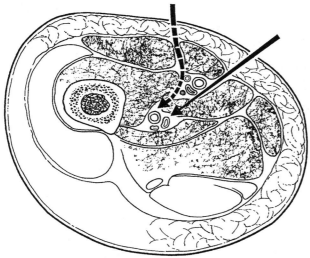

Figure 3. Cross-section of the left thigh in its middle third showing the relationship of the deep and superficial femoral arteries and the neighboring muscles. Dashed arrow: anterior approach lateral to the sartorius muscle. Solid arrow: anterior approach medial to the sartorius muscle and the superficial femoral sheath.

Figure 4. Cross-section of the middle third of the thigh showing the posteromedial approach to the deep femoral artery. Exposure follows the plane between the abductor longus in front and the abductor grevis and magnus muscles in the back. This approach avoids the superficial arteries and Hunter's canal.

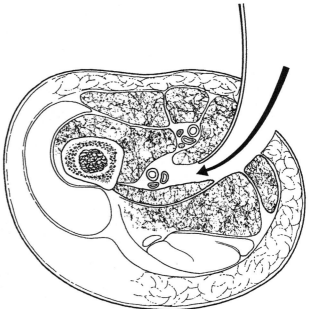

superficial femoral artery and accompanying veins and nerves. Deeper than this neurovascular bundle is a well-defined fibrous junction between the sheaths of the vastus medialis and the adductor longus muscles (Figs. 3 and 4). Deeper than the deep femoral artery is the pectineus muscle proximally and the adductor brevis and adductor magnus muscles distally.

Surgical Techniques

An incision is made parallel to either the medial or lateral border of the sartorius muscle

(Fig. 2, inset). An effort is made to make this incision inferior to any previous surgical scar or infection in the groin. In general, we have used the anteromedial approach along the medial border of the sartorius muscle to access the upper middle zone of the artery. The more anterior approach lateral to the sartorius muscle has been used to access the lower middle and distal zones of the artery. This anterior approach is particularly valuable in patients with postoperative scarring or infection of the medial segment of the middle third of the thigh. The anterior approach also makes it possible to preserve the sartorius blood supply, which enters via its medial border.

After the incision is deepened beyond the sartorius muscle, the superficial femoral vascular bundle is mobilized and reflected medially in the anterior approach (dashed arrow in Fig. 3), or laterally in the anteromedial approach (solid arrow in Fig. 3). This exposes the fibrous connection or dense fascial union between the sheaths of the adductor longus and the vastus medialis muscles. Incision of this fibrous union for several centimeters exposes the underlying deep femoral vascular structures. Usually a vein is the most superficial of these and it bulges forth when the fibrous union between the adductor longus and the vastus medialis is incised (Fig. 3). Deeper than the vein is the deep femoral artery, which can be carefully dissected free, avoiding injury to the many small friable branches that arise from this vessel. Self-retaining retraction methods can be helpful in holding apart the deeper layers of the wound to provide adequate exposure.

If the deep femoral artery is not pulsatile, it can easily be located by identifying venous branches deep to the incised fascial junction of the adductor longus and vastus medialis. Tracing these branches to one of the main deep femoral veins will permit localization of the adjacent artery even when it is pulseless and soft. Since the surgeon is working in virginal tissue planes and with previously undissected vessels, the approaches that have been described to the two distal zones of the deep femoral artery can be accomplished in 5-15minutes.

In patients who have had previous infection in the subsartorial canal, the distal portions of the deep femoral artery can be reached through uninvolved tissue planes by employing a more posteromedial approach (Fig. 4). To facilitate this approach, the patient's thigh and knee are moderately flexed and the thigh is abducted and externally rotated. An incision is made on the medial aspect of the thigh overlying the portion of the deep femoral artery to be used. This incision is deepened posterior to the adductor longus muscle and the artery is accessed between this muscle and the adductor magnus and adductor brevis muscles.

We have used these direct approaches to the two distal zones of the deep femoral artery to provide outflow or inflow for arterial reconstruction in 85 patients. In 56 of these patients, the middle or distal portions of the deep femoral artery were used as sites for bypass insertion or outflow, whereas in 29 patients, the middle or distal deep femoral artery was used as a site for bypass origin or to provide inflow. Early in our experience,[6] these approaches were used only in patients with surgical scarring or infection of the groin, often coupled with disease or scarring of the common femoral artery and proximal zone of the deep femoral artery. In these patients we found it difficult or impossible to use these vessels for the arterial reconstruction or to trace these vessels inferiorly to a usable distal portion of the deep femoral artery. Patients with *concrete groins* from prior surgery have also been reported by Hershey and Auer[5] and DePalma and his colleagues.[7] We have begun to use these approaches in primary arterial reconstructions as well, because of the ease and speed with which they can be accomplished. These direct approaches have been helpful and appear to be indicated in patients who require a primary bypass and have extensive arteriosclerotic disease in the common and superficial femoral arteries and the proximal portion of the deep femoral artery. These approaches are also indicated in patients who require a distal bypass but who have a limited length of adequate autologous vein.

Lateral Approaches to the Popliteal Artery

Medial and posterior approaches to the popliteal artery have been described and may be considered standard. Lateral access routes to this artery both above and below the knee joint can also be used and are particularly helpful in patients requiring a secondary operation.[8,9]

Surgical Techniques

Above-knee Popliteal Artery

The popliteal artery above the knee joint is approached with a lateral incision between the iliotibial tract and the biceps femoris muscle (Fig. 5). By deepening the incision in the lateral intermuscular septum, the popliteal space is entered and the neurovascular bundle can be palpated within the popliteal fat. The popliteal artery is easily isolated from the adjacent popliteal vein(s), taking care not to injure the common peroneal nerve (Fig. 6). After the popliteal artery is dissected from these structures, gentle traction with silicone vessel loops can elevate it close to the skin level where surgical manipulation and anastomosis can be carried out with the same ease as is usual through the standard medial approach.

Below-knee Popliteal Artery

This is approached via a lateral incision over the head and proximal fourth of the fibula (Fig. 5). This incision is deepened through the subcutaneous tissue and superficial muscular attachments to the fibula, taking care to identify the common peroneal nerve as it courses around the neck of this bone (Fig. 7). This nerve is dissected free so that it can be retracted and protected from injury. The biceps femoris tendon is divided. The ligamentous attachments of the fibular head are incised and the upper fourth of the fibula is freed bluntly from

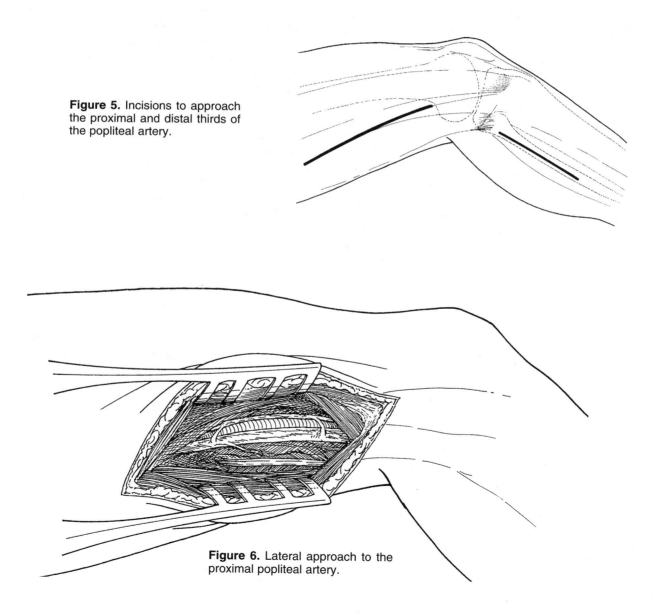

Figure 5. Incisions to approach the proximal and distal thirds of the popliteal artery.

Figure 6. Lateral approach to the proximal popliteal artery.

its muscular and ligamentous attachments, staying as close to the bone as possible. After a retractor is placed deep to the fibula to protect underlying structures, one or two holes are drilled in this bone at its proposed site of transaction. With such holes, a rib shears can cleanly transect the bone without leaving sharp spicules. After the bone is divided, any remaining deep attachments can be exposed and cut. With the upper fibula removed, the entire below-knee popliteal artery, tibio-peroneal trunk, anterior tibial artery, and the origins of the peroneal and posterior tibial artery lie just deep of the excised bone and can easily be dissected from their adjacent veins (Fig. 8). After mobilization these arteries

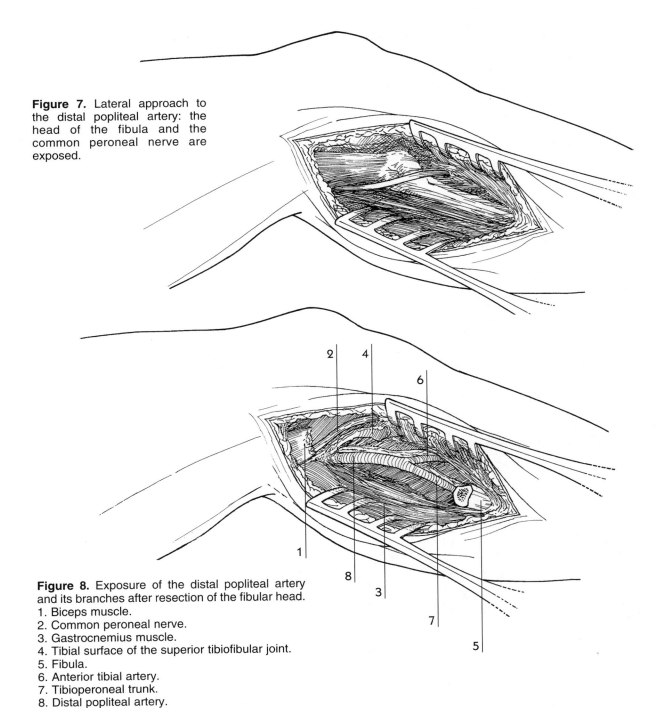

Figure 7. Lateral approach to the distal popliteal artery: the head of the fibula and the common peroneal nerve are exposed.

Figure 8. Exposure of the distal popliteal artery and its branches after resection of the fibular head.
1. Biceps muscle.
2. Common peroneal nerve.
3. Gastrocnemius muscle.
4. Tibial surface of the superior tibiofibular joint.
5. Fibula.
6. Anterior tibial artery.
7. Tibioperoneal trunk.
8. Distal popliteal artery.

are more superficial in the wound than via standard medial approaches, and surgical manipulation and anastomotic suturing can be performed with greater ease.

Tunneling for Grafts

To conduct grafts to or from a popliteal artery that is approached laterally, tunnels are constructed in a subcutaneous plane. For grafts from the femoral arteries approached via a standard groin incision, the course should be across the anterior aspect of the mid-thigh and then down the lateral aspect of the lower thigh to the popliteal fossa. If the external iliac artery, the axillary artery, or the thoracic aorta provides graft inflow, the tunnel follows a gradual curve from the inflow artery to the lateral aspect of the thigh and then inferiorly to the popliteal fossa.

Approaches to Leg Arteries

The standard medial approach to the posterior tibial and peroneal arteries in the leg is well known,[10] as is the standard anterolateral approach to the anterior tibial artery.[10] If these access routes are scarred or infected, all three vessels can be easily reached via a lateral approach with fibula resection,[11] and the anterior tibial artery can be accessed from a medial approach with division of the interosseous membrane.[12]

Inframalleolar Arteries

In the last decade, as more of our patients have required reoperation with very limited lengths of remaining autogenous vein, we have been forced to perform a variety of bypasses to inframalleolar arteries.[13,14] These include the posterior tibial and dorsal pedal (dorsalis pedis) arteries below the ankle joint and their main terminal branches. The latter consist of the medial and lateral plantar branches of the posterior tibial and the lateral tarsal and deep plantar or deep metatarsal arch branches of the dorsal pedal artery (Fig. 9).

Surgical Technique

The technical principles involved in the bypasses below the ankle joint are similar to those for all infrapopliteal bypasses in the leg.[10] The most important adjuncts for achieving technical success are the use of headlights to ensure optimal illumination of the surgical field and a commitment to the time and effort that is required.

It is also critical to obtain a dry field without injuring these small and sometimes diseased arteries. To this end, it is essential to minimize trauma to these little vessels, and spring-loaded microclips (Weck) can be helpful.[10]

Exposure of the Lateral and Medial Plantar Branches

These branches are the continuation of the posterior tibial artery in the foot. The lateral plantar artery ends in the main or deep plantar arch and is usually larger than its medial counterpart (Fig. 9). The medial branch gives off small collateral vessels to the intrinsic muscles of the first, second, and third toes. However, when the lateral branch is occluded, the medial branch may enlarge and conjoin with the plantar arch through collaterals. The initial skin incision is made sufficiently long to permit exposure of the retromalleolar portion of the posterior tibial artery (Fig. 10), which extends inferiorly and laterally onto the sole of the foot (Fig. 11). After the posterior tibial artery is isolated, the dissection is progressively extended across the sole of the foot. A direct approach to the individual branches is not advisable for several reasons. First, the skin of the sole of the foot is not easily retracted. Therefore, adequate exposure is difficult to obtain when the incision does not follow the exact course of the arterial branch. Second, these plantar branches tend to lie deep within the foot, which, coupled with their small diameter, further hinders their localization. Finally, the dissection of the bifurcation of the posterior tibial artery is recommended because it can aid in distinguishing the lateral from the medial plantar branch. The lateral plantar branch is usually located inferiorly when the

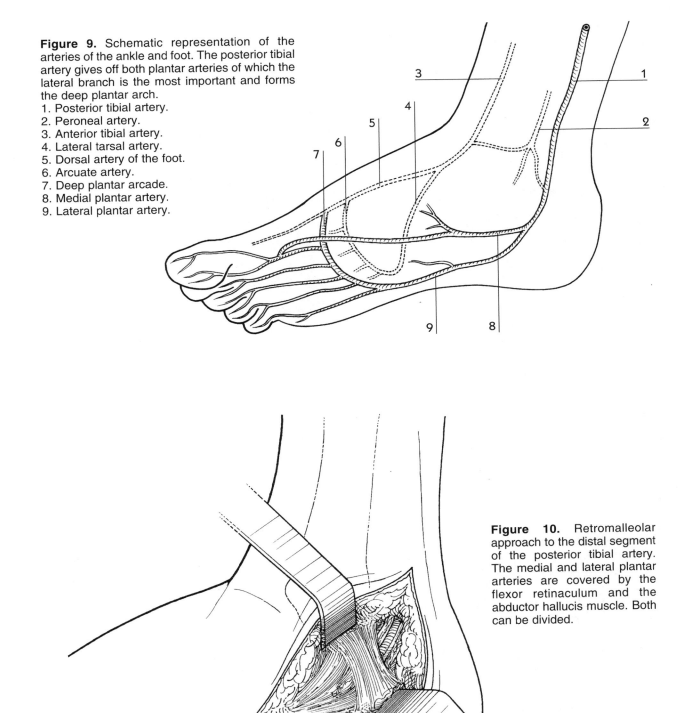

Figure 9. Schematic representation of the arteries of the ankle and foot. The posterior tibial artery gives off both plantar arteries of which the lateral branch is the most important and forms the deep plantar arch.
1. Posterior tibial artery.
2. Peroneal artery.
3. Anterior tibial artery.
4. Lateral tarsal artery.
5. Dorsal artery of the foot.
6. Arcuate artery.
7. Deep plantar arcade.
8. Medial plantar artery.
9. Lateral plantar artery.

Figure 10. Retromalleolar approach to the distal segment of the posterior tibial artery. The medial and lateral plantar arteries are covered by the flexor retinaculum and the abductor hallucis muscle. Both can be divided.

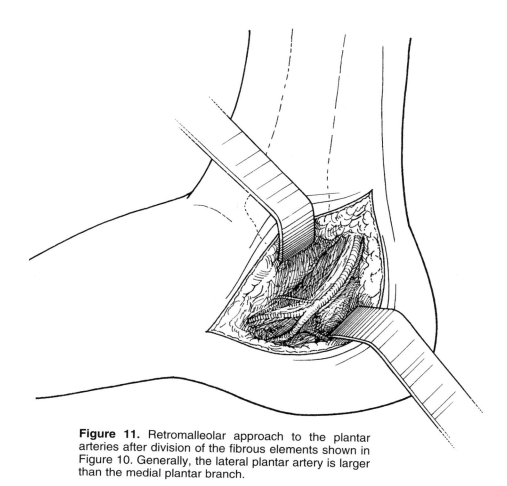

Figure 11. Retromalleolar approach to the plantar arteries after division of the fibrous elements shown in Figure 10. Generally, the lateral plantar artery is larger than the medial plantar branch.

foot is externally rotated on the operating table. Exposure of the proximal 2-3 cm of the plantar branches is accomplished by incision of the flexor retinaculum and transection of the abductor hallucis muscle (Figs. 10 and 11). If necessary, more distal exposure of these branches can be obtained by division of the medial border of the plantar aponeurosis and the flexor digitorum brevis muscle.

Exposure of the Deep Plantar or Deep Metatarsal Arch Branch

The deep plantar branch is the main extension of the dorsalis pedis artery (Figs. 9 and 12). It originates at the metatarsal level where it descends into a foramen bounded proximally by the dorsal metatarsal ligament,

distally by the dorsal interosseous muscle ring, and medially and laterally by the base of the first and second metatarsal bones (Fig. 12). As the deep plantar branch exits from this tunnel, it connects with the lateral plantar branch to form the deep pedal arch (Fig. 9).

A slightly curvilinear, longitudinal 3-4 cm incision over the dorsum of the mid-portion of the foot permits the dissection of the dorsalis pedis artery down to its bifurcation into the deep plantar and first dorsal metatarsal branches (Fig. 12). The extensor hallucis brevis muscle is retracted laterally, or transected if necessary, and the dorsal interosseous muscle ring is split to allow better exposure of the proximal portion of the deep plantar branch. The periosteum of the proximal portion of the second metatarsal bone is then incised and

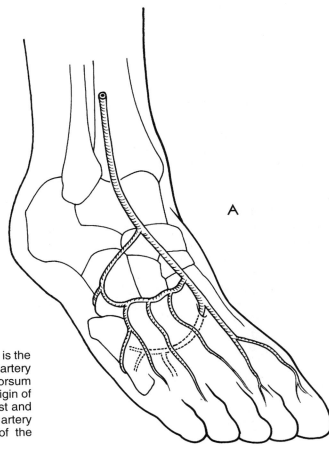

Figure 12. A. The deep plantar arch is the main terminal branch of the dorsal artery of the foot. B. An incision over the dorsum of the foot allows exposure of the origin of the arcade that runs between the 1st and 2nd metatarsals. Exposure of this artery is facilitated by lateral retraction of the short extensor of the hallux.

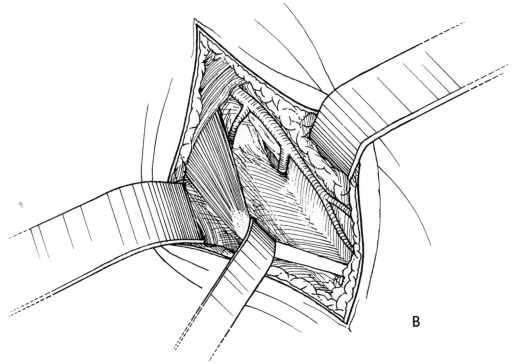

elevated. A fine-tipped rongeur is used to excise enough of the metatarsal shaft to allow for ample exposure of the deep plantar branch (Fig. 13).

Exposure of the Lateral Tarsal Branch

The lateral tarsal artery arises from the dorsalis pedis artery at the level of the navicular bone and runs laterally toward the 5th metatarsal bone and under the short extensor muscle of the toes (Fig. 12). This branch is an important source of blood supply to the dorsal aspect of the foot and anastomoses with the arcuate artery of the foot.

To expose the lateral tarsal artery, the dorsalis pedis artery is dissected at the level of the ankle joint after division of the inferior extensor retinaculum. Dissection then continues distally to the origin of the lateral tarsal branch. Further mobilization of the latter artery

can be achieved by lateral retraction of the long extensor tendons of the toe. If additional exposure of the lateral tarsal branch is necessary, division of the first and second long extensor tendons of the toes may be performed.

Conclusion

Use of the nonstandard, alternative approaches to infrainguinal arteries described in this chapter has made possible the salvage of many ischemic lower extremities that would otherwise be extremely difficult or impossible to revascularize. Most of these reoperations were in the increasing proportion of patients whose limb-threatening ischemia occurred after a primary arterial reconstruction failed. In this setting, the unusual alternative approaches facilitated secondary operation that could be performed without the need to redissect arteries through a scarred or infected wound.

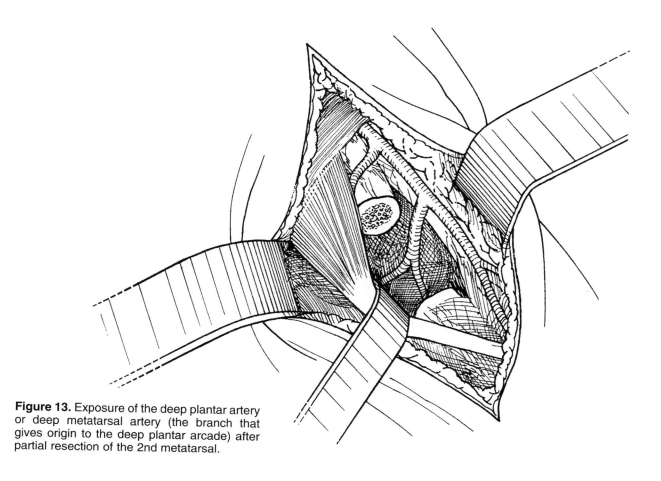

Figure 13. Exposure of the deep plantar artery or deep metatarsal artery (the branch that gives origin to the deep plantar arcade) after partial resection of the 2nd metatarsal.

These approaches have also permitted shorter bypasses and thereby allowed us to use autogenous vein in patients who might otherwise have required a prosthetic graft. This is particularly important for bypass procedures which extend to infrapopliteal arteries since vein graft patency is so much better in this location.[15] Therefore, the importance of these alternative approaches has assumed increasing emphasis and utility in our practice. We believe that they will be equally helpful to others as more vascular surgeons accept the premise that most limb-threatening lower extremity ischemia can and should be treated by arterial reconstruction rather than amputation.

References

1. Veith FJ, Gupta SK, Samson RH, et al. Progress in limb salvage by reconstructive arterial surgery combined with new or improved adjunctive procedures. *Ann Surg* 1981; 194: 386-401.

2. Bartlett ST, Olinde AJ, Flinn WR, et al. The reoperative potential of infrainguinal bypass: Long-term limb and patient survival. *J Vasc Surg* 1987; 5: 170-179.

3. Samson RH, Veith FJ, Janko GS, et al. A modified classification and approach to the management of infections involving peripheral arterial prosthetic grafts. *J Vasc Surg* 1988; 8: 147-153.

4. Stabile BE, Wilson SE. The profunda femoris popliteal artery bypass. *Arch Surg* 1977; 112: 913-918.

5. Hershey FB, Auer AI. Extended surgical approach to the profunda femoris artery. *Surg Gynecol Obstet* 1974; 138: 88-90.

6. Nunez AA, Veith FJ, Collier P, et al. Direct approaches to the distal portions of the deep femoral artery for limb salvage bypasses. *J Vasc Surg* 1988; 8: 576-581.

7. De Palma RG, Malgieri JJ, Rhodes RS, Clowes AW. Profunda femoris bypass for secondary revascularization. *Surg Gynecol Obstet* 1980; 151: 387-390.

8. Veith FJ, Ascer E, Gupta SK, Wengerter KR. Lateral approach to the popliteal artery. *J Vasc Surg* 1987 6: 119-123.

9. Danese CA, Singer A. Lateral approach to the popliteal artery trifurcation. *Surgery* 1968; 63: 588-591.

10. Veith FJ, Gupta SK. Femoral-distal artery bypasses. In: Bergan JJ, Yao JST, eds. *Operative Techniques in Vascular Surgery.* New York, Grune & Stratton, 1980, pp 141-150.

11. Dardik H, Dardik I, Veith FJ. Exposure of the tibial-peroneal arteries by a single lateral approach. *Surgery* 1974; 75: 377-382.

12. Dardik H, Elias S, Miller N, et al. Medial approach to the anterior tibial artery. *J Vasc Surg* 1985; 2: 743-746.

13. Veith FJ, Ascer E, Gupta SK, et al. Tibiotibial vein bypass grafts: A new operation for limb salvage. *J Vasc Surg* 1985; 2: 552-557.

14. Ascer E, Veith FJ, Gupta SK. Bypasses to plantar arteries and other tibial branches: An extended approach to limb salvage. *J Vasc Surg* 1988; 8: 434-441.

15. Veith FJ, Gupta SK, Ascer E, et al. Six-year prospective multicenter randomized comparison of autologous saphenous vein and expanded polytetrafluoroethylene grafts in infrainguinal arterial reconstructions. *J Vasc Surg* 186; 3: 104-114.

31

Veins of the Lower Limb

Michel Perrin, Jean-Louis Calvignac

Surgical access to veins of the lower limb is necessary in a variety of circumstances. Superficial veins are accessed in the treatment of chronic venous insufficiency, medial and lateral saphenous veins for arterial restoration grafts, and deep veins in trauma, tumors, thrombophlebitis, and primary or secondary valve incompetence.

Anatomic Review

The greater saphenous vein (GSV) is a continuation of the medial marginal vein which lies anterior to the medial malleolus. It ascends vertically along the medial side of the leg, a few centimeters posterior to the posteromedial edge of the tibia, traverses the medial surface of the knee, and continues across the medial surface of the thigh. In the upper two-thirds of the thigh, the GSV is in direct contact with the fascia so it lies relatively fixed, is at the level of the groin, and generally reaches the level of the common femoral vein (CFV).[1-3] Numerous tributaries enter the saphenous vein at this level (Fig. 1).

The lesser saphenous vein (LSV) follows from the lateral marginal vein to the level of the peroneal malleolus. It passes equidistant from the inferior extremity of the fibula and the calcanean tendon and then rises obliquely inward towards the posterior midline. Initially lying subcutaneously, it traverses the fascia in the middle of the leg to run superficially over the midline. It penetrates the popliteal fossa between the lateral and medial heads of the gastrocnemius muscle. The lateral saphenous nerve travels with the LSV from the malleolus to the inferior third of the leg. The LSV normally terminates on the posterior wall of the popliteal vein or in its lateral or medial wall in the popliteal fossa. In approximately one-third of cases, the gastrocnemius veins join the LSV before its termination; this results in a short common trunk that joins the popliteal vein. Variations in LSV termination may be simplified into six main types[4] (Fig. 2).

Most frequently, the gastrocnemius veins empty into two trunks: the medial and the lateral gastrocnemius veins. The former is the

From Vascular Surgical Approaches, edited by Alain Branchereau and Ramon Berguer. ©1999, Futura Publishing Co., Inc., Armonk, NY.

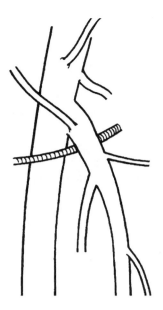

Figure 1. Saphenofemoral junction showing the arch of the GSV and its affluents. Note crossover of the superficial lateral pudendal artery.

Figure 2. Variations in the termination of the LSV (shaded in diagram)
1. Common femoral vein.
2. Greater saphenous vein.
3. Popliteal vein.

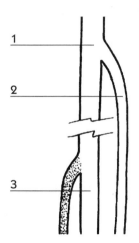
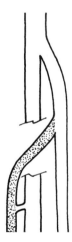
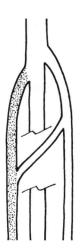
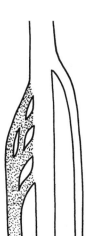
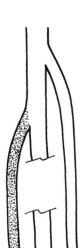
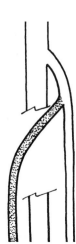

larger of the two. In two-thirds of cases, the two trunks join the popliteal vein separately. This termination generally lies below the termination of the lesser saphenous vein. In a third of the cases the gastrocnemius veins terminate in the LSV shortly before the latter empties into the popliteal vein.

The anatomy of the perforating veins has been extensively described in the literature.[5,6] For the treatment of chronic venous disease the most frequently accessed veins are: at the femoral level, the perforating described by Dodd; and at the leg level, the median perforating veins of the ankle, and the perforating of the lateral network (lateral perforating of the ankle and median posterior perforating).

Deep Veins

The popliteal vein originates at the ring of the soleus muscle and terminates at the ring of the great adductor muscle.[8] Acting as confluent of the leg veins, it receives the gastrocnemius veins, several articular veins, and most frequently, the bulb of the LSV at approximately the interarticular line of the knee. In more than one-third of cases it is double, especially in the inferior two-thirds, and even triple in 2% of the population. In 90-95% of cases it has a valve just below the ring of the great abductor muscle. The superficial femoral vein (SFV) is a continuation of the popliteal vein and may be double or triple. It spirals upwards around the artery from its lateral to its medial wall crossing it posteriorly. There are three or four valves; the fourth is present in 90% of cases and generally lies 1-2 cm below the junction of the vertical branch of the deep femoral vein (DFV). The level of the junction with the DFV varies and gives rise to the common femoral vein. The DFV[9] may communicate directly at its origin with the popliteal vein. This vein terminates in a single trunk in only 16% of cases.[12] Consequently, there are frequently several DFVs; the largest and most important, both anatomically and surgically, is the vertical DFV. This vertical branch has a valve, usually located in the upper third and situated 1-2 cm before its junction with the SFV.[10] The CFV lies under the inguinal ligament where it continues

as the external iliac vein. In more than 75% of cases the CFV or the external iliac vein has one single valve above the saphenofemoral junction.

Greater Saphenous Vein

The patient is placed in dorsal decubitus. The leg is elevated at an angle of 20-30 degrees. The lower extremity rests on the buttock and heel and is in slight abduction and lateral rotation. The surgeon is located on the contralateral side facing the skin incision and the assistant. The table is inclined 20 degrees towards the surgeon. The saphenofemoral junction is accessed by a skin incision centered on a point situated 2.5 cm outside and below the pubic tubercle (Fig. 3). The incision is 3-5 cm long and lies just within the femoral artery, which is identified by its pulse. When making the incision, the inguinal cutaneous fold should be avoided, especially in obese patients. We prefer to use a parallel incision above this fold, especially in females. The subcutaneous cellular tissue and superficial fascia are cut along a transverse axis. Retractors

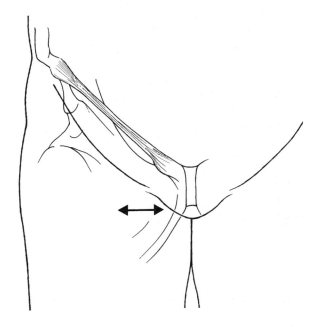

Figure 3. Incision to access the bulb of the GSV.

are installed perpendicular to the axis of the incision. The GSV lies within the fat, where it is easily identified. When dissecting this vein, transversal dissection is to be avoided to prevent injuring lymphatic channels, instead, longitudinal dissection should be performed. Dissection of the GSV towards the proximal part of the member leads to the saphenofemoral junction. This is identified as soon as the anterolateral and medial walls of the CFV are exposed on either side of the presumed saphenofemoral junction. In certain cases, the lateral pudendal artery may be situated below the terminal portion of the arch of the GSV and thus hinder exposure. In case of difficulties, it may be sectioned, although in males it should be mobilized and transposed. Access to the GSV trunk is easy along its entire length. The GSV is easily identified after dividing the skin and subcutaneous cellular tissue. Access to the GSV is simplified by preoperative duplex scan which is highly recommended for obese patients.

Lesser Saphenous Vein

The patient is placed in lateral decubitus for a unilateral approach; the operated limb is uppermost and the table is inclined 30 degrees towards the assistant. For a bilateral approach the patient is prone. The dorsal decubitus position is justified only for vein stripping involving both the medial and lateral saphenous veins, or when the LSV terminates in the GSV or SFV without a connection with the popliteal fossa (types 4 and 5, Fig. 2). The approach to the termination of the LSV and the level of the skin incision are determined by the topography of the saphenopopliteal junction, previously identified by a duplex scan. This incision is transversal, slightly downwardly concave, and measures 4-6 cm. Its midpoint is over the ascending course of the trunk of the previously identified LSV. Subcutaneous cellular tissue is incised transversally down to the superficial fascia of the leg and detached around the incision, using a finger (Fig. 4). A 5 cm longitudinal fasciotomy exposes the fat tissue of the popliteal fossa. The LSV is identified: it is the most superficial vascular element of the popliteal cavity and generally in

contact with the deep surface of the lateral edge of the previously dissected fascia. The anastomosis between the GSV and LSV may be a valuable guideline. The proximal dissection of the LSV is performed with scissors and gauze (Fig. 4); all branches are tied before dividing them. A common trunk of the LSV-gastrocnemius vein may exist and should be freed as far as its popliteal junction. At its termination the wall of the LSV is fairly thin and fragile and should be dissected with care. The termination of the LSV is not necessarily on the posterior wall of the popliteal vein. It may be postero- or anterolateral and occasionally anterior. In addition, the arch of the LSV may be directly linked to the sciatic nerve bifurcation from which it may need to be disengaged. To access the LSV at its origin, a short (1 cm) transversal skin incision is performed at the level of the fossa created by the posterior edge of the lateral malleolus and the Achilles tendon. Lying in the subcutaneous cellular tissue, it can be depressed and is supple; it should not be confused with the firmer and pearly lateral saphenous nerve to which it closely adheres. Preoperative ultrasound identification facilitates dissection of the LSV in the leg. It lies subcutaneously in the inferior two-thirds, and consequently it is easily accessed by a 2 cm or 3 cm posterior medial incision. The fascia must be sectioned in its proximal third: the LSV is easily identified in contact with the deep surface of the fascia.

Gastrocnemius Veins

These veins are surgically accessed for ligation at the level of their termination. Prior to surgery, their topography should be established by duplex or, in certain cases, phlebography. The approach is identical to that described for exposure of the LSV-popliteal vein junction. Once the popliteal vein is identified, it is dissected for several centimeters exposing its posterior, lateral, and medial walls, particularly in the lower half of the popliteal fossa. The gastrocnemius veins, once identified, need only to be freed for a short segment where they emerge from the gastrocnemius muscles. They have fragile walls and

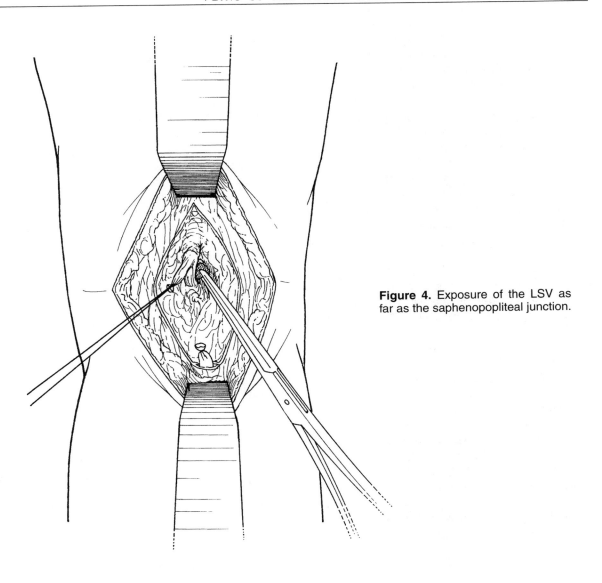

Figure 4. Exposure of the LSV as far as the saphenopopliteal junction.

often adhere to the artery of the same name which must be preserved.

Perforating Veins

These are exposed in order to perform elective or extensive ligation. In elective surgery, the 2-4 cm skin incision is centered on the previously identified perforating vein. It is preferable to perform an oblique incision in the same direction as the skin fold. The perforating vein may be exposed in either its supra- or subfascial segment after incision of the fascial defect. De Palma suggests performing several parallel transversal skin incisions.[11] These veins may also be semielectively exposed[12] with the patient in dorsal decubitus using a vertical, straight skin incision performed 2 cm behind the posteromedial edge of the tibia. It begins 3 cm above the medial malleolus and terminates in the middle of the leg. In order to identify the perforating veins, the subcutaneous cellular tissue is incised and freed from the fascia. A subfascial approach is systematically used for extended access to the perforating veins. In Linton's technique, the previous skin incision is extended upwards as far as the proximal third of the tibia. The fascia of the leg is divided for the complete length of the incision, parallel to the skin. It is freed in front as far as the posteromedial edge of the tibia, and behind as far as the intermuscular wall separating the posterior and anterolateral compartments. In Felder's technique, the patient is prone. The vertical posterior skin incision begins 2 cm above the malleolar level and continues to within a few centimeters above the fold of the knee. The incision may be medial or, preferably, slightly displaced away from the LSV. The fascial incision is parallel to the skin incision. By following the detachment in front of the fibula, the perforating veins exiting from the anterolateral compartment are exposed.

A recently described technique uses a video device for accessing the perforating veins.[13] A 1-2 cm initial skin incision is performed in the upper third of the leg, 10 cm below the tip of the patella, and the leg fascia is then incised for a few millimeters. A soft-ended device, linked to an inflating apparatus, is introduced between the muscular plane and the fascia. The muscle is detached from the fascia at the level of the posterior cavity by pressurizing it to about 30 mm Hg. The device is replaced by the autofocus optical instrument that allows the perforating veins to be identified on a screen. A second identical incision is performed level with the first, but 5 cm posteriorly, which allows introduction of a soft trochar for surgical access.

The Popliteal Vein

The popliteal vein is accessible using a posterior or a medial approach (Fig. 5). In the posterior approach, the patient is prone or in lateral decubitus.[14] The limited access to the popliteal vein has been previously described in relation to the saphenopopliteal junction. For extended popliteal vein exposure, the skin incision is S-shaped with an upper vertical segment, a horizontal segment lying in the skin fold of the knee, and a lower vertical segment, laterally close to the axis of the limb (Fig. 5E). The fascia is incised slightly lateral to the axis of the limb. In the upper part of the incision, the sciatic nerve is identified and isolated along with the femoral biceps muscle (crural

biceps) from which it emerges; the semitendinous muscle is retracted medially (Fig. 6). The tibial (medial sciatic popliteal) and common peroneal nerves (lateral sciatic popliteal) lie in the inferior part of the incision. Retractor compression must be avoided. The gastrocnemius muscles are retracted along with their vascular supply. The plantar muscle is also retracted; its tendon may be divided where it crosses the lower corner of the incision (Fig. 6). The nerve of the medial gastrocnemius muscle is the only motor branch that originates from the medial edge of the sciatic nerve; during an extended vascular procedure, cutting it may occasionally be unavoidable. The LSV, Giacomini's vein, and the gastrocnemius veins may all be systematically tied. There is a limited risk of thrombosis in ligating the latter. Identification of the neurovascular elements may be complicated by the thick layer of fat tissue, which is abundant in the upper part of the incision. Usually the vein is exposed before the artery with which it may be confused due to its thickness.

A medial approach allows the popliteal vein to be accessed from above and below the knee. The patient is in decubitus. A longitudinal incision is performed 1 cm behind the posterior edge of the femur and tibia (Fig. 5, C and D). This approach encounters only fatty tissues and, then, above the knee, the sartorius and medial gastrocnemius muscles, and below the knee, the medial gastrocnemius muscle and the tendons of the gracillis, semitendonous, and semimembranous muscles, all of which are retracted. The vein is lateral and slightly posterior in relation to the artery that partially hides it (Figs. 7 and 8). Complete exposure of the popliteal vessels using a medial approach is a traumatic procedure: the tendons of the gracilis, sartorius, gastrocnemius, semimembranous, and the medial gastrocnemius muscles need to be sectioned and, eventually, reconstructed.

The posterior approach to the popliteal vein is the preferred one particularly if there are morphologic anomalies or when the operation is performed because of trauma or for resection of a tumor. A medial approach is preferable for surgical treatment of recent deep vein thrombosis or when performing extensive thrombectomy on a patient in the dorsal

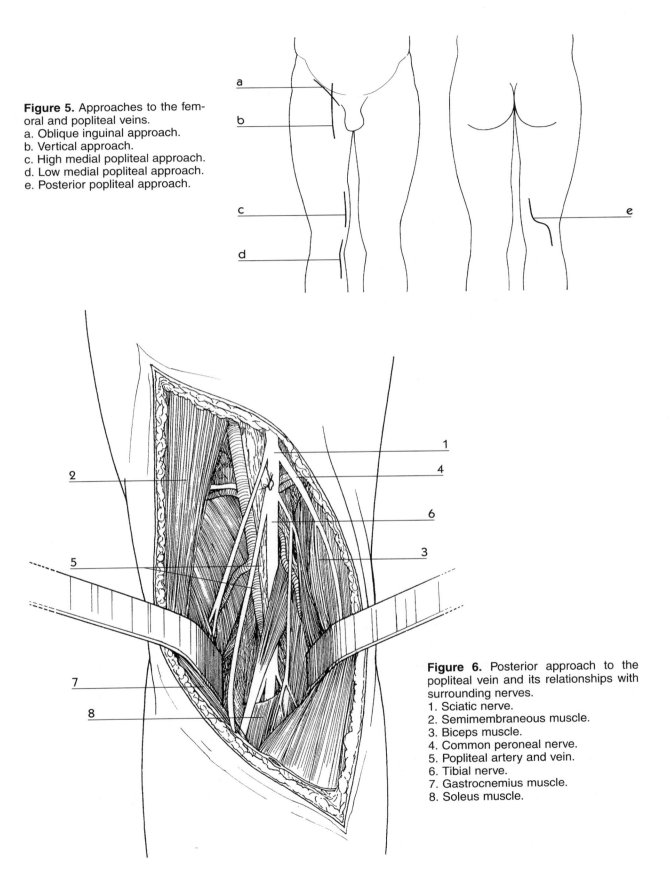

Figure 5. Approaches to the femoral and popliteal veins.
a. Oblique inguinal approach.
b. Vertical approach.
c. High medial popliteal approach.
d. Low medial popliteal approach.
e. Posterior popliteal approach.

Figure 6. Posterior approach to the popliteal vein and its relationships with surrounding nerves.
1. Sciatic nerve.
2. Semimembraneous muscle.
3. Biceps muscle.
4. Common peroneal nerve.
5. Popliteal artery and vein.
6. Tibial nerve.
7. Gastrocnemius muscle.
8. Soleus muscle.

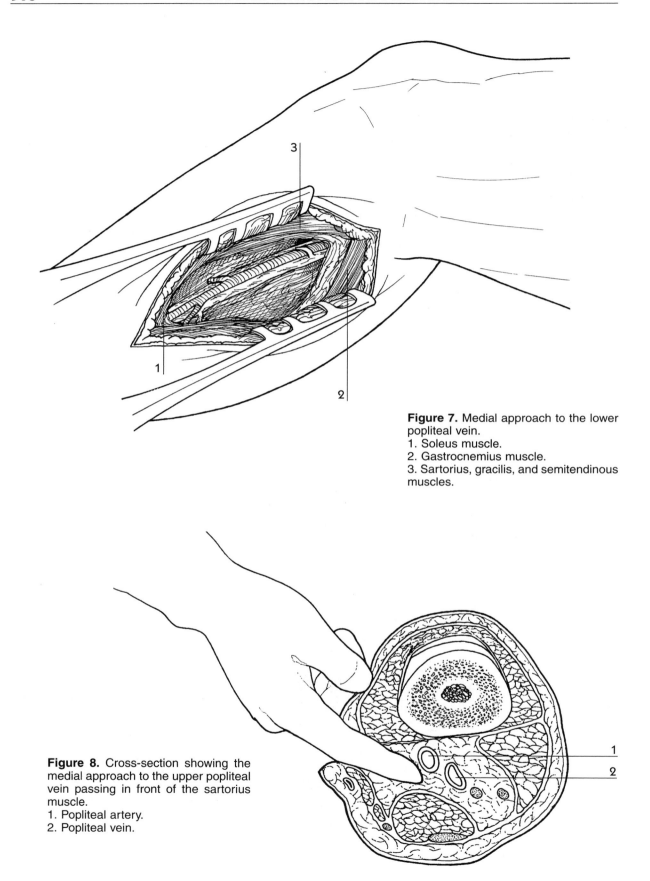

Figure 7. Medial approach to the lower popliteal vein.
1. Soleus muscle.
2. Gastrocnemius muscle.
3. Sartorius, gracilis, and semitendinous muscles.

Figure 8. Cross-section showing the medial approach to the upper popliteal vein passing in front of the sartorius muscle.
1. Popliteal artery.
2. Popliteal vein.

decubitus position. The medial approach is also preferable in surgery for post-thrombotic syndromes because one may need to perform an extended thrombectomy with the patient lying supine on the operating table. The medial approach is also preferable when operating for venous thrombosis because the lesions in the wall of the vein found at operation may require exposure at a higher level than the popliteal vein.[15]

Common Femoral Vein[14]

Vascular surgeons routinely use the vertical approach to the femoral vessels (Fig. 5B). It is debated whether a direct or lateral approach is preferable; the latter permits avoidance of the lymph nodes at the groin (Fig. 5A). With the patient in dorsal decubitus, the operated limb is slightly flexed in abduction and lateral rotation. A roll supports the lateral aspect of the knee. The 10-15 cm incision is more or less arched and inwardly concave (Fig. 9). Its upper end lies approximately 2.5 cm above the middle of the line that runs from the anterosuperior iliac spine to the pubic tubercle (Fig. 9). The dissection begins at the superolateral angle of the femoral triangle by freeing the inguinal ligament and the sartorius muscle. It continues along the medial edge of the latter muscle down to the vascular sheath. Above, disinserting the iliopsoas muscle from the inguinal ligament avoids damage to the latter. A retractor gives sufficient exposure of the

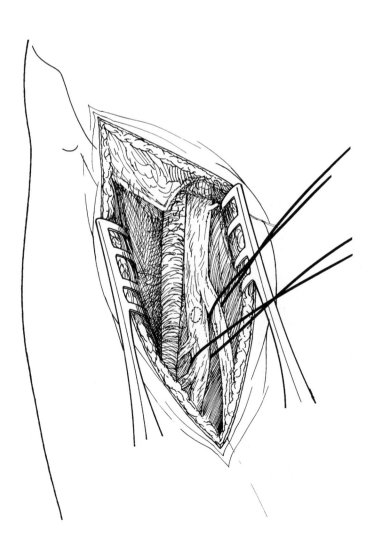

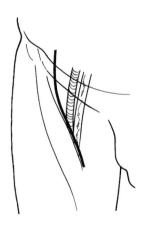

Figure 9. Approach to the common femoral vein and junction of the superficial and deep femoral veins at the groin.

iliofemoral venous junction (Fig. 9). Careful dissection is required because of the presence of several circumflex and/or epigastric branches. Freeing of the CFV close to its two originating branches is performed from top to bottom in order to avoid damage to the latter. Dissection must avoid damage to the femoral nerve laterally and the GSV medially.

Superficial Femoral Vein

This is a distal extension of the approach to the femoral triangle described above. The skin incision is parallel to the sartorius muscle of which the SFA and SFV are satellites. The lower the approach, the more practical it becomes for the surgeon to change sides, from the lateral to the medial side of the operated limb. In order to preserve the GSV its location must be established beforehand. At the top, the sartorius muscle is retracted laterally; below, it is retracted medially (Fig. 10). The sheath of

the sartorius is incised in front of and/or behind the body of the muscle. The approach to the femoropopliteal junction requires dissecting the tendon of the adductor magnus muscle (Fig. 10). The farther down the dissection proceeds towards the bottom of the SFV, the more nerve and vascular branches are encountered. Whenever possible these branches must be preserved.

Deep Femoral Vein

Extension of the approach to the femoral triangle is more difficult over the DFV because of vessels and nerves that cross the path of dissection. The medial femoral approach allows access to the DFV far from the femoral bifurcation (see Chapter 26). A 12 cm vertical incision follows the outline of the lateral edge of the vast medial muscle in the middle third of the thigh. The opening in the aponeurosis leads to a muscular interstice widened by

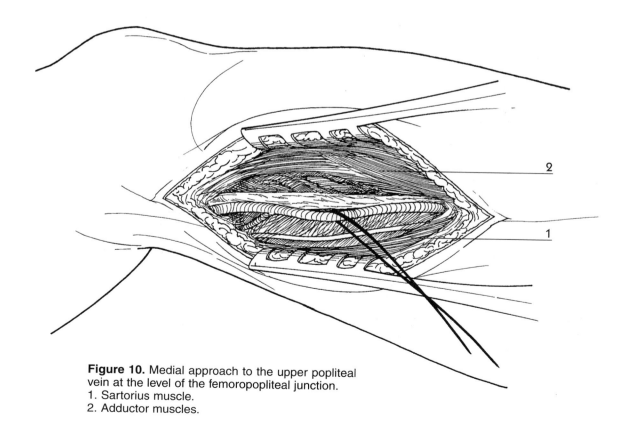

Figure 10. Medial approach to the upper popliteal vein at the level of the femoropopliteal junction.
1. Sartorius muscle.
2. Adductor muscles.

lateral retraction of the anterior rectus and vastus medialis muscles and medial retraction of the sartorius and middle adductor muscles. The DFV, in contact with the deep femoral artery, is generally found in a fatty trench at the bottom of this interstice.

References

1. Furderer CR, Marescaux J, Pavis D'Escrurac X, Stemmer R. Les crosses saphéniennes. Anatomie et concepts thérapeutiques. *Phlébologie* 1986; 39: 3-14.

2. Henriet JP. Le confluent veineux saphéno-fémoral et le réseau artériel honteux externe. Données anatomiques et statistiques nouvelles. *Phlébologie* 1987; 40: 711-715.

3. Gillot C. La crosse de la veine saphène interne. Bases anatomiques et techniques de la crossectomie. *Phlébologie* 1994; 47: 117-113.

4. Mercier R. Quelques points d'anatomie de la veine saphène externe. *Phlébologie* 1973; 26: 1991-196.

5. Gillot C. Les veines perforantes internes de la jambe, de la cheville et du pied. *Phlébologie* 1994; 47: 76-109.

6. Van Limborgh J. L'anatomie des veines communicantes. *Phlébologie* 1965; 1: 361-365.

7. Perrin M. Insuffisance veineuse chronique des membres inférieurs. Généralités. Rappel anatomique et physiologique. *Encycl Med Chir.* Paris. Techniques chirurgicales. Chirurgie Vasculaire, 43-160, 1994, 12 p.

8. Cadenat FM. *Les voies de pénétration des membres (3ème ed).* Paris, Doin, 1978, pp 262-274, 287-291, 303-306.

9. Perrin M. *L'insuffisance Veineuse Chronique.* Paris, Arnette, 1994 p 6.

10. Perrin M. *L'insuffisance Veineuse Chronique.* Paris, Arnette, 1994 p 10.

11. De Palma RG. Surgical therapy for venous stasis: Results of a modified Linton operation. *Am J Surg* 1979; 137: 810-813.

12. Dodd H, Cockett FB. *The Pathology and Surgery of the Veins of the Lower Limb. 2nd ed.* Edinburg, Churchill-Livingstone, 1976, pp 280-284.

13. O'Donnel TF. Surgical treatment of incompetent communicating veins. In: Bergan JJ, Kistner RL, eds. *Altas of Venous Surgery.* Philadelphia, WB Saunders, 1992, pp 111-124.

14. Rutherford RB. *Atlas of Vascular Surgery.* Philadelphia, WB Saunders, 1993, pp 112-147.

15. Perrin M. *L'insuffisance Veineuse Chronique.* Paris, Arnette, 1994 pp 114-119.

INDEX